Diseases and disorders.

DISEASES and DISORDERS

VOLUME 2

Emphysema—Obesity

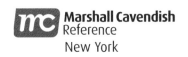

Marshall Cavendish
Reference
New York

Marshall Cavendish
99 White Plains Road
Tarrytown, New York 10591

www.marshallcavendish.us

Library of Congress Cataloging-in-Publication Data
Diseases and disorders
    p. cm.
  Includes bibliographical references and index.
  ISBN 978-0-7614-7770-9 (set: alk. paper)
-- ISBN 978-0-7614-7771-6 (v. 1) -- ISBN 978-
0-7614-7772-3 (v. 2) -- ISBN 978-0-7614-7774-
7 (v. 3)
  1. Diseases. 2. Medicine. I. Title.

  RC41.D57 2007
  616--dc22

2007060867

Printed and bound in Malaysia

12 11 10 09 08 07 1 2 3 4 5 6

Marshall Cavendish
Publisher: Paul Bernabeo
Production Manager: Michael Esposito

The Brown Reference Group
Project Editors: Anne Hildyard, Jolyon Goddard
Editor: Wendy Horobin
Development Editor: Richard Beatty
Designer: Seth Grimbly
Picture Researcher: Becky Cox
Illustrator: Peter Bull
Indexer: Kay Ollerenshaw
Managing Editor: Bridget Giles
Senior Managing Editor: Tim Cooke
Editorial Director: Lindsey Lowe

Contents

Emphysema

Emphysema is a progressive, irreversible, and degenerative disease of the lungs. In emphysema, the alveoli, the air sacs in which carbon dioxide in the bloodstream is exchanged for oxygen in the air, become damaged by tobacco smoke and other air pollutants, such as dust.

In emphysema, the alveoli lose their elasticity and break down, eventually destroying the body's ability to acquire sufficient oxygen. As the disease progresses, the ability to exhale becomes more difficult, further undermining the ability to acquire sufficient oxygen.

Causes and risk factors

The primary cause of emphysema is smoking. Although the risk is higher for smokers, nonsmokers chronically exposed to secondhand smoke are also at risk. In the past, men were more likely to develop emphysema than women, but as the number of women smokers has increased, the prevalence rate of emphysema in women has begun to approach that of men.

Other air pollutants besides tobacco smoke will also cause damage to lung tissue that leads to emphysema. For example, the World Health Organization (WHO) reports that there are 400,000 deaths from chronic obstructive pulmonary disease (COPD) caused by burning of biomass fuels (such as wood) each year. It takes years for the lung damage to accumulate before it becomes noticeable; thus more than 90 percent of people diagnosed with the disease are age 45 or older.

Genetic factors influence the risk of developing emphysema in a small percentage of individuals. Research has shown that a hereditary deficiency of the protein alpha-1-antitrypsin, which protects the elasticity of lung tissue, increases the risk of lung damage and leads to emphysema.

In addition, HIV infection and some connective tissue disorders, such as Marfan syndrome, may make affected individuals more susceptible to developing emphysema.

Symptoms and signs

The first signs of emphysema are usually shortness of breath during moderate exercise, such as during walking. Dry or productive coughs and wheezing also indicate the presence of the disease. The symptoms intensify as the disease progresses.

Inability to breathe adequately leads to chronic fatigue. Fatigue while breathing may trigger a loss of

KEY FACTS

Description
A disease of the lungs that reduces the body's ability to get adequate oxygen.

Causes
The alveoli or air sacs in which gas exchange occurs are irreversibly destroyed; as they are destroyed, the lungs' ability to exchange carbon dioxide in the bloodstream for oxygen in the air is reduced.

Risk factors
Tobacco smoking, air pollution, and age all increase the risk of the disease.

Symptoms
Shortness of breath, coughing, wheezing, and reduced ability to exercise are the primary symptoms; they may also include sudden weight loss, swelling of lower limbs, fatigue, and anxiety.

Diagnosis
A physical examination, coupled with tests of breathing efficiency, chest X-rays, or measurements of blood gases.

Treatments
The most important treatment by far is to quit smoking; drugs such as bronchodilators and corticosteroids may boost ease of breathing; supplemental oxygen may be administered; in severe cases, lung reduction surgery or lung transplants may be required.

Pathogenesis
Exposure to tobacco smoke as well as other air pollutants damages the walls of the alveoli, which become brittle and break down; as the lungs lose their elasticity, it becomes more difficult to exhale stale air.

Prevention
Quitting smoking, avoiding tobacco smoke, and limiting exposure to other lung irritants.

Epidemiology
Emphysema develops slowly; thus it is seen most often in older individuals. More than 90 percent of emphysema patients are age 45 or older. Years of exposure to tobacco smoke typically precedes the onset of the disease, but it is also seen in coal miners affected by dust.

PULMONARY EMPHYSEMA

As well as smoking, exposure to air pollution and dust can cause emphysema. (1) shows normal bronchioles and alveoli; (2) shows a distended bronchiole; and (3) shows distended air sacs or alveoli. The distension is typical of pulmonary emphysema suffered by coal miners, who continually breathe in coal dust.

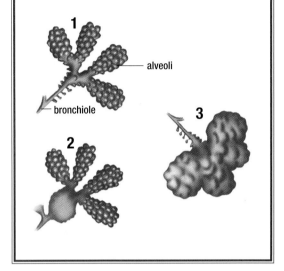

appetite, which in turn leads to weight loss. In advanced cases, even breathing leads to fatigue, since much energy is spent trying to forcibly expel stale air from the lungs. Emphysema may also be accompanied by swelling of the lower limbs and anxiety.

Treatments and prevention

There is no way to reverse the damage to the lungs caused by emphysema; therefore, the best way to treat emphysema is to prevent it. The best way to prevent emphysema is to quit smoking tobacco. Other preventive measures are to find ways to reduce exposures to secondhand smoke and other air pollutants, and to maintain good health and resistance to infection by regular exercise, good nutrition, and adequate rest. Once the effects of emphysema begin to manifest themselves, the symptoms can be managed by a variety of methods. Bronchodilator drugs may be administered to relieve coughing, shortness of breath, and difficulty breathing by relaxing bronchial passages, thus increasing the efficiency of air flow into and out of the lungs. Inhaled or oral corticosteroids may be also administered to help combat inflammation of lung tissues, but long-term use may trigger a number of adverse side effects, such as brittle bones or high blood pressure. Breathing exercises may also help emphysema patients breathe more efficiently.

To prevent infections that may aggravate symptoms, emphysema patients should keep their vaccinations up to date, especially against influenza (which needs to be updated every year) and against pneumonia (which needs to be updated every five to seven years.) Antibiotic treatment may be required to cure existing infections or may be administered as a prophylactic to prevent the onset of secondary infections.

Supplemental oxygen may be administered in severe cases in which a patient's blood oxygen levels are low. The duration and timing of oxygen administration will vary, depending on the severity of disease. Portable oxygen delivery systems make it possible for emphysema patients to engage in many activities once considered impracticable.

In some cases, surgery may be required. Lung reduction surgery, in which portions of the lung are removed, reduces overall lung volume but increases breathing efficiency (at least for some months after the operation). Lung transplants may be the only option in extreme cases of emphysema.

Epidemiology

Global statistics on prevalence of and mortality from emphysema specifically are difficult to obtain. Emphysema is frequently combined with chronic bronchitis and irreversible forms of asthma as COPD. The disease is often described as a contributing factor to the death of a patient but may not be credited as the cause of death. Nevertheless, the World Health Organization (WHO) reports that COPD is the fourth leading cause of death worldwide, with 2.7 million deaths in 2000. Likewise, COPD is the fourth leading cause of death in the United States, claiming more than 120,000 lives annually.

In 2003 about 1.7 percent of adults in the United States (3.6 million individuals) had been diagnosed specifically with emphysema. Nearly 14,000 people in the United States died from the disease that year. Extrapolation of emphysema prevalence rates from nations in which emphysema data are available indicates that more than 40 million persons worldwide may suffer from the disease.

David M. Lawrence

See also
• Aging, disorders of • Cancer, lung • COPD
• Environmental disorders • Smoking-related disorders

Endometriosis

Endometriosis is a condition in which fragments of the tissue normally found in the lining of the uterus appear elsewhere in the body. It affects many women during childbearing years. The disease can cause pain and irregular menstruation and can lead to infertility.

Endometriosis occurs when tissue called endometrium, which is usually restricted to the lining of the uterus, appears in other parts of the body. Pieces of this tissue can be found anywhere in the pelvic area: on the ovaries, on the fallopian tubes, and on the wall of the pelvic cavity. In rare cases, the tissue has been found inside the vagina, inside the bladder, on the skin, and even in the lungs, spine, and brain. If endometriosis affects the fallopian tubes, it can cause infertility; the tissue can block the tubes and prevent an egg from passing from the ovary to the uterus. About 30 to 40 percent of women with endometriosis are infertile.

Causes

The causes of endometriosis are unknown. A number of theories exist. Retrograde menstruation may lead to seeding of the pelvic cavity. Another theory suggests that the endometrial tissues are taken up by the lymphatic fluids that drain the uterus. The tissues are transported to other sites, where they grow. Another theory proposes that a type of normal tissue found outside the uterus is, for reasons unknown, transformed into endometrium. Both environmental and genetic causes are under investigation.

Symptoms

The most common symptom of endometriosis is pain in the pelvic area, which can be severe. Other symptoms may include diarrhea or constipation and abdominal bloating, especially at the time of menstruation, heavy or irregular periods, and fatigue.

Diagnosis

Endometriosis is difficult to diagnose, and a physical exam often yields no telltale signs. A characteristic finding that can suggest a diagnosis is a nodule that is extremely tender to the touch, which is felt in the ligament behind the uterus. Laparoscopy, in which the pelvic cavity is examined with a viewing instrument under general anesthesia, may also be performed.

Treatment

Management and treatment of endometriosis depends on the severity of symptoms, the extent of the disease, and the age and family plans of the woman. Hormonal treatments may be suggested to suppress production of the female sex hormone estrogen, which exacerbates symptoms. Hormonal therapies that are effective include birth control pills, progestins, gonadotropin-releasing hormone (GnRH)-agonists, and aromatase inhibitors. Hysterectomy may be recommended, although endometriosis can recur even after surgery until menopause occurs. Rarely, if endometriosis is widespread, further surgery is needed to treat other affected areas.

Diana Gitig

KEY FACTS

Description
Uterine tissue is found elsewhere, often in the pelvis.

Causes
Unknown.

Risk factors
Women who have children after the age of 30, or who never give birth, are more likely to have endometriosis.

Symptoms
Pelvic pain and infertility.

Diagnosis
Laparoscopy, a procedure in which the pelvic cavity is examined with a viewing instrument, usually confirms the diagnosis.

Treatments
Painkillers may be sufficient. Hormonal therapy to suppress production of the female sex hormone estrogen can relieve symptoms. Surgery is an option in severe cases.

Pathogenesis
Infertility, but pregnancy may bring about an improvement in the condition.

Prevention
Difficult to prevent as its cause is unknown.

Epidemiology
In the United States, the prevalence of endometriosis is estimated to be 10 percent.

See also

- Female reproductive system • Infertility
- Menstrual disorders • Pregnancy and childbirth

Environmental disorders

Environmental disorders are caused by environmental hazards such as microorganisms, parasites, air and water pollution, radiation, and occupational risks. What makes them of interest as environmental disorders is the pathway of infection or exposure.

Many environmental disorders are caused by abiotic, or nonliving, agents. These include radiation as well as air, soil, and water pollution. Pollution can be caused by organic chemicals, such as petroleum products, and by inorganic chemicals, such as hydrochloric acid. Even substances not normally thought of as pollutants, for example, milk, can trigger environmental illness in some situations. Radiation and pollutants can come from natural sources as well as human sources.

Though nature may appear benign, risks abound, even in the most idyllic settings. A relaxing day at the beach can lead to weeks of misery as a result of sunburn. A drink of water from a clear mountain stream can lead to days of gastrointestinal agony. Intense, lingering pain can result from touching a poisonous plant. A minor scrape on a football field can lead to death from an untreatable infection, for example, methicillin-resistant *Staphylococcus aureus* (MRSA).

Environmental risks are compounded when one considers how humans have modified the landscape. Grit from urban air pollution can irritate the nose and throat and cause respiratory infections. Untreated sewage in streets serves as a source for waterborne infections. Even the air conditioner, a staple of modern human life in the developed world, may serve as a conduit for lethal disease.

The World Health Organization (WHO), in its 2006 report *Preventing Disease through Healthy Environments*, defined the environment as "all the physical, chemical and biological factors external to the human host, and all related behaviours, but excluding those natural environments that cannot reasonably be modified." Factors that one cannot modify at the source, such as sunlight, but to which one can modify exposure, for example, by wearing sunscreen, were considered to be environmental factors. The WHO report includes accidents, depression, suicide, and violence among the group of environmental health threats.

Disease burden can be measured using a statistic called disability-adjusted life year (DALY), which measures the number of years of potential life lost due to premature mortality and the years of productive life lost due to disability. The WHO report estimated that about 24 percent (354 million DALYs) of the global

RELATED ARTICLES

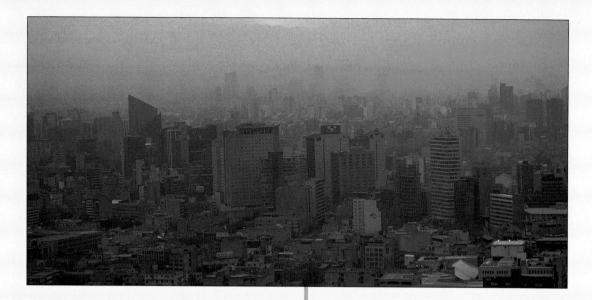

annual disease burden is caused by some form of environmental factor. Likewise, about 34 percent of the disease burden in children under the age of 15 is caused by some form of environmental exposure. The report found that the proportion of deaths (in terms of premature mortality because of environmental factors) is as high as 23 percent overall; the proportion of deaths attributable to environmental causes among children less than 15 years of age is 36 percent.

The toll exacted by environmental disorders is highest in developing countries. The WHO report found that the highest burden is borne in parts of Africa, with more than 100 DALYs per 1,000 population and more than 350 deaths per 100,000 population. The burden in most of the rest of Africa, the former Soviet Union, parts of eastern Europe, and southern and southwestern Asia is more than 50 DALYs per 1,000 and more than 200 deaths per 100,000. The disease burden in much of the developed world (western Europe, Australia, Canada, Japan, and the United States) is less than 20 DALYs per 1,000, with fewer than 150 deaths per 100,000.

The differences in health burden from environmental causes between developed and developing countries stem from a number of factors, including: differences in infrastructure, such as in sanitation and water supplies and insect vectors of disease; differences in governmental regulation of industrial activity, such as food processing or emissions of pollutants; and differences in social development, such as education. Environmental disorders can be caused by both biotic

Mexico City is one of the most polluted cities in the world. The main source of the pollution is the exhaust fumes from 4 million motor vehicles. The government of Mexico City is attempting to solve the problem with innovative measures.

(living) and abiotic (nonliving) agents. Biotic causes of environmental disorders include pathogens, such as bacteria, fungi, worms, and other parasites. Poisonous plants and animals, even biting and stinging animals, cause what can be considered environmental disorders. Abiotic causes include radiation and chemicals, both of which have natural and human sources.

Disease from water, soil, and food

While pathogens and parasites are specifically infectious diseases, they can be considered environmental diseases under certain circumstances: for instance, if the primary pathway of exposure is a vector other than person-to-person contact, or if exposure could be controlled by modifying the environment or behavior that makes exposure likely.

Water- and food-borne diseases that result in diarrhea or dysentery are the leading cause of environment-related health problems in the world. The primary diarrheal diseases include: amoebiasis; cholera; giardiasis and other protozoal diseases; salmonellosis; shigellosis; typhoid and paratyphoid fevers; and viral diseases. Collectively, they are the cause of more than 16 percent of the global environmental disease burden (58 million DALYs per year) and

13 percent of deaths (1.7 million per year). Overall, this represents more than 94 percent of all cases of diarrheal disease, according to WHO estimates. Children under 15 are most affected, with 54 million DALYs per year and 1.5 million deaths. Among environmental disorders, diarrheal diseases cause 29 percent of total disease burden and 36 percent of all deaths in that age group.

The primary pathway of infection is fecal-oral exposure via contaminated water, poor sanitary conditions, or poor hygiene. Inadequate clean water supplies are the primary cause, since water is readily contaminated by fecal waste from humans and animals. In the developing world, high populations, often depending on a limited water supply, coupled with limited infrastructure for wastewater collection and sewage treatment, create a recipe for disaster. In the developed world, inadequate hygiene is a major contributing factor, although aging infrastructure may pose problems in long-urbanized areas. Almost all (99 percent) of the environmental disease burden from diarrheal diseases falls upon developing nations.

Other water-, soil-, and food-borne diseases considered in the WHO analysis include ascariasis, hookworm, schistosomiasis, trachoma, and trichuriasis. Ascariasis, hookworm, and trichuriasis are intestinal nematode diseases. They are primarily contracted via the ingestion of food and contact with soil or other media contaminated with fecal matter. These diseases are responsible for 2.9 million DALYs. The health burden from trachoma is 2.3 million DALYs and that from schistosomiasis is 2.2 million DALYs. These diseases are almost exclusively developing world phenomena.

Airborne diseases

Upper and lower respiratory tract infections (excluding tuberculosis) comprise the second-largest cause of environment-related disorders. According to WHO estimates, upper and lower respiratory tract infections cause 11 percent of the global environmental health burden (38 million DALYs) overall, and 16 percent (31 million DALYs) of the global burden among children less than 15. Respiratory infections are responsible for 12 percent of all environment-related deaths (1.5 million), with 830,000 of those deaths among children younger than 15.

While respiratory tract infections are often caused by pathogens, a number of other factors increase the risk. Air pollution plays a significant role. Sources of pollutants include: tobacco smoke (with an obvious risk to smokers themselves, but also to nonsmokers inhaling tobacco smoke); solid fuels such as wood and coal; industrial sources; automobile exhaust; and housing conditions.

As with water- and food-borne diseases, the heaviest toll falls upon developing nations, with 97 percent of the global burden (37 million DALYs). One of the reasons for the disparity is the heavy reliance of solid fuels for cooking and heating. As much as 36 percent of lower respiratory tract infections worldwide may be attributed to this practice.

Tuberculosis (TB) is responsible for 1.8 percent (6.3 million DALYs) of the global disease burden and 2.2 percent (285,000) of deaths. Although TB is primarily an infectious disease spread by human-to-human contact, environmental conditions, such as overcrowding, contribute to its spread. About 89 percent (6.1 million DALYs) of the burden from tuberculosis is felt in the developing world.

Asthma and chronic obstructive pulmonary disease (COPD) are also triggered largely by airborne pathogens and pollutants. COPD is responsible for 3.3 percent of the global environmental disease burden (12 million DALYs) but 9.9 percent (1.3 million) of deaths. Asthma causes 1.9 percent (6.7 million DALYs) of the global burden but only 0.8 percent (106,000) of deaths. Both diseases are more prevalent in the developed world. Because of its progressive nature, COPD is mainly an adult phenomenon, while 41 percent of the asthma burden is borne by children less than 15 years of age.

Lung cancer is also linked to exposure to airborne pollutants such as tobacco smoke. The disease accounts for 1 percent of the environmental health burden (3.4 million DALYs) and 2.9 percent of deaths (380,000). The distribution of the health burden from lung cancer is about evenly split between the developed and developing world.

Insect-borne diseases

Insect-borne diseases, such as malaria, Chagas' disease, filariasis, river blindness (onchocerciasis), leishmaniasis, dengue, and Japanese encephalitis, are considered environmental diseases because humans can control exposure to the insect vectors. The risk of contracting the diseases is reduced by modifying the environment to permanently eliminate or reduce habitats favorable to the insect vectors; by altering the environment to temporarily reduce conditions favorable to the insect vectors; or by changing housing conditions or behavior to reduce contact with the insect vectors. These diseases are mainly problems of the developing world.

Malaria, filariasis, Japanese encephalitis, and dengue are transmitted by the bites of infected mosquitoes. Malaria, which is caused by protozoan parasites of the genus *Plasmodium*, is the most costly of all the insect-borne diseases, accounting for 5.4 percent of the global environmental disease burden with 19 million DALYs and 530,000 deaths per year. More than 90 percent of the disease burden and death falls upon children under 15 years of age. Filariasis, caused by nematode worms of the genera *Brugia* or *Wucheria*, accounts for 1.1 percent of the global environmental disease burden, with 3.7 million DALYs. The toll from the viral diseases Japanese encephalitis and dengue are 670,000 DALYs and 590,000 DALYs per year, respectively.

Leishmaniasis is caused by protozoan parasites of the genus *Leishmania*, which is transmitted primarily by the bites of sand flies. River blindness is caused by nematode worms of the genus *Onchocerca*, via the bites of black flies. The burden from the two diseases is 550,000 DALYs and 56,000 DALYs per year, respectively. Chagas' disease, caused by protozoan parasites of the genus *Trypanosoma*, is spread by "assassin" or "kissing" bugs. Chagas' disease is responsible for 370,000 DALYs per year.

Radiation, toxic chemicals, and cancer

Radiation and toxic chemicals are responsible for many environmental diseases. They contribute to susceptibility for some of the diseases discussed above. Radon gas, for example, is emitted naturally from rocks and soils, so it can be inhaled. The gas is inert, but it decays to radioactive polonium and lead and is a major cause of lung and other cancers.

The most prevalent source of radiation affecting humans is sunlight. Ultraviolet and other shortwave radiation are very damaging to cell components such as DNA. DNA damage typically results in mutations, and mutations may trigger development of cancerous tumors. Too much sun for a day may trigger sunburn, but over a few decades it may result in skin cancer.

Toxic chemicals, particularly mutagens (chemicals that cause mutations), often play an important role. Chemicals in food may increase the risk for stomach and colon cancers. Inhalation of asbestos fibers greatly increases the risk of contracting mesothelioma, an otherwise rare form of lung cancer.

Cancers other than lung cancer account for 3.1 percent (11 million DALYs) of the global environmental health burden and 7.7 percent (1.0 million) of deaths per year. Cancer is a disease primarily of adults, although 5 percent of the disease burden is borne by children under the age of 15. About two-thirds of the cancer burden is in the developing world.

Lead affects the mental development of children, leading to mild to severe mental retardation. Lead, because of its use as an octane booster in gasoline as well as a component of many paint products, was a common contaminant in urban areas. Concerns over the effects of lead on child development resulted in prohibitions of its use.

Food supply and climate change

Food production requires favorable environmental conditions. Most crops require moderate temperatures and adequate water. When conditions do not favor food production, shortages ensue, but often there is a lack of financial capital to import food supplies. This leads to undernourishment, in which a person does not receive enough calories in the diet, as well as malnourishment, in which a person receives a diet lacking in one or more essential nutrients. In either case, health is harmed, as malnourished persons— especially children—are more susceptible to diseases such as diphtheria, measles, meningitis, poliomyelitis, tetanus, and whooping cough. The total global health burden from malnutrition and related problems is 18 million DALYs and 370,000 deaths per year. More than 99 percent of the cases are in children under 15.

Finally, climate change may affect all of the factors discussed, including the ability to raise food. Water supplies and the habitats of organisms that harbor or transmit disease may also be affected. Accurate predictions of where effects will be felt, and if those effects will be harmful, are difficult to make.

David M. Lawrence

Epilepsy

A brain disorder in which clusters of nerve cells, or neurons, in the brain exhibit abnormal electrical activity, epilepsy causes disturbance of emotions and behavior and sometimes convulsions, muscle spasms, and loss of consciousness.

When ancient Babylonians or Egyptians saw a person having a seizure, they believed that the condition was of supernatural origin and that the gods were visiting that person. Egyptian papyri show people with a "sacred disease" that is now recognized as epilepsy. However, Hippocrates (c. 460 to c. 380 BCE), disagreeing with these beliefs, scoffed at the idea of a divine origin for epilepsy. In his treatise *On the Sacred Disease*, he sarcastically addressed each of the different gods supposed to produce seizures and declared that there was no evidence for these notions. He insisted that the disease was a disease of the brain. The idea of supernatural causes did persist, however, and during the Middle Ages acquired a demonic twist. Medieval paintings depict people with ghastly demons coming out of the body at the end of a seizure.

Myths and stigmas concerning epilepsy are still prevalent in many places. Epilepsy is feared as a terrible and puzzling disease. But researchers are fitting together pieces of the epilepsy puzzle, and scientists now know that epilepsy is not one disease but many conditions with a common thread.

Epilepsy has been described as an electrical storm in the brain during which groups of nerve cells fire rapid electrical impulses. The type of seizure depends on which parts of the brain are affected.

Types of epilepsy

Hundreds of epilepsy syndromes as well as several types of seizures exist. Each disorder has a specific set of symptoms. While some appear to be hereditary, others are traced to specific events, such as a blow to the head or a stroke. However, for most cases, the cause is idiopathic (unknown). The areas of the brain in which the syndromes originate usually give the conditions their names. The more common types are described below.

In absence epilepsy, people have momentary lapses of consciousness or brief blackouts. At one time called *petit mal* (from the French, meaning "little sickness"), the symptoms begin in childhood or adolescence. The child may not even be aware that he or she has had a

seizure; teachers may perceive that the child is staring into space or not paying attention. The child may experience a jerking arm or rapidly blinking eyes. Childhood absence epilepsy usually stops during puberty, but occasionally it may develop into a more serious form of epilepsy. These occurrences tend to run in families, and faulty genes may be responsible.

KEY FACTS

Description
A brain disorder that may cause seizures or other undesirable behaviors.

Causes
An electrical storm in the brain, in which groups of nerve cells rapidly fire electrical impulses.

Risk factors
Some cases appear to be hereditary; some are traced to an event such as a blow to the head or a stroke; most causes are unknown.

Symptoms
Vary with the type of epilepsy and depend on the section of the brain that is affected.

Diagnosis
Electroencephalography (EEG), in which electrodes are attached to the head to study electrical activity of the brain; magnetic resonance imaging (MRI); and computed tomography (CT).

Treatments
No cure exists at present; drug therapies are designed to remedy seizures and control undesirable behaviors; surgery may be recommended when drugs do not control seizures.

Pathogenesis
Can be life threatening, especially if seizures are not controlled.

Prevention
No specific prevention; general caution to avoid injury or blows to the head.

Epidemiology
An estimated 42 million people worldwide are afflicted; around 2.5 million Americans are affected by epilepsy and seizures.

Psychomotor epilepsy is characterized by strange or purposeless movements. This type of epilepsy originates in a region of the brain called the temporal lobe. The child may get up out of his or her seat in school and walk around the room as if in a daze, pulling at clothing or making other unusual movements. This type of epilepsy is also called recurrent partial seizure.

Temporal lobe epilepsy (TLE) is a common type of epilepsy. It usually begins in childhood. An aura—a "warning" sensation—may accompany this seizure. Repeated TLE seizures can cause the hippocampus in the brain to shrink, affecting memory and learning. Recognizing this type for early treatment is critical.

Frontal lobe epilepsy involves a cluster of short seizures with sudden onset and termination. Many types of these seizures exist; the symptoms depend on where in the frontal lobe the seizures occur.

Occipital lobe epilepsy usually begins with visual hallucinations, since this area of the brain is related to vision, rapid eye blinking, and other eye-related symptoms. Otherwise, the symptoms are similar to TLE.

Parietal lobe epilepsy tends to begin in the parietal lobe but spreads to other parts of the brain and closely resembles the symptoms of other kinds of epilepsy.

Lennox-Gastaut syndrome is a type of severe epilepsy that begins in childhood. The syndrome is characterized by sudden attacks resulting in falls. It is very difficult to treat.

Rasmussen's encephalitis is a condition that begins in childhood and is progressive. Half of the brain shows continual inflammation. It may be treated with a radical surgical procedure called hemispherectomy.

Ramsay Hunt syndrome type II is a rare and progressive type of epilepsy that begins in early adulthood and leads to reduced muscle coordination and cognitive ability in addition to seizures.

Infantile spasms is a type of epilepsy that begins in infancy with clusters of seizures before the age of six months. The infant may bend or cry out during an attack.

A complication associated with epilepsy is status epilepticus, which is a severe, life-threatening condition in which the person has prolonged seizures for over five minutes or does not fully regain consciousness between seizures. Rarely, death may occur for no discernible reason in people with epilepsy.

Whereas any type of seizure is a major concern, a seizure in isolation does not mean a person has epilepsy. People exhibit seizures with several other conditions such as high fever, narcolepsy, Tourette's syndrome, cardiac arrhythmia, and eclampsia.

Causes

Recent advances in molecular genetics, molecular biology, and electrophysiology have increased the knowledge and understanding of the basics of electrical discharge in the nervous system that is assumed to underlie epilepsy. Neurotransmitters, the chemicals that regulate electrical charges in the brain, are involved. Alterations in the levels of excitatory neurotransmitters or the inhibitory neurotransmitter gamma-butyric acid (GABA), or both, are believed to play a role in epilepsy. Genes may control the process. Knowing how new nerve cells migrate to their proper locations has led to the identification of faulty genes (mutations) that disrupt the normal pattern. For example, a gene called doublecortin may cause migrating nerve cells to stop short of the destination.

Symptoms and signs

Two major categories, partial and generalized, include more than 30 different types of seizures. Partial seizures occur in only one area of the brain and comprise about 60 percent of all seizures. Partial seizures are divided into simple and complex.

During a simple partial seizure the person remains conscious but may have unusual or unexplainable feelings of joy, anger, sadness, or nausea. They may hear, smell, taste, see, or feel things that are not there.

Complex partial seizures last only a few seconds, and the person just blanks out or has strange movements called automatisms. Violent behavior, such as hitting the wall or throwing a book across the room, may lead others to conclude that the person has a mental illness. The person may have an aura that indicates the seizure is coming. Another term for these partial seizures, especially those centered in the temporal lobe, is *psychomotor seizures*.

Generalized seizures result from abnormal neuronal activity in many parts of the brain, and these are of several types. During absence seizures the person has momentary loss of consciousness and may stare into space for several moments or have jerking or twitching movements. In tonic seizures the victim stiffens muscles of the body, generally the arms, back, and legs. In clonic seizures both sides of the body experience jerking movements. Myoclonic seizures cause the person to experience sudden jerking movements or twitches of the upper body, arms, or legs. In atonic seizures the person loses normal muscle tone and may fall down, nodding the head involuntarily like a rag doll. Tonic-clonic seizures include a mixture of symptoms such as loss of consciousness, stiffening of the body,

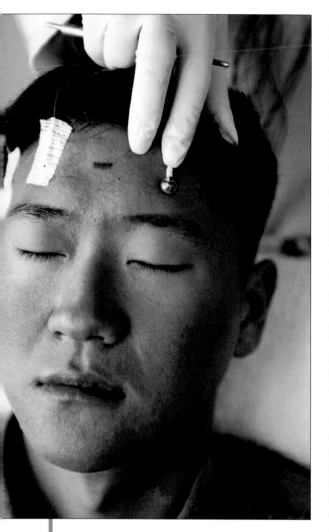

An electroencephalograph can help to diagnose epilepsy. Electrodes are attached to the patient's scalp; these electrodes are connected to a machine that amplifies brain impulses, which are measured as electrical activity. The results are recorded on a monitor. Any abnormal electrical activity is shown on the wave patterns, and different types of epilepsy can be identified.

and repeated jerking of arms and legs. The older name for this type is *grand mal* seizure.

Diagnosis

While some symptoms of epilepsy are obvious, others may be subtle, and discovering which type of epilepsy a patient is suffering from is essential before treatment can begin. The physician begins with an extensive medical history of the patient and family. He or she performs an electroencephalograph (EEG), in which

16 to 30 small electrodes are attached to the scalp with a special paste or with a special cap. A light is flashed in the eyes, and impulses or brain waves are recorded on a moving sheet of paper. Another important test is magnetic resonance imaging (MRI). One new version of MRI called fluid-attenuated inversion recover (FLAIR) may reveal important information about the processes deep in the brain. FLAIR can show abnormalities in the hippocampus and other internal regions. Other tests include blood tests and a spinal tap.

Treatments

Drugs are used to combat convulsions. Several drugs that have been on the market for several years, including phenytoin, valproate, and carbamazepine, are drugs of first choice. For the 30 percent of people with epilepsy who do not respond well to the drugs of first choice, newer drugs called antiepileptic drugs are approved as monotherapy (treatment by means of a single drug) or in combination with other drugs. These newer drugs include tiagabine, lamotrigine, gabapentin, topiramate, levetiracetam, felbamate, zonesimide, and oxcarbamazepine. However, all these drugs are powerful and have side effects.

Intractable epilepsy occurs when a person continues to experience seizures despite treatment with drugs. In such cases, doctors may recommend evaluation for surgery. A team of doctors, usually at a university medical center, looks at the type of seizures and at the brain region involved. Surgery may reduce or halt some seizures, but it is not without risk. Radiosurgery, in which ionizing radiation is used to destroy brain tissue, is being used experimentally in some medical centers to treat epilepsy. Other new treatments include stem-cell transplants and transplanting GABA-producing neurons from the fetuses of pigs into the brains of patients. Future treatments may include gene therapy to counter the effects of faulty genes.

Epidemiology

About 200,000 new cases of epilepsy occur in the United States each year; 10 percent of the population of the United States will have a seizure in their lifetime, and 3 percent will develop epilepsy by the age of 75. Men are slightly more likely to develop epilepsy than women. In addition, African Americans have a higher incidence of the disorder.

Evelyn Kelly

See also
• Brain disorders • Diagnosis

Epstein-Barr infection

Epstein-Barr virus is the most frequent agent of infectious mononucleosis, and it is known to cause cancer of the head and neck in children, especially in Africa. The virus was discovered by Michael Epstein and Yvonne Barr in 1964, while they were researching cancer that primarily affected the head and neck of children.

Epstein-Barr virus (EBV) belongs to the herpes family of viruses; it is also called herpes virus type 4. EBV is transmitted through the saliva of infected people during kissing, sharing food, or other intimate contact. After entry, EBV invades the cells lining the throat (epithelial cells). In the epithelial cells, EBV multiplies, and numerous particles of the virus are released, destroying the epithelial cells in the process. The released viral particles then invade B lymphocytes (a type of white blood cell), which triggers a potent response by "killer" T lymphocytes that attempt to defeat the infection. However, Epstein-Barr infection usually remains inactive in B lymphocytes. The formation of coinlike structures called "episomes" allows EBV to reside in the nucleus of infected cells.

EBV is not spread as easily as some other viruses, such as the virus that causes the common cold, but it is common worldwide. In the United States and Great Britain, 50 percent of the population have positive blood tests for Epstein-Barr infection at the age of five and up to 90 percent in the adult population. Lower socioeconomic groups tend to acquire the virus at an earlier age. However, during early childhood and pre-adolescence the infection does not cause symptoms.

Symptoms and signs

Clinical signs of acute Epstein-Barr infection (mononucleosis) occur mostly in people exposed to the virus after the second decade of life, such as college students and military recruits. Typical signs include sore throat, fever, and swollen glands of the neck. In severe cases, there is also significant spleen enlargement. Although the spleen's primary function is to filter blood, many white cells, particularly lymphocytes, are located in this organ. When there is an inflammatory reaction against the virus, the spleen can become quite large, and there is a risk of rupture. In normal people, the symptoms of acute infection usually resolve in 4 to 6 weeks. However, the virus can remain dormant, establishing a lifelong carrier state. Epstein-Barr infection is spread by the excretion of viral particles in the saliva of people chronically infected with the virus, who are otherwise healthy and symptom free.

Pathogenesis

Epstein-Barr infection remains dormant and chronic in more than 95 percent of infected people. However, in people with altered immune systems, the virus may activate and result in malignancy. Examples include Burkitt's lymphoma, the most common childhood cancer in central Africa, lymphoma after transplant surgery, and leukoplakia (raised white patches in the mouth) in AIDS patients.

Edward Cachay and Sanjay Mehta

KEY FACTS

Description
A type of herpes virus that causes infectious mononucleosis and other disorders.

Causes
A virus invading the lymphocytes.

Risk factors
Epstein-Barr infection is transmitted through exposure to saliva of infected people.

Symptoms
Signs of infection are mostly the result of the body trying to eradicate the virus.

Diagnosis
Clinical symptoms and laboratory tests, such as white cell count and antibody tests.

Treatments
No specific treatment or vaccine is available.

Pathogenesis
In people with weak or abnormal immune systems, the infection may lead to development of cancer.

Prevention
Avoiding close contact with infected people.

Epidemiology
Common worldwide. In the United States 90 percent of adults aged 35 to 40 have been infected.

See also
• Cancer • Hepatitis infections • Infections, viral • Lymphoma • Mononucleosis

Eye disorders

The cornea is the transparent, dome-shaped window covering the front of the eye. It is a powerful refracting surface, providing two-thirds of the eye's focusing power. The cornea consists of five discrete layers: epithelium, Bowman's layer, stroma, Descemet's membrane, and endothelium. When healthy, the endothelial cell layer is a single stratum of hexagonal cells that keeps the cornea dehydrated and clean. Following trauma or injury, the surrounding endothelial cells slide over to the injured area. If excessive, the cornea becomes swollen and cloudy.

Corneal dystrophies are important disorders because they can greatly reduce vision. There are over 20 corneal dystrophies that affect all parts of the cornea; however, many are extremely rare. They are genetic in nature and may be present at birth, but more frequently they occur during adolescence and progress gradually throughout life. Some forms are mild, while others can be severe.

Corneal dystrophies may be categorized as epithelial, stromal, lattice, and endothelial. They are also classified based on inheritance pattern, including dominant granular dystrophies, recessive macular dystrophy, and dominant lattice-like dystrophies. The most common corneal dystrophies are keratoconus and Fuchs' dystrophy.

Keratoconus

Keratoconus, which literally means "conical or cone-shaped cornea," is an endothelial dystrophy in which the normally round dome-shaped cornea progressively thins, causing a conelike bulge to develop, resulting in severe optical deterioriation. In its earliest stages, keratoconus causes slight blurring and distortion of vision and increased sensitivity to glare and light. These symptoms usually first appear in early adulthood and affect each eye differently. Keratoconus can progress for 10 to 20 years and then slow or stabilize.

Despite considerable research, the etiology of keratoconus remains uncertain. It can be inherited, but it can be associated with several general abnormalities of connective tissue and eye disease. Within any individual keratoconic cornea, there may be found regions of degenerative thinning coexisting with regions undergoing wound healing.

A genetic predisposition to keratoconus has been observed, with frequency of occurrence within families ranging from 6 to 19 percent. The specific gene or genes responsible for this heredity have not yet been identified; however, most genetic studies agree on a dominant autosomal model of inheritance. Keratoconus

---

RELATED ARTICLES

is also diagnosed more often in people with Down syndrome, although the reason for this link has yet to be identified. Keratoconus has been associated with asthma, allergies, and eczema. A number of studies suggest that vigorous eye rubbing may contribute to the progression of keratoconus, and that patients should be discouraged from the practice.

Keratoconus can be difficult to detect because it usually develops so slowly. However, in some cases, it may proceed rapidly. Myopia and astigmatism may accompany this disease, creating additional problems with distorted and blurred vision. Glare and light sensitivity may also be experienced. Keratoconic patients often have frequent prescription changes each time they visit their ophthalmologist or optometrist.

Diagnosis of keratoconus involves a standard opthalmological examination, including a Snellen visual acuity test. Measurement of the curvature of the cornea is performed using a keratometer, with a detection of irregular astigmatism suggesting the possibility of keratoconus.

Further testing may be done using a retinoscope in which a high beam of light is passed through the patient's retina and the reflection is observed as the light source is tilted back and forth. Keratoconus exhibits a "scissor reflex" in which the two bands of light move toward and away from each other like the blades of a pair of scissors. Slit lamp examination may also be performed to further observe the corneal epithelium. A handheld keratoscope can provide a noninvasive visualization of the surface of the cornea by projecting a series of concentric rings of light onto the cornea.

Finally, corneal topography, or mapping of the surface of the cornea, can provide a definitive diagnosis of keratoconus. This technique projects an illuminated pattern onto the cornea and determines its topology by analyzing the digital image. The "map" that is produced reveals distortions in the cornea, with keratoconus appearing as a steepening of curvature. Corneal topography can also be used to benchmark the disease and assess rates of progression.

Treatment of keratoconus usually begins with the use of rigid contact lenses, although soft contact lenses or eyeglasses may still be suitable in the early stages. The rigid contact lenses help to provide the best possible vision by providing a smooth spherical anterior surface that fills in behind the lens, but they do not affect the rate of progression of the condition.

As the condition progresses, good vision may be difficult to maintain, and contact lens tolerance may vary. "Intacs" or corneal inserts, placed just under the eye's surface in the periphery of the cornea, help achieve a flatter cornea, leading to clearer vision. Another new procedure for treating keratoconus, known as corneal collagen cross-linking riboflavin (C3-R), is a noninvasive method of strengthening corneal tissue to halt bulging of the eye's surface. Eye drops containing riboflavin (vitamin B_2) are placed on the cornea and then are activated by a special light to strengthen connective tissue within the eye. C3-R may be combined with Intacs to treat keratoconus.

Finally, in keratoconus patients who cannot tolerate a rigid contact lens, or for whom contact lenses or other therapies no longer provide acceptable vision, a corneal transplant procedure, replacing the weakened, bulging tissue with normal tissue, may be required. Refractive surgery procedures such as laser surgery can further weaken the cornea and are contraindicated.

Keratoconus cannot be prevented. Some specialists believe that patients with keratoconus should have aggressive treatment of ocular allergy and should be instructed not to rub their eyes.

According to the National Eye Institute, keratoconus is the most common corneal dystrophy in the United States, affecting 1 in every 2,000 individuals. There is a slightly higher prevalence in females than males. Keratoconus is usually bilateral, affecting both eyes. It is common for keratoconus to be diagnosed first in one eye and not until later in the other eye.

Fuchs' dystrophy

Fuchs' dystrophy is an inherited condition that affects the delicate inner layer (endothelium) of the cornea. The endothelium functions as a pump mechanism, constantly removing fluids from the cornea to maintain its clarity. Patients gradually lose these endothelial cells as the dystrophy progresses. Once lost, the endothelial cells do not grow back, but instead excrescences, or abnormal outgrowths, form over the Decement's membrane, which gradually becomes abnormally thick. The pump system becomes less efficient, causing corneal

STRUCTURE OF THE EYE

The eyeball has three layers, which in turn are composed of different structures. The outermost layer includes the sclera (white of the eye) and transparent cornea. The middle layer comprises the iris (colored part of the eye), ciliary body (muscles that alter the shape of the lens), and the choroid (which contains blood vessels). The inner layer forms a light-sensitive membrane called the retina, upon which rays of light converge to form images. The front of the eye is filled with aqueous humor and the back cavity with vitreous humor. The humors provide nutrients as well as pressure to maintain the shape of the eyeball.

The eye can be affected by many disorders. These include detached retina, in which the light-sensitive retina lifts away from the back of the eye, and diabetic retinopathy, in which the blood vessels in the eye swell as a result of high blood pressure or diabetes.

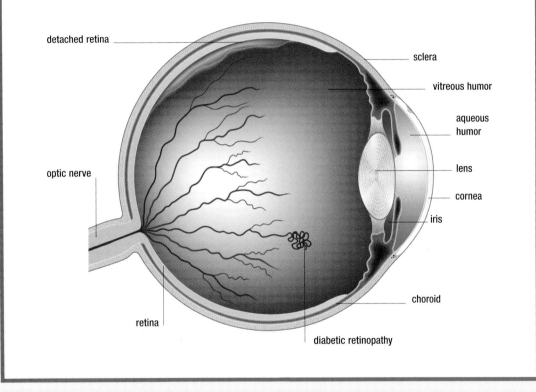

clouding, swelling, and, eventually, reduced vision. Fuchs' dystrophy progresses in three clinical stages, which usually span 10 to 20 years: cornea guttata, stromal and epithelial edema or swelling, and corneal scarring.

Cornea guttata. The earliest sign of Fuchs' dystrophy is cornea guttata, in which the cornea has a "beaten metal" or "orange peel" appearance. Occasionally, a diffuse brown pigmentation of the central posterior surface is also seen. The endothelial cells show degeneration, and Descemet's membrane thickens. The patient usually has no complaints at this stage. Some very observant patients notice that the quality of their 20/20 vision is not the same as before.

Stromal and epithelial edema. As cornea guttata progressively grow over time, the endothelial cells are disrupted, halting the pump system that removes fluids from the cornea. Fluid seeps into the cornea, producing stromal and epithelial edema. As edema increases, the stroma thickens centrally, the cornea becomes opaque, or cloudy, and this opacity spreads, reducing vision. The epithelium develops blisters known as bullae. The bullae rupture, causing pain, and expose the cornea to the danger of infectious keratitis. As stromal edema increases, Descemet's membrane develops wrinkles, termed striae. Pain and sensitivity to light develop as the edema spreads to the epithelium.

The exact cause of Fuchs' dystrophy is unknown. Hereditary plays a role. The inheritance pattern is autosomal dominant, which means that half of the offspring of an affected individual (both male and female) will receive the gene for Fuchs' dystrophy and are at risk for developing this corneal deterioration. Hormonal and inflammatory factors are also believed to play a role.

Fuchs' endothelial dystrophy develops later in life, usually in the fifth or sixth decade. Women are at higher risk for developing the disorder, and members of families with the dystrophy are at higher risk. In general, corneal dystrophies exhibit familial patterns and have no association with systemic or environmental factors. Fuchs' is also associated with a slightly increased prevalence of open-angle glaucoma.

Initially, a patient with corneal guttata has no symptoms. With the progression of the disorder to the stromal and epithelial edema phase, patients experience decreased vision upon wakening and, later, foreign body sensation. Microscopy reveals thickening of the Descemet's membrane, corneal guttata, corneal stromal edema, wrinkles in Descemet's membrane resulting from corneal edema, fine pigment "dusting" on the corneal endothelium, and bullae.

Slit lamp microscopy, which magnifies the endothelial cells, is used to diagnose Fuchs' dystrophy. Confocal microscopy is an imaging technique with better contrast than conventional microscopy, which is capable of producing three-dimensional images. It is also useful in diagnosing Fuchs' dystrophy. The endothelium is also evaluated and monitored using pachymetry, which shows the thickened cornea, and specular miscroscopy, which visualizes the number, density, and quality of endothelial cells that line the back of the cornea.

The treatment for Fuchs' endothelial dystrophy varies, depending upon the severity of the disease. Corneal guttae do not need to be treated if the cornea has not been damaged and if there is no sign of stromal or epithelial edema. If edema exists, salt solutions such as sodium chloride drops or ointment are often prescribed to draw fluid from the cornea and reduce swelling. Some patients use a hair dryer held at arm's length to help evaporate small amounts of edema and decrease blur.

A bandage soft contact lens can be beneficial in reducing discomfort in patients who have advanced corneal edema with bullae. If severe pain is present and good vision is not required, electrosurgery (cautery) of the Bowman's layer can be done, or a conjunctival flap can be made. To improve vision, penetrating keratoplasty is performed. Cataracts are common in patients with Fuchs' dystrophy, and combining penetrating keratoplasty and cataract extraction is recommended. Corneal grafts for Fuchs' dystrophy account for approximately 10 percent of all corneal grafts performed. Generally, if the graft is performed before there is involvement of the peripheral cornea, there is an 80 percent likelihood that the graft will remain clear for two years.

Fuchs' dystrophy cannot be prevented. Early detection via a comprehensive eye examination can lead to treatment options that will be beneficial as the disorder progresses.

The exact incidence of Fuchs' dystrophy is unknown. After age 40, approximately 70 percent of patients with Fuchs' dystrophy have corneal guttata; however, only 0.1 percent of these patients have epithelial edema and bullae formation.

The disorder is three times more likely to occur in women than in men, according to a 30-year study done in the United States; however, no race is immune from the disorder. Patients usually develop the disorder in their 60s and 70s, although it is possible to develop Fuchs in the 30s or 40s.

Ocular movement disorders

Ocular movement and vision are inseparable. The eye has six muscles, known as extraocular muscles, which control movement: the inferior oblique, the superior oblique, the lateral rectus, the medial rectus, the inferior rectus, and the superior rectus.

The primary function of the four rectus muscles is to control the eye's movements from left to right and up and down. The two oblique muscles move the eye to rotate the eyes inward and outward. All six muscles work in unison to move the eye. As one contracts, the opposing muscle relaxes, creating smooth movements. In addition to the muscles of one eye

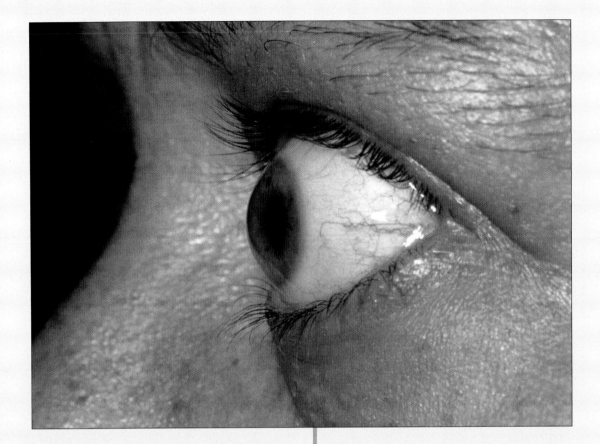

working together in a coordinated effort, the muscles of both eyes work in unison. The brain controls the eye muscles, which ensure proper alignment of the eyes. It is critical that the muscles function together in order for the brain to interpret the image from each eye as a single one. If one eye is misaligned, two different images are sent to the brain. The brain often responds by ignoring one of the images. If this occurs in childhood, development of vision is limited. If untreated, permanent visual impairment and loss of depth perception can occur because the visual system in the eye and the brain never develops properly.

Strabismus

Strabismus is a visual defect in which the eyes are misaligned and point in different directions. Also referred to as "squint," strabismus can occur early in childhood or later in adulthood, although the causes of the eye misalignment are different. Strabismus can be the first sign of a serious vision problem. Estropia, or convergent strabismus, occurs when one eye is turned in toward the center. This condition is the most

In a person suffering from thyrotoxicosis, the eye bulges from its socket (exophthalmos). Swelling of the soft tissue in the eye socket causes the eyeball to be pushed forward.

common form of strabismus. Exotropia occurs when one eye turns out away from the center of the face. Hypertropia occurs in which one eye turns up toward the forehead. Hypotropia occurs when one eye turns down toward the cheek. The two most common types of strabismus are esotropia and exotropia.

Amblyopia. Strabismus must be detected early in children as it can cause amblyopia, or "lazy eye." Amblyopia refers to a reduced vision in one of the eyes because the eye and the brain are not working together properly. The eye itself can look normal, but it is not being used normally because the brain is favoring the other eye. If a child sees double, his or her brain quickly learns to ignore one of the images to maintain single vision. Because of improper stimulation of the involved eye, the portion of the brain serving that eye does not develop properly. In a very short time, the brain permanently suppresses vision from the turned eye. Adults with acquired strabismus typically see double, unlike children.

The causes of strabismus are not well understood. Strabismus tends to run in families, but no specific genes have been linked to the disorder. Furthermore, it is not possible to predict if a child will develop strabismus based on family history. Strabismus of all types is more common in children with developmental problems such as prematurity, cerebral palsy, Down syndrome, and other genetic conditions, and as a consequence of vision loss of any cause. Common causes of strabismus in adults include stroke, Graves' disease, nerve weakness, trauma, vision loss, and recurrent or residual childhood strabismus.

Several syndromes have been associated with strabismus, including Brown's syndrome, Duane's syndrome, Mobius syndrome, and sixth nerve palsy.

Brown's syndrome is caused by an impairment of the trochlear tendon's ability to pass through the trochlea. The result is that the affected eye cannot be fully elevated when the eye is looking toward the nose. Brown's syndrome may be congenital or acquired, unilateral, or bilateral. Severe cases require surgery.

Duane's syndrome occurs when certain nerves of the extraocular muscles become misdirected during fetal development. The result is that the eyes may be straight, esotropic, or exotropic. There is limited eye movement, and the affected eye retracts into the eye socket with attempted movement. In most cases, both eyes are affected, and severe cases require surgery.

Mobius syndrome is characterized by the inability of one or both eyes to move outward. This condition often needs to be corrected with surgery.

Sixth nerve palsy refers to a weakness of the nerve that supplies the lateral rectus muscle, which moves the eye outward. This is usually an acquired condition, associated with the gradual or sudden onset of eye crossing, double vision, and an inability of the eye to move outward. In children, sixth nerve palsy is thought to be caused by a viral illness, herpes zoster virus, which also causes chicken pox. Other causes in the young age group include head trauma and other brain disorders. Sixth nerve palsies generally improve over the course of several months, but may require surgery.

Strabismus is a common condition among children, but it can also occur later in life. It occurs equally in males and females and may run in families. However, many people with strabismus have no relatives with the condition. Hyperopia, or farsightedness, is thought to be a contributing factor. In children, several disorders are associated with strabismus, including retinopathy of prematurity, retinoblastoma, traumatic brain injury, hemangioma near the eye, and cerebral palsy. Some disorders associated with strabismus in adults include diabetes, stroke, ocular trauma, traumatic brain injury, Guillain-Barré syndrome, and botulism. It is vital to test children's vision, preferably by age 3, to ensure that both eyes are used in order to prevent amblyopia.

Signs associated with strabismus include crossed eyes, eyes that do not align in the same direction, uncoordinated eye movements, double vision, and vision in one eye with loss of depth perception. Abnormal head posture, which helps the patient accommodate, is often exhibited.

The diagnosis of strabismus includes all areas of the evaluation of a comprehensive adult or pediatric eye and vision examination. Routine vision screening for young children includes testing for strabismus, usually using the light reflex for infants, and cover testing for preschool-age children. Some health care professionals screen for vision problems with a fundus camera that takes instant pictures of a child's eyes. Crescents of light reflected off the eyes can indicate strabismus.

Strabismus cannot be prevented. However, complications of strabismus can be prevented if the problem is detected early and treated properly. Children should be monitored closely during infancy and the preschool years to detect potential eye problems, particularly if a relative has strabismus. The American Association for Pediatric Ophthalmology and Strabismus, the American Academy of Pediatrics, and the American Academy of Family Physicians recommend that at a minimum all children be screened for eye health before age 6 months and again between 3 and 5 years of age by a pediatrician, family practitioner, or ophthalmologist.

The treatment for strabismus depends on several factors, including the patient's age, the cause of the problem, and the type and degree of the eye turn. Treatment may include patching, corrective glasses, prisms, or surgery. With patching, the better eye is covered, forcing the child to use the weaker eye. Over time, the brain adjusts to using the weaker eye, and vision gradually improves. For this treatment to be effective, it must be done at a young age before the child can develop amblyopia.

Surgery is sometimes performed for both adults and children to straighten a crossed eye. Strabismus surgery involves making a small incision in the tissue covering the eye, which allows the ophthalmologist access to the underlying eye muscles. The eyeball is never removed from the socket during this kind of eye surgery. Which eye muscles are repositioned during the surgery depends upon the direction the eye is turning. It may be necessary to perform eye muscle surgery on both eyes.

Strabismus affects 2 to 4 percent of both the child and adult population. It accounts for 50 percent of all amblyopia cases.

Lid disorders

The eyelids are vital to the health of the surface of the eye because of their protective function and their contribution to the production and dispersal of the tear film, which cleans and lubricates the eye. Eyelid problems range from benign, self-resolving processes to malignant, possibly metastatic, tumors. Lid disorders, such as blepharitis, can interfere with the eyes' ability to produce tears and, therefore, protect the eye. If untreated, this can lead to a condition known as "dry eye," which can result in irreversible damage to the eye and vision.

Bacterial infections of the outer eye are common and usually respond rapidly to treatment with antibiotics; however, under certain circumstances, complications may occur. These infections may be difficult to manage because they frequently recur in some patients. Malignant eyelid tumors may be associated with lash loss and erosion of normal eyelid structures. Most eyelid disorders are not vision-threatening or life-threatening.

Blepharitis

Blepharitis, or chronic inflammation of the eyelid, is a common ocular condition. Symptoms include redness of the eyes and eyelids, itching, burning, and a feeling that something is in the eyes. Some patients complain that their eyelids form crusts and stick together in the morning. Blepharitis always involves the eyelid margin (edge), but in some cases it may also affect the conjunctiva (inner lining of the eye), cornea (clear outer layer of the eye), and eyelid skin.

Anterior blepharitis refers to inflammation of the front layer of the eyelid. Although there are many possible causes of anterior blepharitis, it is most often related to bacterial infection or seborrheic dermatitis, a chronic inflammatory skin condition.

This condition leads to oily secretions, eyelid swelling, scaling, and flaking; they produce ocular itching and burning that can be severe. Both layers of the eyelid may be affected.

Posterior blepharitis affects the inner eyelid and occurs when the small (meibomian) glands in the inner layer of the eyelid either become inflamed or secrete an excessive quantity of their normal product. These glands produce an oily substance, an important part of the normal tear film that bathes the surface of the eye. Overproduction of this substance can produce an irritating burning sensation of the eyes, although the eyelids may remain normal in appearance.

Complications from blepharitis include stye and chalazion. A stye (external hordeolum) is an abscess, which occurs when a lash follicle becomes infected. A stye develops rapidly, producing an elevated, painful, red, swollen area on the eyelid. When there is an inflammation of a meibomian gland, a firm nodule may form, which is referred to as a chalazion (internal hordeolum). Chalazia may occur suddenly or may appear gradually over time. They may be painful, red, and swollen, or may simply produce a firm mass.

Skin disorders can cause posterior blepharitis: acne rosacea, which leads to red and inflamed skin; and scalp dandruff (seborrheic dermatitis). The most common causes of anterior blepharitis are bacteria, including staphylococcus and scalp dandruff. Bacterial infection or plugging of the glands by abnormally thick secretions is thought to play a role.

Adults are affected more often than children. The condition may occur at an increased frequency within certain families and in children with Down syndrome. Chronic blepharitis is often linked to occupations in which the hands are dirty for much of the day. Poor hygiene is also a risk factor. Seborrheic dermatitis of the face or scalp is also a common risk factor. Dermatitis caused by herpes simplex, varicella-zoster virus, allergies, and staphylococcus may also cause blepharitis. It has also been associated with rosacea. Drugs and allergens can cause acute blepharitis. Chronic cases can be aggravated by environmental irritants such as exposure to chemical fumes, smoke, and smog.

Symptoms of blepharitis include a feeling of a foreign object in the eye or a burning sensation, excessive tearing, itching, sensitivity to light (photophobia), red and swollen eyelids, redness of the eye, blurred vision, frothy tears, dry eye, or crusting of the eyelashes on awakening.

Routine examination of the eyelids and eyelashes is done to diagnose blepharitis. Examination with a slit lamp microscope is used for more detailed inspection. This apparatus is a microscope with an attached light that allows the doctor to examine the eye under high magnification; it is used for examination of the cornea, iris, and lens.

Blepharitis is a chronic condition. Treatment of anterior blepharitis, including stye, includes removal of the infected hair follicle and topical antibiotics. For posterior blepharitis with significant meibomian gland involvement, some physicians may recommend treatment with oral antibiotics or steroids. Both anterior and posterior blepharitis are treated with warm compresses (warm, moist wash cloth applied to the eyelid) followed by lid cleansing (using a moist cotton swab to gently clean the eyelid margin) two to three times each day.

Keeping the eyelids, scalp, and face clean is the most effective way to prevent blepharitis and its recurrence. Avoiding exposure to smoke and chemical fumes and obtaining treatment for skin disorders like rosacea and seborrhea also help prevent blepharitis. Blepharitis is a common, noncontagious eye disorder throughout the world. It affects people of all ages, but blepharitis caused by seborrhea is seen more frequently in older patients and is associated with dry eyes.

Basal cell carcinoma

Basal cell carcinoma is the most common eyelid malignancy. About 75 percent of cases occur on the lower lid or on the skin of the nasal side of the eye. This cancer is locally invasive and usually distinguished by its pearly white borders and ulcerated center, and bleeding in some cases. Often, this tumor is discovered during routine slit lamp evaluation. There is usually no associated pain or discomfort.

The cause of the tumor is associated with sun exposure and sunburns and is most common among older, fair-skinned individuals. In addition, exposure to ionizing radiation and environmental exposures, such as hydrocarbons or pesticides, has been implicated as a potential cause. Genetic determinants such as inherited defects in DNA replication or repair, or both, can also be a factor. People commonly at risk are fair-skinned people over age 50; it is rare among those with dark skin. The incidence increases significantly with sun exposure. Those who work outdoors or live in sunny climates or areas with high sun exposure are at greater risk.

Basal cell carcinoma typically appears on the lower eyelid. It begins as a small, raised growth and classically appears as a nodule with a pitted center. The tumor may have a "pearly" appearance. Basal cell carcinoma of the eyelid progresses very slowly. Metastasis is rare, but if left untreated, the disease can spread to and destroy surrounding tissue. Complete recovery is possible with surgical excision, but it can recur.

If left untreated, the growth may gradually invade the surrounding tissue. However, basal cell carcinomas rarely metastasize (spread to other parts of the body). Diagnosis is made by microscopic examination of the tumor cells.

The most common treatment for basal cell carcinomas is surgical removal. The tumor does not metastasize (spread to other parts); therefore, systemic therapy is not required. However, if the tumor is large, reconstructive surgery, including skin grafting, may be required. If surgical removal of the tumor is not an option, cryotherapy (freezing) or radiation therapy may be used.

Individuals at risk, especially the fair-skinned, should avoid overexposure to sunlight. Sunglasses should be worn to protect the delicate skin around the eyelids from UV light. Protective clothing, headgear, and sunscreen are advisable when spending time outdoors.

In the United States, the prevalence of basal cell carcinoma is around 1 million, with more than 900,000 cases developing in the head or the neck. Basal cell carcinomas represent 20 percent of eyelid tumors and 90 percent of eyelid malignancies.

Herbert Kaufman and Josephine Everly

Female reproductive system

The female reproductive system consists of all the organs necessary for ovulation, sexual intercourse, and the sustenance of the fertilized ovum until childbirth. The female reproductive system starts functioning at the onset of puberty and continues until menopause, when the ability to reproduce naturally is no longer possible. As with any complicated body system, there is a potential for error during development before birth and afterward in the mature system.

In the developing embryo, regardless of sex, two systems, the Müllerian and the Wolffian ducts, coexist until about week eight. The Müllerian system gives rise to female genital organs, while the Wolffian system gives rise to the male organs. In the first step, the embryo's genotype, XY or XX, determines whether ovaries or testes form. The Müllerian and Wolffian systems form the rest of the genital organs. Once the appropriate gonads develop, they begin to secrete hormones: estrogen in females and testosterone in males. In a male, Müllerian Inhibiting Substance causes regression of the Müllerian system, and testosterone causes further differentiation of the Wolffian system into male genitalia and phenotype. The Müllerian system does not require such a hormonal stimulus. In fact, the female phenotype is the default status in the embryo. That is, any embryo, regardless of being XY or XX, will develop female internal organs unless Müllerian Inhibiting Substance is present to inhibit the Müllerian system and testosterone is available to promote the differentiation of the Wolffian system. In both the male and female, secondary sex characteristics such as hair pattern or breast development depend on exposure to hormones such as testosterone and estrogen, which occur normally during puberty.

The Müllerian system consists of bilateral paired ducts that migrate to and fuse in the midline of the embryo to form the uterus, cervix, fallopian tubes, and upper part of the vagina. The fused ducts are solid and need to canalize (become hollow again). Anatomic anomalies may result from either faulty fusion or recanalization.

Müllerian anomalies occur in about 3 to 6 percent of women but are more common in women who have recurrent miscarriages. Some of the most common anatomic abnormalities of the female reproductive tract include an imperforate hymen, a longitudinal or transverse vaginal septum, uterine septum, bicornate uterus, and vaginal agenesis (lack or failure of development).

Many of these patients present around the age of sixteen with normal growth and secondary sexual characteristics but with the absence of menarche (beginning of the menstrual cycle), otherwise known as primary amenorrhea. Ovarian dysgenesis usually presents with an absence of secondary sexual characteristics.

RELATED ARTICLES

FEMALE REPRODUCTIVE SYSTEM

The female reproductive organs lie within the pelvic cavity. They comprise the ovaries, fallopian tubes, uterus, cervix, and vagina. Normal functioning of the reproductive system begins at puberty and ceases at menopause. The ovaries produce estrogen, which is essential for the development of female sexual characteristics. An ovum or egg is produced each month and travels down the fallopi-an tubes to the uterus, where it is fertilized, or menstruation occurs. The many parts of the reproductive system can commonly develop complications, for example after childbirth.

The female reproductive organs are situated in the lower part of the pelvic cavity. To allow space for the growth of a fetus during pregnancy, the area is wider than that of a man.

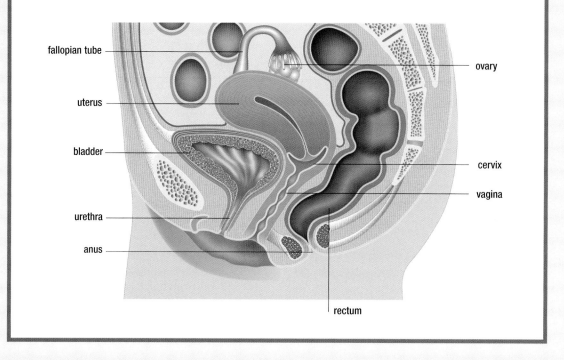

fallopian tube
uterus
bladder
urethra
anus
ovary
cervix
vagina
rectum

Imperforate hymen

An imperforate hymen, or the abnormal persistence of an intact thin sheet of tissue at the level of the vaginal opening, is a simple defect that can result in primary amenorrhea. Classic symptoms are monthly pelvic pain and a mass from a collection of old menstrual blood in the vagina. A surgical incision opening the hymen easily corrects the defect and relieves the symptoms.

Vaginal septa

A vaginal septum is an abnormal thin wall or membrane that connects two opposite walls of the vagina. The septum can be longitudinal (vertical) or transverse (horizontal) and can occur at any level between the hymen and the cervix. Depending on the location, a septum can cause an obstruction similar to an imperforate hymen. Presenting symptoms and treatment choices vary with the location and extent of the septum.

Vaginal agenesis

In utero, the Müllerian ducts give rise to the upper vagina and uterus. Underdevelopment of the Müllerian duct system, known as Müllerian agenesis, will result in an absence of the vagina. Typically, vaginal agenesis is also associated with cervical and uterine agenesis.

Uterine anomalies

Defects in Müllerian duct fusion result in a uterus in which the upper parts remain separated and are referred to as horns. The variation of normal development with one cervix (where fusion has occurred at that level) and two horns is called a bicornuate uterus. Total failure of fusion results in two horns and two cervices and is called a uterus didelphys. Incomplete recanalization of the fused ducts leads to the presence of a septum (residual inner wall) in the uterus and is referred to as a septate uterus. A complete uterine septum refers to total recanalization failure in which the septum extends through the uterus and cervix (occasionally there are two cervices, and sometimes, two vaginas).

Anatomic anomalies are often asymptomatic. If the anomaly results in obstruction of the normal menstrual blood outflow track, the patient often presents with pain or amenorrhea, or both. Anomalies that distort the uterine cavity can contribute to miscarriage, preterm (early) delivery, or breech presentations in which the baby is not in the typical head-downward position.

Imaging studies such as ultrasound or MRI assist in making the diagnosis. Treatment of uterine abnormalities includes doing nothing if the patient has no symptoms, or surgical correction to improve fertility or correct obstructions as necessary. All these conditions require individualized assessment and management plans.

Genetic abnormalities

Most of the body's cells have 46 chromosomes, which are arranged as 23 pairs. However, eggs and sperm cells have only 23 chromosomes; when the father's sperm and the mother's egg combine during fertilization, a cell is produced with 46 chromosomes. Male chromosomes are XY and female are XX.

Chromosomal abnormalities such as gonadal dysgenesis may result in the lack of development or the premature depletion of primordial germ cells that are the starting point for egg production. Without germ cells, ovaries do not develop or have no eggs to release. This condition is referred to as gonadal dysgenesis. Women typically present with primary amenorrhea. Turner's syndrome is the most common cause of gonadal dysgenesis.

Turner's syndrome is a genetic disorder that occurs in approximately 1 in 1,000 births. Classic Turner's syndrome has a 45 X karyotype (chromosomal characteristic). Without two normal X chromosomes

(46 XX), the ovaries cannot develop properly and are replaced with fibrous tissue. These "streak ovaries" consequently produce neither eggs nor estrogen. Because the Müllerian system is the default mechanism, even in the absence of estrogen, the internal and external female reproductive organs will form normally. The secondary sex characteristics will not develop normally, however, nor will the woman menstruate without estrogen. Women with Turner's syndrome typically appear short and stocky and have a webbed neck; they may also have heart and aortic abnormalities. This condition is not associated with mental retardation. Being a genetic disorder, Turner's syndrome is irreversible. Treatment options include hormone replacement therapy to promote secondary sex characteristics as well as to prevent the adverse effects of low estrogen—such as osteoporosis. Pregnancy is possible through donor eggs (when another woman donates her eggs, which are then fertilized and transferred to the patient's uterus). Women with Turner's syndrome who are considering pregnancy by donor eggs should have an imaging study of the heart to ensure there are no abnormalities.

Receptor abnormalities and enzyme deficiencies

Androgens are hormones that promote the development and maintenance of male sex characteristics. Males born with a normal genotype, 46 XY, but with an absence or resistance to androgens, will grow up displaying an outwardly normal female phenotype and lack the internal female organs. As a result, at puberty these 46 XY "females" will have primary amenorrhea.

Examples of these disorders include complete androgen insensitivity syndrome (androgen insensitivity), 5-alpha-reductase deficiency, vanishing testes syndrome, absent testis determining factor (absence of androgen), and adrenal and ovarian dysfunction (overabundance of androgens).

Complete androgen insensitivity syndrome. This is a disorder in which people with 46 XY karotype appear female. Due to a defect in the androgen receptor and thus an inability to effectively bind testosterone, the body does not recognize the testosterone that is present, which is needed for normal internal and external male genital development. As such, these individuals fail to develop typical male characteristics. The external genitalia are female in appearance. Normally functioning, though undescended, testes are present because the genotype is male. Müllerian Inhibiting Substance secreted from the testes leads to the regression of the normal female internal structures including the fallopian tubes, uterus, and upper third of the vagina. At puberty, some androgens are converted to estrogen, which allows breast development to occur despite the absence of ovaries. Menses cannot occur due to the lack of normal female reproductive organs.

Individuals with androgen insensitivity syndrome usually present at puberty with primary amenorrhea. Measuring high (male) levels of testosterone in the blood, along with the absence of the upper vagina, uterus, and fallopian tubes on physical exam or pelvic ultrasound, confirms the diagnosis.

Undescended testes are at significantly higher risk of developing testicular cancer. As such, the testes should be surgically removed after puberty (once breast development is complete). This allows the individual to have a fully female phenotype, which improves the psychological impact of this diagnosis.

5-Alpha-reductase deficiency. Deficiency of 5-alpha-reductase is another syndrome in which a genetically male, 46 XY, person appears phenotypically female. An enzyme called 5-Alpha-reductase is located in many tissues. This enzyme converts testosterone to a more potent male hormone called dihydrotestosterone (DHT).

In the developing male embryo, DHT is responsible for normal development of the male external genitalia. A deficiency of 5-alpha-reductase, therefore, leads to a lack of growth and enlargement of male external genitalia.

At birth, the newborn may appear female or have ambiguous genitalia which are not clearly male or female. At puberty, the normal dramatic rise in testosterone results in an increase in male pattern hair growth, muscle mass, and voice deepening. The external genitalia respond in part to the testosterone surge and mature into genitals that are more identifiably male.

Diagnosis may be made at birth if the child has ambiguous external genitalia, which necessitates further evaluation. However, sometimes the infant may be assigned a female sex based on the genital appearance, and the diagnosis is delayed until puberty

when the above changes occur. Treatment centers on raising the child in a nurturing environment that will minimize the psychological impact during puberty. Hormonal therapy is not usually indicated.

Menstrual cycle and endocrine abnormalities
The normal menstrual cycle functions to select, mature, and typically release a single egg from the ovary (ovulation), and to prepare the endometrium (lining of the uterus) for implantation of a fertilized egg. This process repeats itself on a monthly basis and is tightly regulated by stimulatory and inhibitory signals sent between the ovary, hypothalamus, and pituitary gland.

The average age of menarche in North America is 14.5 years. Lack of menses by the age of 16 is defined as primary amenorrhea, while secondary amenorrhea is defined as the absence of menses for more than three cycles, or six months in women who have previously had menses.

The classic 28-day menstrual cycle is often divided into a 14-day follicular phase and a 14-day luteal phase. Ovulation typically occurs on day 14 and initiates the transition between these two phases. At the beginning of the follicular phase, the uterine lining is thin, having been sloughed off during menstruation, and the hormonal environment is relatively quiescent. Hypothalamic GnRH (gonadotropin releasing hormone) stimulates production of follicle-stimulating hormone (FSH) and luteinizing hormone (LH) from the pituitary. These hormones in turn act on the ovary to stimulate follicular development.

A follicle consists of the oocyte (egg-forming cell) and surrounding support cells. During each cycle, many follicles begin to develop in response to FSH and LH. As the follicles grow and mature, they begin to secrete estrogen. Typically, a single follicle eventually becomes dominant, and the remainder degenerate and are resorbed. The secreted estrogen initially has an inhibitory effect on pituitary FSH and LH secretion. Through a complex interaction, however, estrogen eventually causes a midcycle surge of FSH and LH. The LH surge causes ovulation of the dominant follicle. When the oocyte is expelled, most of the support cells are left behind in the ovary. These cells form a structure called the corpus luteum, hence the luteal phase, which begins to produce progesterone.

Progesterone gradually rises, nourishing and thickening the lining of the uterus known as the endometrium.

If sperm and egg meet, and fertilization is successful, the fertilized egg may then implant in the progesterone-nourished endometrium and continue to grow. If no fertilization occurs, progesterone levels drop, and the endometrium sloughs off when this supporting hormone is withdrawn, leading to menstruation and the start of a new cycle. The average adult menstrual cycle lasts 28 days, with a range from 23 to 38 days, and menstruation typically lasts for 4 to 7 days. Anything outside these parameters is considered abnormal.

Adrenal and ovarian dysfunction

When produced in excess, adrenal steroid hormones can cause menstrual abnormalities by inhibiting gonadotropin-releasing hormone secretion from the hypothalamus. Glucocorticoid excess is often accompanied by androgen excess. Menstrual irregularities, including amenorrhea, are common when there is androgen excess and are often accompanied by excessive secondary sexual hair growth. There can also be temporal hairline recession and a deepening of the voice when significant androgen excess is present.

Androgen-secreting tumors, congenital adrenal hyperplasia, and polycystic ovarian syndrome may all cause varying degrees of adrenal hormone excess. Congenital adrenal hyperplasia and polycystic ovary syndrome (PCOS) will be discussed below.

Polycystic ovary syndrome. Polycystic ovary syndrome (PCOS) occurs when two of the following three abnormalities are present in the absence of other contributing medical conditions: amenorrhea or irregular cycles as a result of failure to ovulate; increased androgens manifested by symptoms such as acne and facial hair, or diagnosed by blood tests; and multiple cysts on the ovaries, noted on ultrasound.

Obesity is a major risk factor for developing PCOS, but PCOS can occur in thin individuals as well. PCOS can be associated with insulin resistance similar to a prediabetic state, high cholesterol levels, high blood pressure, and eventually heart disease. Since women with PCOS do not ovulate, menstruation does not occur and the uterus continues to thicken

the endometrium in the absence of the production and subsequent withdrawal of progesterone. This uninhibited proliferation of the endometrium without menses increases a woman's risk for abnormal thickening of the uterine lining (hyperplasia) and, possibly, endometrial cancer. Frequently, patients with PCOS are not concerned about these menstrual irregularities and do not seek medical care until they are faced with difficulties conceiving.

As many as 75 percent of women who present with infertility, as a result of a failure to ovulate, have PCOS. Diagnosis and evaluation of these patients begins with a careful history, including information about puberty, age at menarche, and the nature of the woman's menstrual cycle. The patient would be asked whether the cycle was regular, the frequency of the cycle, and if there was any bleeding between cycles. The normal menstrual cycle ranges from 25 to 35 days, but in these women the cycle occurs only every 2 to 3 months. Clinically, patients should be examined for signs of androgen excess, such as acne and excessive hair growth. Ultrasound reveals multiple cysts lining the outer edge of the ovaries; these are the follicles that failed to ovulate. Laboratory tests to diagnose PCOS evaluate hormone levels and also look for potentially associated conditions such as lipid changes and diabetes.

Given the multiple symptoms of PCOS, treatment needs to address several problems. Birth control pills are the treatment of choice in a woman who does not want to become pregnant. Birth control pills, which contain the hormones estrogen and progesterone, act on the brain and ovaries to regulate the abnormal hormone levels.

Androgenic effects such as acne and hair growth improve as a result of reduced hormone levels as well as estrogen's induction of increased sex-hormone binding globulin (SHB6), which inactivates androgen activity. Also, the uterine lining no longer grows uncontrollably so that menstrual irregularities and the risk of uterine cancer improve.

Metformin, a drug used also in diabetics, helps regulate blood insulin and androgen levels. This improves ovulatory function and is one option for women attempting to conceive. Alternatively, clomiphene, a medication that directly promotes ovulation, can be used. Clomiphene may be associated with the release of multiple eggs at one time, leading to twins in 5 to 8 percent of clomiphene-induced pregnancies. It rarely results in triplets. Diet and exercise are the two most important interventions for women with PCOS, who should also consult with a physician.

Congenital adrenal hyperplasia (CAH). The human body has two adrenal glands, one located atop each kidney. These glands are significant sources of three important hormones: cortisol, aldosterone, and androgens. Cortisol helps to maintain normal bodily functions during times of stress. Aldosterone regulates the body's salt balance. Androgens promote development and maintenance of certain secondary sex characteristics.

In congenital adrenal hyperplasia, defects in enzymes required for hormone production can cause excessive facial hair in females, acne, weight changes, menstrual irregularities, infertility, and changes in blood pressure. The spectrum of symptoms varies depending on the specific type and severity of the adrenal enzyme deficiency. Severe forms of CAH can change the hormonal environment of the developing fetus. Female newborns may develop external genitalia that appear male, and abnormal development can occur in male newborns. CAH is diagnosed by blood tests for different hormones levels. Then, depending on the type of enzyme deficiency, CAH is treated by replacing the missing hormones to normalize any abnormal changes, including elevated blood pressure and symptoms such as acne and hair growth.

Dysmenorrhea

Dysmenorrhea, a painful cramping sensation in the lower abdomen (pelvis) during menses, occurs in 60 to 93 percent of all adolescent females, making it the most common gynecological complaint among this

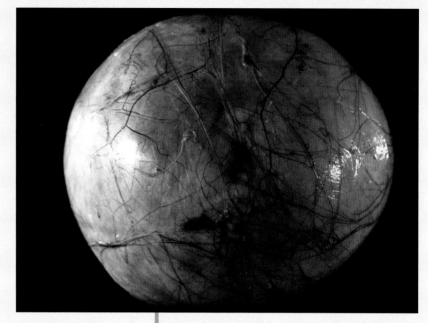

This large ovarian cyst is filled with fluid. Such cysts rarely prove to be malignant.

age group. Dysmenorrhea generally does not begin until ovulatory menstrual cycles are established. In order for ovulatory menstrual cycles to occur, the hypothalamic-pituitary-ovarian axis needs to mature. This usually occurs by two to four years after menarche (the first menses).

Symptoms of dysmenorrhea may start prior to the onset of menses and continue for a period of one to three days. The pelvic cramps may be accompanied by other symptoms such as sweating, tachycardia (rapid heartbeat), headaches, nausea, vomiting, and diarrhea. Uncoordinated uterine contractions, hypercontractility, increased uterine muscle tone leading to uterine ischemia (inadequate blood flow and poor oxygenation), and prostaglandin release from the uterine lining are the principal causes of the pain of dysmenorrhea.

A complete medical and menstrual history (including questions regarding age at menarche; duration of menstrual cycles and interval between them and the onset and duration of cramps; the severity of symptoms of nausea, vomiting and diarrhea; medications; and sexual history), as well as a complete physical exam, including a pelvic exam, should be performed. Nonsteroidal anti-inflammatory drugs (NSAIDs) such as ibuprofen should be used first in the treatment of dysmenorrhea. These usually relieve pain in 70 to 90 percent of patients. NSAIDs should be started immediately at the onset of menses or pain and continued for the first one or two days of the menstrual cycle or for the duration of the pain. If symptoms are severe, patients may take the NSAIDs a day or two prior to the onset of menses.

Birth control pills are tried next if NSAIDs fail. Birth control pills contain estrogen and progesterone and prevent ovulation. In doing so, they also affect the uterine lining and production of other molecules called prostaglandins, which play a role in pain production.

All patients should be followed closely for the first few months after treatment has started, in order to evaluate their response to therapy. If these treatment options fail, the patient has recurrent pain, or symptoms worsen, the patient should be reevaluated, and other possible causes may be investigated.

Pelvic inflammatory disease

Pelvic inflammatory disease (PID) is an infection involving the uterus, fallopian tubes, or ovaries, or all three organs. PID usually results from infection by sexually transmitted bacteria such as chlamydia or gonorrhea. PID affects approximately 2.5 million American women per year at a cost of $5 billion. Risk factors for developing PID include unprotected intercourse, multiple sexual partners, and being younger than 35 years of age. PID rarely occurs in pregnant women.

Most women present with lower abdominal pain that worsens with intercourse or jarring movements. The pain frequently begins during or shortly after menstruation and may last less than two weeks. Other symptoms can include abnormal uterine bleeding, vaginal discharge, fever, and chills. On pelvic examination, the patient experiences abdominal pain when the cervix is moved by the physician. This important physical finding is known as cervical motion tenderness.

PID is difficult to diagnose because the symptoms and their severity vary from woman to woman and can mimic symptoms of other diseases such as appendicitis. Most frequently, the doctor may make the diagnosis based just on the discussion with the patient and the physical exam. One way to definitively diagnose PID is to visualize the reproductive organs

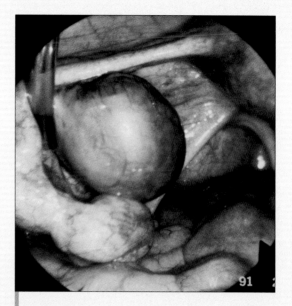

A laparoscopic view inside a woman's abdomen shows a follicular cyst of the ovary. The cyst is the large round structure at center left; the uterus is partly seen at the upper right, with a fallopian tube passing above the cyst.

using a laparoscope. A laparoscope is a small telescope with an attached camera that is inserted into the abdomen through a small surgical incision. An ultrasound can show changes in the pelvic organs consistent with PID. Laboratory tests on blood or the cervix may identify bacteria or other signs of infection. Since bacterial infection causes PID, antibiotics are necessary for treatment.

Female circumcision

Female circumcision (FC), a practice seeped in tradition, culture, religion, and socioeconomic pressures, dates as far back as the fifth century BCE, and has been practiced in some form virtually throughout the world.

There are four classifications of the procedure that is carried out during female circumcision: type I—excision of the clitoral hood, with or without part or all of the clitoris; type II—excision of the clitoris with partial or total excision of the labia minora; type III—excision of part or all of the external genitalia and stitching or narrowing, or both, of the vaginal opening (infibulation); type IV—pricking, piercing, stretching or burning of the clitoris or labia, or both.

Approximately 140 million girls and women across Africa, Asia, Middle East, Europe, and North and South America have been circumcised. An additional 2 million are at risk each year. As a result of immigration patterns, nearly 170,000 girls in the United States are at risk for or have undergone FC. FC spans a range of different ethnic, cultural, and socioeconomic groups as well as most religions, including Christian, Muslim, Jewish, and indigenous African religions. As few as 5 percent of women are affected in some areas, while more than 90 percent are affected in other areas. The girls are usually between the ages of 6 to 12, but they may be circumcised at any time from infancy to adulthood.

Traditionally, the practitioners of FC tend to hold matriarchal roles in the society, or they may be related to the girl. Traditional beliefs hold that FC ensures a girl's desirability for marriage, and that perception perpetuates this custom. FC functions as a rite of passage in many societies and is thought to preserve virginity and fertility and to be more hygienic.

Nonmedical personnel usually perform female circumcision without anesthesia or sterile conditions, and this procedure thus can be very dangerous. Risks include hemorrhage, death, injury to other nearby organs, infection, anemia from prolonged bleeding, and possible fractures from being held down. Late complications include chronic pelvic pain, dysmenorrhea, infertility, chronic urinary tract infections, difficult labor and delivery, pain with intercourse, and psychological trauma.

Clinical history and physical exam reveal the extent of circumcision and its impact on the woman. The choice to pursue treatment depends on the type of circumcision, whether the woman wishes to attempt reversal, and if reversal is needed for the safe birth of a child. Type I and II are difficult to reverse, since tissue that has been removed cannot be replaced. Fortunately, types I and II are frequently asymptomatic. Type III FC, which involves cutting the labia and sewing them together to make a smaller vaginal opening with a thin flap of tissue closing off the rest of the vagina, is the most frequently reversed process because it causes the most complications. During the reversal process, the thin flap of tissue is removed to enlarge the vaginal opening. The labia will still be absent.

Endometriosis

Endometriosis is a noncancerous condition that occurs when endometrial tissue, which normally lines the endometrial cavity and causes menstruation when shed, instead grows outside the uterus. This tissue can implant virtually anywhere in the body but usually is located in the pelvis. It is not entirely clear why or how the endometrial cells become located outside the uterus. Endometriosis affects somewhere between 5 to 20 percent of women in the United States. It is more common in white and Asian women, women with a family history of endometriosis, and in women who have never been pregnant. The displaced endometrial cells still respond to the hormones estrogen and progesterone. As such, this tissue grows and bleeds during the menstrual cycle in the same way that endometrial tissue does in the uterus. However, endometriosis tissue has no way to drain out as in normal menses. The trapped tissue can cause severe pain, which typically begins shortly before menses and resolves at the end of the cycle. The classic presentation of endometriosis is pain with menses, intercourse, and defecation. Other associated symptoms include infertility, abnormal uterine bleeding, and endometriomas. An endometrioma is a fluid-filled cyst in the ovary that contains endometrial tissue. These cysts (often called "chocolate cysts") contain old menstrual blood, which looks like chocolate syrup. Many women have no symptoms at all, even with extensive endometriosis. Since hormonal stimulation drives the functioning of the tissue, endometriosis generally occurs in reproductive age.

Endometriosis is often diagnosed based on the woman's clinical history and her physical exam. A definite diagnosis requires visualizing the displaced tissue with a laparoscope and confirmation with a biopsy (tissue specimen of affected tissue).

Multiple treatment options exist; these include no treatment, especially if symptoms are mild; pain medication; birth control pills, which suppress endometrial growth; preventing menstruation with other drugs; and surgery to treat the endometrial lesions and the affected pelvic organs. The chosen therapy depends on symptom severity and whether or not a woman wishes to retain reproductive capacity.

Hilary Smith, Moune Jabre Raughley, and Gary Frishman

Fetal alcohol syndrome

Alcohol use in pregnancy has a negative effect on the fetus and newborn. In February 2005, the U.S. Surgeon General issued an updated Advisory on Alcohol Use and Pregnancy, asserting that there is no established "safe" level of alcohol consumption in pregnancy. The update recommended that women who are pregnant or are considering pregnancy should not consume alcohol.

Recent studies have shown poor outcomes for children who are exposed to small amounts of alcohol before birth. The amount of drinking in pregnancy that is thought to potentially damage the fetus is typically more than 1 drink per day ($\frac{1}{2}$ ounce), or less if binge drinking occurs (more than five drinks per episode). However, new research indicates that even children prenatally exposed to 0.5 drinks daily may have poor outcomes. Alcohol use in pregnancy results in a known spectrum of disorders. Among these is fetal alcohol syndrome (FAS).

Diagnosis

FAS refers to a set of physical malformations and central nervous system abnormalities seen in the offspring of women who use alcohol during pregnancy. The reported prevalence of FAS in developed countries varies widely, but the average is around 1 in 3,000 live births. Although there is no precise dose response relationship between the amount of alcohol consumed and perinatal outcome, the prevalence of FAS among moderate to heavy drinkers may be as high as 20 to 40 percent.

The diagnosis of FAS is based on three criteria. The first is growth problems, that is prenatal or postnatal height or weight, or both, at or below the 10th percentile, documented at any one point in time. Height documentation must be adjusted for age, sex, gestational age, race, or ethnicity. The second criterion is specific facial features: a smooth area between the nose and upper lip (smooth philtrum), a thin upper lip (thin vermilion border), small eye opening (small palpebral fissures), and underdeveloped mid-face features (hypoplastic midface). The third criterion is central nervous system abnormalities: decreased head circumference, sleep disturbances, attention deficits, decreased response to noise, hyperactivity, and problems with speech development, learning, and visual focus. Other alcohol-related birth defects that may occur are those related to the eyes, heart, ears, kidneys, and limbs. It is important to remember that there is no exact dose-response relationship between the amount of alcohol consumed and infant outcome.

Treatments and prevention

True treatment lies in preventive strategies. Identifying women of childbearing age and screening them for alcohol use is of great importance. No conventional treatment exists because the diagnosis of

---

KEY FACTS

Description
FAS is a specific recognizable pattern of malformations that include prenatal and postnatal growth deficiency, central nervous system abnormalities, and craniofacial abnormalities.

Causes
Alcohol exposure of the fetus.

Risk factors
Maternal alcohol use before or throughout pregnancy, or both.

Symptoms
A spectrum of findings after delivery and as the child develops.

Diagnosis
Diagnosis can be suspected with poor growth in the fetus or other associated ultrasound findings.

Treatments
There is no effective treatment for FAS. As such, every effort should be focused on prevention. All women should be screened for alcohol use in pregnancy.

Pathogenesis
This is complex and incompletely understood. Alcohol and its metabolites easily cross the placenta. Animal models suggest interferences with protein synthesis, and problems with placental transfer of glucose and amino acids.

Prevention
Prenatal and antenatal screening for alcohol use and exposure.

Epidemiology
The reported incidence of FAS varies from 1 in 50 to 1 in 2,500 live births. In the Western world, the incidence has been reported as 0.33 in 1,000 live births. The incidence among those women who are heavy drinkers is significantly greater, possibly as high as 20–40 percent.

FAS is made after delivery. Prenatal ultrasound can only suggest a diagnosis, as most fetuses with FAS appear normal on ultrasound. In addition to growth problems noted above, congenital anomalies that can be seen on ultrasound and that have been associated with FAS include heart defects, central nervous system abnormalities (small head, neural tube defects), facial abnormalities (small chin, cleft lip and palate), truncal and skeletal abnormalities (diaphragmatic hernia, vertebral malformations), and urogenital malformations (small genitalia). The placenta usually appears normal, although the amount of amniotic fluid around the baby may be low. Many of these features may be subtle and may only be seen late in pregnancy.

It is important to note that most of the features mentioned cannot be seen until the late second trimester, and even then, what can be seen on ultrasound may not be so obvious. Additionally, one may not see all of the above features together. Separate findings may be seen, while others may not. Also, any single anomaly may have an alternate cause.

Early recognition is key so that known complications of FAS can be identified and support mechanisms for the family and child can be put into place. Known outcomes include: school failure, difficulties with peers, conduct problems, and mental health disorders. Long-term problems such as crooked teeth, inner-ear tube infections, problems in language, motor, learning, visual-spatial functioning, and cognition have been associated with FAS. Additionally, screening and good follow-up care can help with the identification of newborns at risk for alcohol withdrawal syndrome: symptoms are tremors, agitation, metabolic acidosis, low blood sugar, and seizures. These have been described in the infants of mothers who were intoxicated at the time of delivery. Even in the absence of a history of alcohol use in pregnancy, newborn babies who show symptoms or signs suggestive of possible alcohol withdrawal (such as tremors, agitation, metabolic acidosis, hypoglycemia, and seizures) should be screened for FAS. Treatment lies in recognizing that FAS is present and handling problems noted individually.

Pathogenesis

Exactly how FAS causes these problems is complex and incompletely understood. Alcohol and its metabolites, which are toxic to a fetus, can cross the placenta. How they exert their effects is still unknown. Animal models suggest an interference with protein synthesis, as well as problems with placental transfer of glucose and amino acids. Low blood sugar and a decrease in

---

T-ACE SURVEY

The T-ACE is a survey developed to assess drinking habits. It comprises four questions and takes less than one minute to administer:

Tolerance
  Q: "How many drinks does it take to make you feel high?"
Annoyed
  Q: "Have people annoyed you by criticizing your drinking?"
Cut down
  Q: "Have you felt you ought to cut down on your drinking?"
Eye opener
  Q: "Have you ever had a drink first thing in the morning to steady your nerves or get rid of a hangover?"

Scoring: The first question is scored positive if the respondent answers that he or she has had more than 2 drinks. A positive response gets 2 points for this question. The last 3 questions are scored 1 point each if answered affirmatively. A total score of 2 or more is considered positive for risk drinking.

---

fetal thyroid hormones and liver glycogen stores have also been demonstrated; these can all affect overall fetal growth and neonatal growth.

Epidemiology

The 2003 National Survey on Drug Use and Health reported that of women aged 15 to 44 years, 9.8 percent used alcohol and 4.1 percent reported binge drinking in the month before the T-ACE survey (see box).

The reported incidence of FAS varies from 1 in 50 to 1 in 2,500 live births. In the Western world, the incidence has been reported as 0.33 in 1,000 live births. The incidence among women who are chronic heavy drinkers is significantly greater, possibly as high as 20 to 40 percent. With screening and counseling of women to avoid alcohol during pregnancy or to stop its use during pregnancy, FAS can be prevented.

Antonette T. Dulay

See also
- Alcohol-related disorders • Birth defects
- Learning disorders • Nervous system disorders • Neural tube disorders

Fibroids

Fibroids are noncancerous tumors of the uterus. They are the most common pelvic tumors in women. In very rare cases, fibroids may change to a cancerous condition. Fibroids affect women during their reproductive years, beginning as small growths in or attached to the uterine wall.

Fibroids may spread and in severe cases completely fill the uterus. In other cases, the growths may hang outside the uterus via a stalk attached to the outer wall of the organ. They do not usually affect fertility, but may create complications during pregnancy that may require delivery by cesarean section.

Causes

The cause of fibroids is unknown, although a genetic link may be involved in some cases. The growth of fibroids is encouraged by the presence of the female sex hormone estrogen; thus the tumors usually do not begin growing until a girl begins menstruating and estrogen production increases. They will continue to grow until the woman reaches menopause and estrogen production drops. In many cases, fibroids do not cause any symptoms, but in other cases fibroids may be indicated by feelings of abdominal fullness or pressure, severe cramping or pain during periods, heavy menstrual bleeding, or frequent urination.

Risk factors

The growth of fibroids is stimulated by hormonal changes during pregnancy. Fibroids may lead to premature births or may cause complications serious enough to warrant delivery of the baby by cesarean section. Sudden growth of fibroids, especially in postmenopausal women, may indicate changes leading to cancer.

Treatments and prevention

Asymptomatic cases often require nothing more than periodic examinations to monitor the condition of the fibroids. In other cases, the treatment required depends on the nature and severity of symptoms present.

Since the growth of fibroids is encouraged by estrogen, management of hormone levels is often used to treat the tumors, but hormonal therapy must be main-tained to have lasting effects. Oral contraceptives are effective in reducing menstrual bleeding. Nonsteroidal anti-inflammatory drugs (NSAIDs) may be used to treat pain and cramping caused by the tumors. In severe cases, surgery may be necessary to remove the fibroids, or even the uterus itself.

David M. Lawrence

KEY FACTS

Description
Noncancerous tumors of the wall of the uterus.

Causes
Unknown.

Risk factors
Exposure to the hormone estrogen encourages growth of fibroids.

Symptoms
Fibroids often cause no symptoms, but abdominal fullness or pressure, cramping or pain during periods, heavy menstrual bleeding, or frequent urination may signal the presence of fibroids.

Diagnosis
Pelvic exam, sometimes accompanied with ultrasound imaging.

Treatments
Hormonal therapy to shrink fibroids, oral contraceptives to reduce menstrual bleeding, or nonsteroidal anti-inflammatory drugs to treat pain and cramping; in severe cases, surgery may be necessary to remove the fibroids.

Pathogenesis
Fibroids begin as small growths in or attached to the wall of the uterus, then spread; they may cause complications during pregnancy; in rare cases, they may lead to cancerous conditions.

Prevention
No known means of prevention at present.

Epidemiology
Fibroids affect as many as 20 percent of women of reproductive age, with the percentage increasing to as many as 40 percent of women over the age of 30. African American women are two or three times more likely to develop fibroids than Caucasian women.

See also
• Female reproductive system • Genetic disorders • Menopause • Menstrual disorders

Fifth disease

Fifth disease, or *Erythema infectiosum*, is so called because it was classified as the fifth among six causes of fever and rash in children. It is caused by a virus called parvovirus B19. This disease is common in children attending day care or school, where there is a chance of contamination of the surroundings with respiratory secretions. Therefore, hygiene is very important in the prevention of the disease.

The viral infection fifth disease is most commonly seen in children between the ages of 5 and 14 years, but it can occur in adults as well. It is easily transmitted from person to person in droplets from coughs and sneezes from the infected person, and may also be transmitted through transfusion of unscreened blood or blood products or from mother to fetus through the placenta during pregnancy. The incubation period of fifth disease is from 4 to 20 days. Each person infected with this virus may infect up to one-third of the persons around him or her. Infected children develop a rose-red rash on the face that starts as separate spots, which merge into the red "slapped face" appearance. In a few days, the rash spreads to the limbs and very lightly on the trunk. Children usually recover in a few days, but adults may develop joint disease or anemia that could either resolve within weeks or last for a very long time. Persons with low immunity, such as those with cancer or those being treated with steroids or chemotherapy, are at particular risk. If the infection occurs in pregnant women, there is a risk of miscarriage. A condition called *hydrops fetalis* may occur, which results in the death of the fetus.

Diagnosis and treatments

Diagnostic tests are necessary if the clinical picture is unclear. These may include tests for IgM (immunoglobulin M) antibodies, which are produced against the virus, or PCR (polymerase chain reaction), which tests for viral particles in the blood.

There is no specific treatment, and in most cases, the infection is self-limiting. Blood transfusions may be necessary if the anemia is severe. In persons with low immunity, treatment with intravenous immunoglobulin is helpful. A vaccine for fifth disease is currently being developed.

Epidemiology

The distribution of this virus is worldwide. Cases can occur sporadically or in small outbreaks. The disease occurs most commonly during the spring and early summer. Although it is most commonly seen in children between the ages of 5 and 14 years, it can occur in adults as well. Although many people are unaware that they have had fifth disease, approximately 60 percent of adults have antibodies against parvovirus B19, and one attack confers lifelong immunity.

Pranavi Sreeramoju

KEY FACTS

Description
An acute, communicable disease.

Causes
Infection with parvovirus B19.

Risk factors
Being in a day care or school; having low immunity; having a blood disorder; pregnancy.

Symptoms
Fever and rash. Anemia may occur. Adults may develop joint pains and swelling.

Diagnosis
Mostly based on clinical features; sometimes, antibody tests or polymerase chain reaction.

Treatments
No effective drug against the virus. Patients with anemia may need blood transfusion and intravenous IgG (immunoglobulin G).

Pathogenesis
The virus initially infects the lining of the respiratory tract and then circulates in the blood, causing fever and body aches. Later, a rash appears, and there may be joint pains or swelling.

Prevention
Washing hands; avoiding contact with respiratory secretions of an infected person; cleaning contaminated surfaces.

Epidemiology
Worldwide distribution. Most commonly affects children between the ages of 5 and 14 years but can occur in adults as well. About 60 percent of adults have antibodies against parvovirus B19.

See also
- Anemia • Cancer • Childhood disorders
- Immune system disorders

Filariasis

Filariasis refers to a group of diseases caused by infection with a family of parasitic nematodes (roundworms). Filariae are long threadlike worms that parasitize extraintestinal tissues in man and in a variety of other vertebrates. Elephantiasis and river blindness are the most dramatic forms of filariasis.

Filarial parasites have complex life cycles that require transmission by arthropod vectors (insects that transmit bacteria or viruses). These nematodes do not have any free-living stages, and transmission to new hosts requires parasite development in the vector.

Causes and risk factors

Two major diseases are caused by filarial parasites: lymphatic filariasis and onchocerciasis. Lymphatic filariasis results from infections with *Wuchereria bancrofti*, *Brugia malayi*, or *B. timori*. All three of these parasite species are transmitted by mosquitoes. When infected mosquitoes feed on a host, they deposit the infective, third-stage larvae of the parasite. These larvae enter the skin of the host and migrate into the lymphatic vessels, where they ultimately develop to adult worms of many centimeters in length. The adult parasites can live for many years, and they generate hundreds of first-stage larvae daily by sexual reproduction. These larvae, or microfilariae, enter the host's bloodstream and can be ingested by feeding mosquitoes for transmission to new hosts. New human infections are dependent entirely on contact with infected mosquitoes.

Onchocerciasis, or river blindness, results from infection with *Onchocerca volvulus*, which is transmitted by blackflies. Infective third-stage larvae enter the host following bites by an infected blackfly. The larvae migrate and develop into adult parasites that form subcutaneous nodules. The adults produce large numbers of microfilariae by sexual reproduction, and these larvae migrate through the skin, where they can be picked up by biting flies to continue the cycle of transmission.

Other filarial parasites in humans include *Loa loa* (the eyeworm, transmitted by tabanid flies), *Dipetalonema* species, and *Mansonella ozzardi*, all of which account for far less disease than lymphatic filariasis and onchocerciasis.

Symptoms and pathogenesis

For lymphatic filariasis, the most significant symptom is elephantiasis, or swelling of the limbs or genitalia, which results from loss of function in the lymphatic vessels, where the adult parasites live. Some patients also develop nocturnal wheezing (tropical pulmonary eosinophilia). Lymphatic filariasis does not lead to high mortality, but the disfigurement and disability threaten economic welfare and social order in endemic regions. Many infected individuals remain free of obvious symptoms, but these patients often have suffered undetected damage to their lymphatics and kidneys.

KEY FACTS

Description

Lymphatic filariasis is a parasitic roundworm infection transmitted by mosquitoes.

Causes

Infection with *Wuchereria bancrofti*, *Brugia malayi*, or *B. timori*; the adult parasites lodge in host lymphatic vessels.

Risk factor

Exposure to multiple bites from infected mosquitoes, found in tropical regions worldwide.

Symptoms

Elephantiasis (swelling of limbs, genitals, scrotal sac); swollen and painful lymph nodes; fever; nighttime wheezing; and cough.

Diagnosis

Circulating microfilariae or parasite antigens.

Treatments

Annual dosing with combinations of albendazole and either DEC or ivermectin; management of affected limbs to decrease fluid accumulation in tissues and to prevent secondary bacterial infections. Global eradication efforts center on preventing transmission by reducing microfilarial levels in the blood of infected hosts.

Pathogenesis

Infections may remain asymptomatic, but infected tissues can progress to irreversible elephantiasis when lymphatic function is compromised.

Epidemiology

Close to 120 million people are infected; 1 billion are at risk in regions of active transmission throughout southern and southeastern Asia, Africa, the Pacific, Latin America, and the Caribbean.

The symptoms of onchocerciasis result from migrating microfilariae and host inflammatory responses. Tissue damage in the eye and skin leads to blindness and dermatitis, with devastating economic and social consequences for individuals and communities.

Diagnosis

Many infected patients remain asymptomatic, so lymphatic filariasis can be difficult to diagnose. Circulating microfilariae may be detected in the blood only at night, coincident with peak vector biting times. Infected patients may have no detectable microfilariae. Accurate diagnosis is best done with blood tests that use antibodies to detect parasite-specific proteins or antigens, which reflect total parasite burden.

In areas of onchocerciasis transmission, the presence of skin nodules and other skin changes can help diagnosis onchocercal infections, and skin snips can be used to detect microfilariae. Antigen detection is also used to confirm the presence of living parasites.

Treatments and prevention

For lymphatic filariasis, infections result entirely from contact with infected mosquitoes; yet elimination of mosquitoes in endemic regions may be impractical or ecologically unsound. However, by reducing or eliminating the microfilariae in infected patients' blood, transmission to mosquitoes can be blocked, and new human infections will be prevented. Two drugs are known to eliminate parasites from the circulation, and these effects last for at least a year. Diethylcarbamazine (DEC) is one such drug; it has been distributed combined with cooking salt to stop transmission in many communities. Currently, the WHO-sponsored global program to eliminate lymphatic filariasis distributes combinations of two drugs, either albendazole with DEC, or albendazole with ivermectin, for annual treatment of infected patients. Treatment must continue for up to six years, because adult parasites may continue to live and reproduce.

Elephantiasis can also be remediated by preventing secondary bacterial infections that often result in affected limbs. Meticulous cleaning of affected regions, as well as efforts to promote lymph flow and tissue drainage (elevating limbs, support bandages), can stop further swelling and tissue damage. Prevention efforts for onchocerciasis have focused on reducing vector populations with insecticides and on reducing microfilarial loads in infected patients. Treatment of onchocerciasis with ivermectin has the combined benefits of blocking transmission to the blackfly vec-

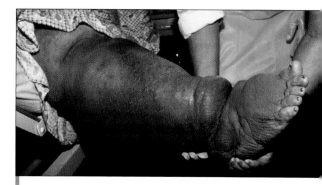

A woman with severe lymphatic filariasis has a hugely swollen leg that is filled with fluid because of inflammation of the lymph vessels and accumulation of fluid.

tor and relieving symptoms and disease in the patient. New research has shown that most filarial species contain bacterial endosymbionts (organisms that live in the body or cells of another organism) called *Wolbachia*. When these bacteria are eliminated with antibiotics, such as tetracycline, the filarial parasites can no longer reproduce and may also die. This discovery has opened the door to new therapeutic possibilities.

Epidemiology

More than 1 billion people are at risk for lymphatic filariasis worldwide because they live in areas of active transmission. Close to 120 million people are infected, although many remain asymptomatic. *W. bancrofti* is endemic in many parts of Asia, Africa, and Latin America. *B. malayi* occurs primarily in Asia, and *B. timori* is restricted to regions of Indonesia. *O. volvulus* is transmitted primarily in Africa, but some infections occur in Latin America and Yemen. Close to 18 million people are currently infected with onchocerciasis, which is the second leading cause of infectious blindness. More than 500,000 people suffer impaired vision or blindness from this parasite, and close to 6 million are afflicted with debilitating skin disease.

For both lymphatic filariasis and onchocerciasis, the efficiency of transmission is low, and infective stage parasites do not multiply in the host. Therefore, multiple bites are required to establish infection, so short-term travelers are at lower risk than those living in areas of transmission.

Juliet Fuhrman

See also
- Infections, bacterial • Infections, parasitic
- River blindness • Roundworm infections

Food intolerance

Food intolerance manifests as an adverse reaction, either physiological or behavioral, or both, in response to certain foods. Reactions can occur in the gastrointestinal, skin, urogenital, musculoskeletal, neurological, or respiratory systems. Unlike food allergies, food intolerances do not involve the immune system, but because symptoms are similar, the two may be confused. Although not life threatening, food intolerance can affect the quality of life.

Food intolerance can develop toward any naturally occurring or artificial food or food ingredient that is ingested. When a particular food item causes irritation in different systems of the body, such as the gastrointestinal, skin, urogenital, musculoskeletal, neurological, or respiratory systems, without the presence of an immune reaction, it is defined as food intolerance. On the other hand, food allergy occurs when the body has an immune reaction, such as the release of histamine, in response to food. Because symptoms of both food intolerance and food allergy are similar, they are difficult to distinguish from each other. For example, peanut ingestion may cause similar symptoms in both conditions, but an allergy to peanuts can be deadly, while intolerance to peanuts may be merely uncomfortable.

Causes and risk factors

Why some foods cause an intolerable reaction in some people is unknown. Common intolerances have been observed to dairy, carbohydrate, gluten, yeast, dyes, flavor enhancers, and preservatives. Carbohydrate intolerance includes intolerance to lactose, the predominant sugar in milk. Those who are lactose intolerant lack the necessary enzyme to digest lactose. Thus, the ingestion of milk products for those people results in digestive discomfort. Lactose intolerance is the most common type of food intolerance. Other substances called sulfites, occurring naturally in red wines or as additives in various foods to prevent mold growth, are another source of intolerance for some people and can cause headaches. A broad group of plant chemicals called salicylates, found naturally in many fruits, vegetables, nuts, coffee, juices, beer, and wine, may trigger other symptoms. Given that aspirin also is a compound of the salicylate family, foods containing salicylates may trigger symptoms in people who are sensitive to aspirin. Furthermore, some people may react psychologically or behaviorally to foods such as caffeine and sugar. Digestive symptoms can also be caused by any food that is consumed in excessive quantities.

Another factor contributing to food intolerances is the quantity of the food ingested; that is, food intolerances are often dose related. People with food intolerance may not have symptoms unless they eat a large portion of the food, or eat the food frequently. For example, a person with lactose intolerance may be able to drink milk in coffee or a single glass of milk, but becomes sick if he or she drinks several glasses of milk or eats a large bowl of ice cream. On the other hand, food allergies can be triggered by even a small amount of the food and occur every time the food is consumed.

KEY FACTS

Description
A physiological or behavioral reaction in response to certain foods.

Causes
Specific foods.

Risk factors
Eating foods that may cause the symptoms of food intolerance.

Symptoms
Digestive problems, runny nose, breathing problems, itching skin, hives, eczema, rash, headaches, insomnia, hyperirritability, anxiety, depression, and concentration problems.

Diagnosis
Eliminating immune involvement that would indicate food allergy rather than intolerance.

Treatment
Depending on the type of food intolerance, enzymes can be taken to aid the digestion of those foods or treatment of symptoms.

Pathogenesis
Unknown.

Prevention
Avoiding foods that cause the symptoms of food intolerance.

Epidemiology
Affects more than 50 million people in the United States.

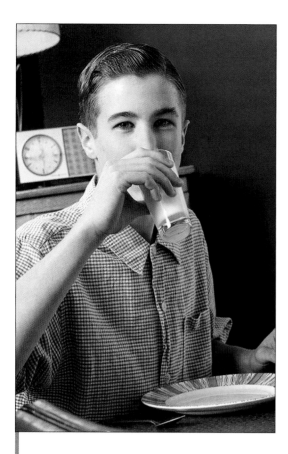

Lactose (the sugar found in milk) intolerance is a common food intolerance. Although someone with a lactose intolerance could probably drink a small amount of milk without ill effect, large quantities would cause digestive problems.

People with food allergies are generally advised to avoid the offending foods completely. Similarly, the highest risk factor for suffering the symptoms of food intolerance is ingesting certain foods.

Food allergies and intolerances are also different from food poisoning, which generally results from spoiled or tainted food and typically affects most people who eat it.

Signs and symptoms

Reactions to foods may be immediate or delayed. Immediate problems may include nausea, vomiting, itching skin, breathing problems, hives, or rashes. Delayed reactions may include digestive problems such as gas, cramps, bloating, runny nose, eczema, headaches, insomnia, heartburn, hyperirritability, anxiety, depression, and concentration problems. All of these symptoms can have a profound effect on the quality of life. Often, if the symptoms are not severe or immediate, the suffering person can rarely distinguish symptoms from some other ailment. For example, dietary components that cause behavioral problems such as irritability and short tempers may not be obvious. Thus, accurate diagnosis is necessary to avoid risk factors and improve the quality of life.

Diagnosis and treatments

Most food intolerances are found through trial and error to determine which food or foods cause symptoms. Keeping a food diary to record what foods are eaten and the symptoms they cause helps to determine what foods are causing problems. Another way to identify problem foods is to go on an elimination diet, completely removing any suspect foods from the diet until a person is symptom free. Reintroducing foods one at a time helps determine which foods cause symptoms. It is important to seek the advice of a health care provider or registered dietitian before beginning an elimination diet to be sure nutritional needs are met. Once it is known which foods are causing problems, treatment is based on avoiding or reducing intake of problem foods and treating symptoms when they arise, such as taking analgesics for headaches. In the case of lactose intolerance, over-the-counter lactase enzyme tablets can be taken to alleviate the symptoms of ingested lactose.

Prevention

Prevention can be simple if certain guidelines are followed. Learning which foods in which amounts cause symptoms, being aware of ingredients and preparation styles while dining out, and reading food labels to check ingredients usually eliminates most symptoms of food intolerance. Prevention of symptoms simply involves avoiding the offending foods.

Epidemiology

The exact number of people who suffer from food intolerance is unknown, but it is thought that the number is greater than those suffering from a true food allergy. Food intolerance affects 1 in 5 people, or 50 million people, in the United States. Lactose intolerance, the most common food intolerance, affects about 10 percent of Americans.

Rashmi Nemade

See also
- Anxiety disorders • Depressive disorders
- Digestive system disorders •Metabolic disorders • Skin disorders •

Food poisoning

Food poisoning is one of the most common illnesses in the United States and worldwide. Food poisoning, which usually arises from contamination of raw foods of animal origin, is characterized by gastrointestinal upsets of varying severity. The illness can be avoided in many cases by following safe food practices.

More than 200 diseases can be transmitted through food. Infectious organisms, present in food through poor hygiene practices, are responsible for most cases of food poisoning. Symptoms, which usually include diarrhea and vomiting, tend to occur suddenly and disappear rapidly, followed by a full recovery. Few people seek medical treatment. However, sometimes more serious illness occurs, leading to widespread symptoms and, rarely, death. People most likely to experience severe symptoms are the elderly, infants and young children, pregnant women, and those whose immune systems are deficient.

Causes

Bacteria, viruses, and parasites can all cause food poisoning. Sometimes illness is caused not by the bacteria themselves but by the toxins they produce, either before or after ingestion.

Worldwide, the leading bacterial cause of food poisoning is *Campylobacter jejuni*, which usually infects raw poultry. One of the most feared food-borne illnesses, called botulism, is caused by bacterial toxins formed by *Clostridium botulinum*. Botulism occurs through improper canning of food and, while rare, is considered a public health emergency. *Salmonella* bacteria are most often associated with eggs; it is estimated that one in 20,000 eggs is contaminated. Infection with *Escherichia coli* (E. coli), a bacterium that produces toxins when it is ingested, is contracted by consumption of contaminated, undercooked ground beef, unpasteurized juice, and raw sprouts. Of particular concern to U.S. travelers is the so-called traveler's diarrhea, caused by a type of E. coli that is transmitted through water or food contaminated with human feces. *Vibrio* bacteria cause food poisoning through contamination of shellfish. Other bacteria responsible for food poisoning include *Staphylococcus*, *Listeria* (particularly found in soft cheeses and prepared foods),

Shigella, and *Toxoplasma*, which is mostly a risk for people with HIV infections.

Two-thirds of reported cases of food poisoning are caused by microorganisms called Norwalk-like viruses. Another common gastrointestinal infection is due to *Crytosporidium*, a parasite that is transmitted by water. An illness called ciguatera poisoning is the result of eating toxins that are sometimes found in large reef fish such as grouper and snapper; similarly, scombroid poisoning can occur when people eat contaminated fish such as tuna and mahi mahi. Hepatitis A, an inflammation of the liver, is a result of eating raw shellfish; and certain fungi contain toxins that produce food poisoning. However, despite an extensive list of potential infectious organisms, the source of most food-borne illnesses is never found.

KEY FACTS

Description
Acute gastrointestinal illness from eating contaminated or toxic food.

Causes
Contamination of food with bacteria, toxins, viruses, or parasites.

Risk factors
Eating food that is improperly washed, stored, or handled.

Symptoms
Stomach upset, nausea, vomiting, diarrhea, and fever; dehydration and death can result.

Diagnosis
Testing of blood and stools for infectious organisms.

Treatments
Anti-infective medicines are given for some bacterial and parasitic infections. Prevention of dehydration.

Pathogenesis
Consumption of food or drink contaminated by toxins or infectious organisms. There is a risk of blood poisoning and, rarely, death.

Prevention
Hygienic handling of food and avoidance of foods that may present a risk.

Epidemiology
In the United States it is estimated that about 76 million people suffer from food poisoning every year; of these, 325,000 require hospitalization and around 5,000 die.

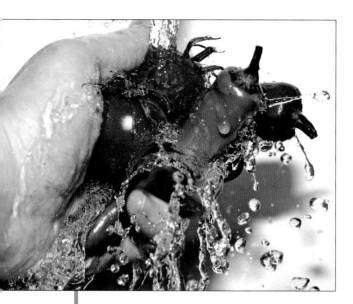

Appropriate handling, preparation, and storage of food are essential to avoid food being contaminated by bacteria. Hygienic practices, such as washing vegetables and fruit under cold running water can help avoid food poisoning.

Symptoms and signs

Stomach pain, nausea, vomiting, diarrhea, and fever are among the most common symptoms of food poisoning; dehydration often follows. In some cases, illness can be severe and even fatal, with widespread symptoms affecting not just the digestive organs but other parts of the body such as the kidneys and nervous system. Hemolytic uremic syndrome, which arises from *E. coli* infection, can result in bloody diarrhea followed by kidney failure and death. Botulism affects the nervous system and can lead to paralysis and death. Food poisoning with *Listeria* bacteria can lead to meningitis or, in pregnant women, spontaneous abortions. Ciguatera and scombroid poisoning produce tingling in the extremities, called paresthesias, and headaches.

The time it takes for symptoms of food poisoning to develop varies, depending on the source of the illness. With bacterial toxins that are formed before ingestion, the onset of symptoms is relatively rapid. Food poisoning caused by bacteria that produce toxins after ingestion, or by organisms that directly infect the gastrointestinal cells, typically takes longer to develop, usually from several hours to a few days. Symptoms of hepatitis A infection may take from 15 to 50 days to appear. The effects of scombroid poisoning appear very rapidly, from only one minute to three hours after ingestion of the toxin.

Depending on the type of poisoning, symptoms can be shortlived or prolonged. In the case of infection with a Norwalk virus, the illness lasts about two days; the symptoms of hepatitis A can continue for weeks.

Diagnosis and treatment

Most cases of food poisoning are never diagnosed because people with this illness often do not seek medical care. Even when they do so, their physician may not order tests to discover the cause. Diagnosis rests on the food history and symptoms followed by specific laboratory testing of suspect foods (if still available), feces, and blood. Treatment in most cases is supportive, involving rest and fluids. Intravenous fluids and hospitalization may be required in severe cases. Some bacterial infections can be treated with antibiotics.

Pathogenesis

Microorganisms associated with food poisoning cause illness by producing toxins prior to ingestion, producing toxins after ingestion, or directly infecting the gastrointestinal lining. When food poisoning is caused by preformed toxins, person-to-person transmission is not possible. *Staphylococcus aureus* food poisoning occurs when a food handler contaminates produce (usually dairy foods, meat, and eggs) with an infected skin sore. With food that has been cooked and left out at room temperature, bacteria can begin to grow in only a few hours. Typically, food infected in this way does not produce any detectable unusual odor or taste.

Prevention

Proper food-handling practices and avoidance of suspect foods such as raw shellfish can reduce the risk of food poisoning. Frozen foods should be defrosted in a refrigerator; raw produce should be thoroughly washed; food should be prepared on clean surfaces with avoidance of cross-contamination of surfaces; meat should be thoroughly cooked. Raw eggs and unpasteurized milk and juices should be avoided. Frequent hand washing is important. Travelers in countries where poor hygiene is likely to be encountered should avoid all raw foods and unbottled water.

Rita Washko

See also
• Diarrhea and dysentery • Digestive system disorders • Gastroenteritis • Infections, bacterial • Infections, parasitic • Infections, viral • Listeria infection • Stomach disorders • Toxoplasmosis

Fracture

A fracture is a break in a bone. A bone fractures when bone tissue under stress fails to withstand a break or tear. A bone usually fractures across its width but may also break along its length or at an angle. Fractures can be the result of sudden impact or prolonged tensile, compressive, or shear stress upon bone tissue.

Fractures are classified by their location or break characteristics. Fractures are displaced if the bone fragments have moved away from one another, or nondisplaced if the bone has not moved. A fracture is described as *open* (compound) if the fracture has broken through the skin, or closed (simple) if the skin is intact. A complete fracture is one that has broken through the bone width, separating the bone into at least two separate pieces. An incomplete fracture is a break on one side of the bone, leaving the bone in one piece. Some fractures have specific names; a common wrist fracture resulting from landing on an outstretched hand is a Colles' fracture.

Causes and risk factors

The direction, speed, and applied force are important determinants in whether bone tissue fails and fractures. Fractures can occur as the result of sudden, direct forces. A common cause of fractures is trauma. Low energy trauma, such as catching a toe along an object, can result in minor fractures with limited soft tissue involvement. High energy trauma, such as a motor vehicle accident, can result in severe fractures with extensive soft tissue damage and damage to internal organs.

Fractures can occur as a result of progressive forces. Athletes often experience stress fractures. As muscles fatigue and their ability to support the skeletal system diminishes, energy is transferred to the bone, making the bone more susceptible to injury.

Osteoporosis is the most common cause of fractures in postmenopausal women and people with underlying bone demineralization conditions. Loss of bone density is often a consequence of the aging process, decreased activity level, and osteoporotic conditions. Decreased bone density affects the strength and elastic properties of bone tissue, reducing a bone's ability to tolerate loading (such as the pull of gravity on the stacked weight of the spinal vertebrae) and increasing the likelihood of fracture.

Hip, pelvis, and femur fractures are most often associated with falls; vertebral fractures are often the result of progressive, long-term loading on spinal vertebrae. Risk factors for fractures associated with osteoporosis include advanced age, female gender, low body mass index, low muscle mass, frailty, low activity level, estrogen deficiency, low calcium intake, history of falls, alcoholism, cigarette smoking, and environmental hazards. Individuals more prone to falling are those with vision deficits, balance and gait problems, and functional limitations.

KEY FACTS

Description
A break in a bone.

Causes
Sudden trauma, osteoporosis, or muscle overuse.

Risk factors
Individuals with osteoporosis or bone demineralization are at higher risk for fractures. Athletes are especially prone to stress fractures.

Symptoms
Pain if pressure is applied. Bone fragments may be felt through the skin or may rupture skin. Bruising and inflammation typically present.

Diagnosis
From symptoms; usually confirmed with X-ray.

Treatments
Depending upon severity, location, and type of fracture, surgery may be necessary. Initially, immobilization is used. Rehabilitative therapy may be needed to regain strength and range of motion.

Pathogenesis
Force or load exceeds bone tissue tolerance; result is tissue break or tear.

Prevention
Fall prevention strategies, including home modification, exercise, and proper shoe wear; prophylactic medication; and training modifications to prevent stress fractures.

Epidemiology
The leading cause of death and disability in persons 65 or older is fall-related injuries, especially hip fractures. Of women 65 years or older, white women are more likely to fracture a hip than are black women. Women are more likely to be hospitalized with a fall-related fracture.

BONE FRACTURES

Fractures can occur in many forms, depending on the force applied and the type of injury. Although fractures tend to occur across the bone, they can also occur in the bone in a spiral form, obliquely, or lengthwise.

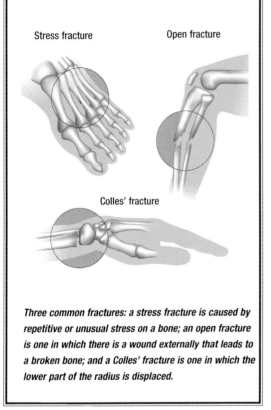

Stress fracture

Open fracture

Colles' fracture

Three common fractures: a stress fracture is caused by repetitive or unusual stress on a bone; an open fracture is one in which there is a wound externally that leads to a broken bone; and a Colles' fracture is one in which the lower part of the radius is displaced.

Signs, symptoms, and diagnosis

Fractures are painful, especially when pressure is applied to the fracture site. Typically, the surrounding tissue is tender, and there is usually swelling within a few hours of injury. With severely displaced bones, there may be limb deformity, a fragment of the displaced bone may be felt through the skin, or the bone may emerge through the skin. Fractures that occur as a result of continuous loading usually cause increasing discomfort. Blood from an injured fracture site may cause a skin bruise, especially with closed fractures. The pooling of blood can cause pain and stiffness in the area around the fracture.

Fracture diagnosis is made based upon signs and symptoms and usually confirmed by X-ray. Hairline or non-displaced fractures are often difficult to confirm by X-ray, and some stress fractures may not be evident by X-ray for several weeks after injury. An MRI (magnetic resonance imaging) scan may be necessary to identify less obvious fractures.

Treatments and prevention

Fracture treatment is highly dependent upon the type, severity, and location of the fracture. Open fractures often require surgery to clean and close the wound and present a greater risk for infection. Closed fractures are usually treated with immobilizers (a cast, brace, or splint) and recommendations for swelling management. The procedure for realigning a bone is called reduction. Surgical reduction for a displaced bone is called open reduction. The nonsurgical reduction of a closed fracture (realigning without penetrating the skin) is called closed reduction. Open reduction is often the sign of a more complicated and severe fracture.

Fixation devices, such as pins and plates, are often necessary to secure bone alignment for proper healing. Fixation devices may be internal (attached to the bone and sutured under the skin) or external (attached to the bone, but with a portion of the fixation device emerging through the skin). Traction may be used to help align bones. After realignment, whether or not surgery is necessary, a period of immobilization is often recommended during the initial healing phases. Immobilization prevents muscle action, helps to keep bones in place, and promotes bone reunification.

During the healing process, there is first tissue inflammation, possibly for several weeks. A hematoma forms, and inflammatory agents respond to the injury. The body cleans up dead tissue and begins to produce collagen for tissue healing. Next, a soft callous forms, often with pain and swelling, owing to increased blood flow to injured areas. Cartilage or early bone tissue begins to form. A natural splint is created to stabilize the fracture. As a result, muscles remain inactive and will often contract into the position of immobilization. Range of motion exercises will lengthen muscles that may have shortened during the immobilization period. Rehabilitation also includes strengthening muscles that have not been used during immobilization.

Bone mineral density assessment using a dual X-ray absorptiometry scan (DXA) can identify those at risk for osteoporosis. For those at high risk, calcium supplements or prophylactic medication. may be indicated.

Patti Berg

See also
• Bone and joint disorders • Osteoporosis

Fragile X syndrome

Fragile X syndrome, the most common form of familial or inheritable mental retardation, is an X-linked genetic disorder in which an unstable region on the X chromosome contains an abnormal number of DNA base pairs. Expression of this syndrome is more common in males and leads to characteristic physical features, developmental delays, and mental retardation.

Fragile X syndrome is an X-linked genetic disorder responsible for more mental retardation and developmental delay than any other familial disorder and is second only to Down syndrome in terms of total number of affected persons. Females, who have two X chromosomes, are less likely to be affected than males, because a random process called X-inactivation turns off one of their X chromosomes, and the other normal copy of the X chromosome compensates to some extent for the abnormal X chromosome. Men have only one X chromosome and one Y chromosome, and X-inactivation does not occur in males. Women with the full mutation can have no clinical problems if all the affected X chromosomes are inactivated to partial expression, based on the percentage of affected cells that are inactivated.

Causes

The disorder is caused by a mutation in the fragile X mental retardation gene 1 (*FMR1*) on the long arm of chromosome X. The effect of this is that the mutated gene cannot produce a certain protein, which is essential to the body's cells, particularly for the cells in the brain. Without this protein, the cells do not develop and function properly.

Symptoms

Having the premutation stage of fragile X syndrome is not without consequences. Individuals with premutations can present with mild cognitive and behavioral deficits. Women with premutations can experience premature ovarian failure. This difficulty with fertility can be the first presenting symptom prompting karyotype testing. For reasons not fully understood, women with the full mutation do not always have premature ovarian failure. Finally, premutation males can present with a fragile X tremor-ataxia syndrome.

Misdiagnosis is common, and the syndrome is often mistaken for Parkinson's disease, cerebrovascular disease, other causes of ataxia, or dementia.

The hallmarks of full fragile X syndrome are the characteristic mental retardation, classic facial features, and behavioral disorders. Males with the disease often have moderate to severe mental retardation. Typical facial features of these patients include a long, thin

---

KEY FACTS

Description
Genetic abnormality causing moderate to severe mental retardation when fully expressed in males and mild to borderline in females, mild retardation to no impairment in the premutation state, and no effect with a normal number of nucleotide base repeats on the X chromosome.

Causes
A defective gene on the X chromosome.

Risk factors
The only known risk factor is a female parent who has the premutation. Males with the premutation or full expression for fragile X syndrome will pass it on to all their daughters but none of their sons.

Symptoms
Males have a characteristic but subtle appearance including a long narrow face, large or protruding ears, attention deficit hyperactivity disorder, and postpubertal macroorchidism (large testes). Females who are premutation carriers or have the full mutation are much less affected than their male counterparts and can have premature ovarian failure and early menopause.

Diagnosis
Made by molecular testing of the *FMR1* gene for the number of CGG repeats.

Treatments
Should focus on supportive therapies for speech or language or both, behavioral therapy, and pharmacological therapy for behavioral disorders in affected individuals. There is no cure for fragile X syndrome.

Prevention
There is no method to predict which patients are carriers without DNA analysis.

Epidemiology
Approximately 1 in 4,500 males and 1 in 6,000 females are affected. It is estimated that 1 in 1,000 males and 1 in 400 women carry the premutation.

face, large ears, and prominent jaw as well as postpubertal macroorchidism in males. The physical features of this disorder are often more pronounced after puberty. The same holds true for developmental milestones. The majority of patients will have normal early development with a subsequent decline with advancing age. Learning disorders become more obvious with age. Behavioral disorders can include autism, including attention disorders, hand biting, shyness, speech disorders, and tactile defensiveness, among others. Affected females will have many of the same features to a lesser degree than their male counterparts.

Diagnosis

Diagnosis is made through DNA analysis. Polymerase chain reaction (PCR) is used to identify the number of CGG (trinucleotide) repeats. The presence of an abnormal number of CGG repeats determines an individual's status, whether it involves the premutation or the full mutation. Southern blot analysis is required for assessment of repeat segment length and methylation status, identifying those with the full fragile X syndrome. Amniocentesis can reliably be used to detect fragile X syndrome prior to birth. Chorionic villus sampling should not be performed as there can be abnormal methylation of the promoter region in placental tissue. This abnormal or partial methylation can result in inaccurate diagnosis, particularly when performed prior to 12 completed gestational weeks.

After birth a high index of suspicion is required to make the diagnosis. Fragile X syndrome should be considered in all children who have unexplained speech or developmental delay, autistic features, or mental retardation, especially if they exhibit any of the physical characteristics of fragile X syndrome.

Particular attention should be given in cases where there are relatives with mental retardation of unknown etiology. Naturally, investigation is warranted in cases with a family history of fragile X or in children of known carrier mothers. As a purely genetic disorder, there is no cure. Once the disorder has developed, symptoms from generation to generation can become worse because there is more likelihood of further CGG repeats.

Treatments

Treatment focuses on maximization of an individual's potential development. Special education, assistance from speech and language therapists and behavioral therapists, and physical and occupational therapy should all be considered. Psychopharmacology is an

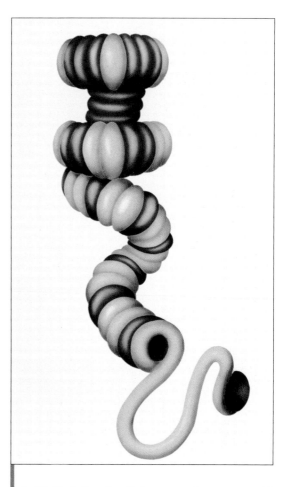

In this illustration of an X chromosome from a person with fragile X syndrome, the fragile area appears at the bottom where the CGG repeat triplet occurs. The repeat is longer in people with the syndrome; once this length reaches a critical dimension, symptoms appear.

adjunct to this, and treatment strategies change frequently. Genetic counseling and emotional support for family members should also be provided. The National Fragile X Foundation can help provide more information about this disorder.

Epidemiology

Around 1 in 4,500 males and 1 in 6,000 females are affected. It is believed that 1 in 1,000 males and 1 in 400 women carry the premutation. Premutation male carriers are at risk of the syndrome after age 50.

Brian Brost

See also
• Autism • Genetic disorders • Language and speech disorders • Learning disorders

Frostbite

Frostbite is injury to body tissues caused by freezing temperatures. It is most common in the winter, in latitudes closer to the North and South poles, and at high altitudes. Risk factors include prolonged activity in freezing temperatures, impaired judgment, such as that due to psychiatric illness or drugs, and an inability to avoid adverse conditions, as might befall very young or old people. Frostbite is more common when the blood supply to the extremities is impaired due to old age, diabetes, peripheral vascular disease, or certain drugs.

Frostbite generally involves parts of the body that are farthest away from the heart, such as the fingers, ears, and nose. The water in the cells becomes frozen and crystallizes, resulting in cell injury or death. Similar to burn injuries, frostbite can be classified by the depth of injury. First-degree frostbite involves the epidermis only and is characterized by redness of the skin. A second-degree or partial-thickness frostbite typically has fluid-filled blisters and is painful. Third-degree frostbite includes all layers of the skin, which is white and has no sensation. Fourth-degree frostbite involves injury to deeper structures such as fat, tendon, and bone and may lead to amputations of the injured toes or fingers. The skin involved is initially pale, firm, cold, and has no sensation. When rewarmed, the area is usually intensely red and painful unless tissue has been destroyed, as evidenced by blisters or gangrene.

Treatment

Treatment should first focus on any life-threatening conditions and include core rewarming if the patient has hypothermia (a low core body temperature). Management of the frostbitten tissue includes initial wrapping in dry clothing, followed by rapid rewarming with water at 104°F to 107°F (40°C–42°C). Rubbing the tissue, dry heat, and hot water should be avoided because they can cause additional injury. Once the injured part is warmed, antibiotic cream can be applied. First- and second-degree frostbite should heal spontaneously, the latter taking 10 to 21 days to form new skin. Third-degree frostbite may require surgical excision of the dead tissue and skin grafting. Fourth-degree frostbite may require amputations.

Prevention

Preventive measures involve protection with appropriate clothing and avoiding risky situations that may lead to prolonged exposure to freezing temperatures. Once numbness of the affected part has developed, the person may not realize that a severe, irreversible injury is occurring. With adequate precautions, most instances of frostbite are preventable.

David Wainwright

KEY FACTS

Description

Injury to the skin and underlying tissues as a result of freezing temperatures.

Causes and risk factors

Frostbite is caused by prolonged exposure to freezing temperatures. Those at higher risk include outdoor workers, winter athletes, and people with poor circulation. Impaired judgment and an inability to escape from the cold may lead to extended exposure.

Symptoms and signs and diagnosis

The diagnosis is made by the history of exposure and the observed skin changes. The skin is pale, firm, cold, has no sensation, and becomes intensely red and painful when rewarmed. Blisters and gangrene indicate a deeper injury with tissue death.

Treatments

The injured tissue should be rapidly rewarmed and an antibiotic cream applied. When tissue destruction occurs, the skin may need to be replaced with skin grafts, or amputations may be necessary.

Pathogenesis

The water in the cells becomes frozen and crystallizes, resulting in cell injury or death.

Prevention

Avoiding prolonged exposure to the cold; wearing appropriate clothing and protection of body areas when exposure is unavoidable.

Epidemiology

Frostbite is most common in outdoor workers and winter athletes. It is an injury observed most frequently in winter, in areas close to the North or South poles and at high altitudes.

See also

- Burns • Environmental disorders
- Occupational disorders

Gallstone

Gallstones are concretions of cholesterol or bilirubin that form in the gallbladder. They are common in Western cultures and result in 500,000 to 700,000 cholecystectomies (surgical removal) annually. Gallstones occur in about three women for every man, and are more common in certain Native Americans, Scandinavians, and native Alaskans. Risk factors for gallstone formation include obesity, weight loss, older age, diabetes, pregnancy, liver cirrhosis, and parenteral (outside the intestine, usually by injection) nutrition.

Gallstones come in two main varieties: cholesterol and pigmented stones. Cholesterol stones comprise 80 percent of all gallstones. Pigmented stones are composed of bilirubin (the breakdown product of heme, the iron-bearing pigment of blood) and are typically black or brown. Black stones occur in diseases that cause red blood cell destruction (hemolysis), such as sickle-cell anemia. Brown stones are typically the result of chronic infections in the channels (ducts) regulating bile flow. Rarely, medications can precipitate in bile and form stones.

Signs and symptoms

The mere presence of gallstones in the gallbladder does not cause symptoms. Pain occurs when a stone causes obstruction of biliary ducts. When this happens, patients complain of right-sided abdominal pain that radiates to the back or the shoulder. In more severe instances, nausea, fever, and jaundice can develop and may progress to life-threatening infection.

Diagnosis and treatments

Diagnosis is made by ultrasonography; it often occurs as an incidental finding. Computerized tomography and magnetic resonance imaging can also detect gallstones but are more frequently used to identify complications of gallstone disease. Abdominal X-ray is not helpful because cholesterol stones often lack calcifications and cannot be seen on X-rays.

Treatment depends on symptoms and whether complications develop. Asymptomatic gallstones require no therapy. Chronic gallstone-related pain is usually treated by laparoscopic removal of the gallbladder. Bile duct obstruction is typically managed by removal of the stone with a nonsurgical endoscope.

Pathogenesis and prevention

Bile is a digestive secretion that is formed in the liver and stored in the gallbladder. A variety of genetic and physiological conditions can result in bile becoming saturated with cholesterol or bilirubin. Gallstone formation begins with deposition of these compounds around a nidus that enlarges over time, especially when the emptying of the gallbladder is impaired. Prevention of gallstones is difficult because many risk factors cannot be modified. When rapid weight loss is anticipated, the bile acid ursodeoxycholate can reduce the incidence of gallstone formation.

Christopher W. Duncan and Stephen D. Zucker

KEY FACTS

Description
Concretions of cholesterol or bilirubin form stones.

Causes
Excess cholesterol or bilirubin in bile, genetic predisposition.

Risk factors
Female gender, race, family history, older age, pregnancy, obesity, hemolytic disorders.

Symptoms
Frequently asymptomatic; abdominal pain, nausea, fever, and jaundice can occur.

Diagnosis
Abdominal ultrasound, computed tomography.

Treatments
Surgery, medication, endoscopy.

Pathogenesis
Precipitation of cholesterol or bilirubin in the gallbladder, poor gallbladder emptying.

Prevention
Medication (ursodeoxycholate).

Epidemiology
More common in women (increases with number of pregnancies), Western cultures, Native Americans, and elderly people. About 11 percent of people in the United States have gallstones.

See also

• Digestive system disorders • Liver and spleen disorders • Obesity • Sickle-cell anemia

Gastroenteritis

The term *gastroenteritis* describes inflammation in the lining of the stomach and intestine leading to a syndrome characterized most commonly by nausea, vomiting, abdominal pain, and diarrhea. Also referred to as the "stomach flu," it is a common problem in the United States and a leading cause of childhood death on a global scale.

There are many causes of gastroenteritis, including bacteria, viruses, and protozoa, all of which can be transmitted through contaminated food as well as from person to person. Such outbreaks continually occur; for example, in 2006 in the United States, an outbreak of gastroenteritis was linked to spinach tainted by the bacterium E. coli 0157:H7.

Causes

There are thousands of different organisms that can cause gastroenteritis. In the United States, it is usually caused by viruses and less commonly by bacteria. Common viral pathogens in the United States include rotaviruses, noroviruses, adenoviruses, and enteroviruses. Bacterial gastroenteritis is usually food-borne or acquired during travel to underdeveloped areas. Leading causes include E. coli (including the strain 0157:H7), salmonella, shigella, campylobacter, and vibrio. In the United States, the protozoa *Giardia lamblia* is most often the cause of gastroenteritis.

Risk factors

Anyone in contact with other people who have gastroenteritis may be at risk for the infection themselves. People who reside in areas of poor sanitation may contribute to the spread of illness from person to person. Those who live in developed nations may also be at risk for bacterial gastroenteritis when they travel to underdeveloped areas where hygienic food preparation and appropriate sanitation may be less common. In doing so, they may inadvertently ingest contaminated food and water. Gastroenteritis acquired in this manner is also known as "traveler's diarrhea."

Symptoms and signs

Symptoms and signs vary, depending on whether the cause of gastroenteritis is bacterial or viral, and the in-cubation period may range from several hours to a few days. In cases of viral gastroenteritis, patients typically report acute onset of nausea, vomiting, abdominal

KEY FACTS

Description
Acute gastrointestinal infection caused by many different types of bacteria, viruses, and protozoa.

Causes
Common causes of viral gastroenteritis include rotaviruses, noroviruses, enteroviruses, and adenoviruses. Among bacteria, common causes include E. coli, shigella, campylobacter, salmonella, and vibrio.

Symptoms
Fever, nausea, vomiting, abdominal pain or cramping, or both, and diarrhea are common symptoms. High fever and bloody diarrhea are more classically associated with bacterial causes. In more severe cases, patients can develop dehydration, electrolyte imbalance, kidney failure, and neurological deficits.

Diagnosis
A cause may be suggested based on history (bacterial vs. viral), although confirmatory testing needs to be performed with stool analysis.

Treatments
Hydration and electrolyte replacement remain the cornerstone of treatment. With severe cases, intravenous hydration may be necessary. Supportive treatment is needed for viral gastroenteritis. In certain situations, antibiotics may be beneficial for treatment of bacterial gastroenteritis. With appropriate treatment, most patients recover after several days.

Pathogenesis
The organism is typically ingested by the host and attaches to the lining of the intestinal wall. The pathogen either produces toxins or will directly invade host cells to cause symptoms.

Prevention
Safe handling of food, clean sanitation habits, and avoidance of ill contacts are the best methods of prevention. In cases of food-borne outbreaks with an identified source, people should avoid the tainted product. A vaccine is also available to prevent gastroenteritis.

Epidemiology
There are 211 million cases, 900,000 hospitalizations, and 6,000–10,000 deaths per year in the United States. It is the leading cause of childhood death worldwide.

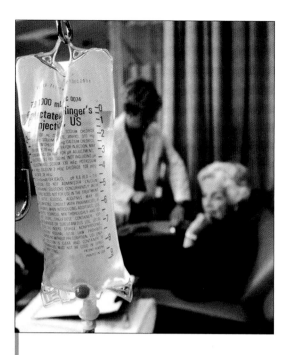

Elderly patients with gastroenteritis usually require hospitalization and intravenous fluid replacement to replace fluid lost from diarrhea and vomiting.

pain, and diarrhea, which is usually nonbloody. Patients afflicted with bacterial gastroenteritis may experience identical symptoms. However, bloody diarrhea and high fever are both more classically associated with bacterial gastroenteritis. Other possible symptoms include muscle aches, headaches, and fatigue. Because of excessive fluid loss (from vomiting and diarrhea), people may develop dehydration and electrolyte imbalances. In very severe cases, patients can also develop kidney damage and neurological complications such as lethargy, seizures, and coma. However, most cases of gastroenteritis are self-limited, and patients usually recover within several days.

Diagnosis and treatments

In cases of bacterial gastroenteritis, various tests can be performed on stool samples to determine the specific cause. In very ill patients, the bacteria can occasionally be found in the bloodstream and grown on laboratory culture. Tests to determine viral causes are available, but they are not commonly used because there is no specific cure for this form of the illness.

The cornerstone of therapy for gastroenteritis is fluid and electrolyte replacement. Patients can often replenish their own fluid supply by increasing their oral intake to match losses from vomiting and diar-

rhea. In more severe cases, patients may require hospitalization and intravenous fluid replacement. In cases of viral gastroenteritis, antibiotics are of no help, and treatment is supportive. In cases of bacterial gastroenteritis, the utility of antibiotics depends on the type of bacteria causing the illness. With bacteria such as campylobacter, shigella, and certain types of E. coli, antibiotics such as ciprofloxacin and levofloxacin are often effective. With other types of bacteria, antibiotics may lead to adverse effects and prolong the period when the organism is shed in the stool, which increases the likelihood of spread to others. Therefore, antibiotic treatment without knowledge of the etiology can potentially lead to more harm than good.

Pathogenesis and prevention

Once the pathogen gains access to the host (typically through ingestion), it attaches to the wall of the intestine, where it may cause damage through several different mechanisms. Some bacteria simply attach to host cells and produce toxins that cause severe diarrhea and dehydration, while other bacteria will actually attach and invade host cells. It is the tissue invasion that results in the bloody diarrhea of bacterial gastroenteritis. Viral pathogenesis is less well understood but is thought to result from viral entry into host cells where they promote fluid secretion into the gastrointestinal tract and subsequent diarrhea.

Prevention includes safe food preparation, appropriate sanitation practices, and avoidance of close contact with those affected. In the United States, a vaccine for infants is available to prevent rotavirus infection.

Epidemiology

It is estimated that 211 million cases of acute gastroenteritis occur in the United States per year, accounting for 6,000 to 10,000 deaths. Global mortality is much greater, and it is estimated that more than 2 million children die per year in Asia, Africa, and Latin America. Infants and children are more commonly affected, although the illness also carries a high mortality rate in the elderly. Although there may be some variation, the majority of illness in temperate climates occurs during winter months due to crowding that promotes spread, especially within households.

Nigar Kirmani

See also
• Cholera • Diarrhea and dysentery • Food poisoning • Infections, bacterial • Infections, parasitic • Infections, viral

Genetic disorders

Genetics is the study of the transfer of characteristics from organisms to their offspring. Humans receive the blueprint for their body encoded in a set of chromosomes from each parent at conception, although further changes can occur in these "instructions" during later development. Each chromosome carries instructions called genes, which are encoded on molecules of deoxyribonucleic acid (DNA). DNA is the "recipe," or formula, for everything the body needs to develop, function, and reproduce over the course of a lifetime. Genetics explores how this information is transferred from parents to offspring, techniques for diagnosis, and methods to correct or minimize the impact of changes on the body and overall health.

Each human body cell contains a total of 46 chromosomes, which fall into 23 pairs. (The exceptions are red blood cells, sperm, eggs, and germ, or reproductive, cells, which are generally not defined as body, or somatic, cells.) One chromosome from each pair is inherited from each parent. Two similar, sometimes called matching, chromosomes in a pair are called homologues. Pairs 1 to 22 are homologues in most people; they are the same in men and women and are called autosomes. The twenty-third pair determines a person's sex. These so-called sex chromosomes are XX in women and XY in men. "X" and "Y" describe the chromosome shape.

These 46 chromosomes, or 23 pairs, comprise the full set, or genome, of genetic information a person requires. The genome provides the necessary instructions on how to grow and function properly by manufacturing proteins. Proteins consist of chains of amino acids (polypeptides) put together in a specific sequence based on the genetic code carried by DNA. Proteins are important structural components of the body, providing its most basic building blocks for all types of tissues, glands, and organs. Proteins are also vital to the body as enzymes (biological catalysts) and hormones (biological messengers). Cells are continuously using their genetic code to function and repair damage to cellular structures.

Cell division

During normal growth, body cells have to divide and reproduce constantly, and worn out or damaged cells are replaced. Cell division is also responsible for the production of sex cells (sperm and egg). The two types of cell division, mitosis and meiosis, ensure that new cells have the required number of chromosomes.

RELATED ARTICLES

DNA STRUCTURE AND FUNCTION

DNA occurs inside the nucleus of almost every cell in the body. A DNA molecule is composed of two strands that tightly intertwine to form a double helix, or twisted ladder shape. Each double helix is composed of two sugar-phosphate "backbones" joined by paired bases that resemble the rungs of a ladder. There are four types of bases: adenine (A), thymine (T), guanine (G), and cytosine (C). Each "rung" is formed by a base pair; adenine always pairs with thymine, and guanine always pairs with cytosine. The sequence, or order, of these four bases in a gene (segment of DNA) supplies the genetic code, or inherited instructions, that dictate the production of a particular type of protein outside the nucleus.

DNA itself, however, never leaves the nucleus. Instead, different molecules of ribonucleic acid (RNA) serve to carry the genetic code outside of the nucleus and then translate the code into the production of amino acids. Messenger RNA (mRNA) facilitates the transport of the genetic message to the outside of the nucleus, where proteins can be constructed, dispersed, and utilized. Messenger RNA builds a temporary template or "mirror image" of a single strand of DNA in a process called transcription. In a similar way to how DNA replicates (copies itself; see artwork), mRNA forms a template by piecing together bases that reflect those on the single parent DNA strand. The same nucleic acids are used except that thymine (T) is replaced by uracil (U). So, where the DNA has guanine, the mRNA has cytosine (and vice versa); and where the DNA has thymine,

the mRNA has adenine; but where the DNA strand has adenine, the mRNA has uracil (instead of thymine).

Once outside the nucleus, this single-stranded mRNA and another type of RNA called transfer RNA (tRNA) work together, using the genetic code to make proteins in a process called translation. The genetic code is "written" in groups of three bases, called codons, on a single strand of DNA or mRNA. The nucleic acids (A, C, G, and T/U) can be grouped into three to make a codon in 64 ways (4 x 4 x 4 = 64 permutations). Sixty-one of these codons are each used to add a specific amino acid to a polypeptide chain, and the other three codons terminate the chain. This sequence of codons (the "triplet code") can be used to construct any protein based on the pattern copied to messenger RNA.

Since there are more codons (64) than amino acids (20), there is redundancy in the code since several codons can code for the same protein. For example, the amino acid leucine can be coded for by the mRNA codons CUU, CUC, CUA, CUG, UUA, and UUG. However, such redundancies are helpful. Should a mutation occur that changes the triplet code, the correct amino acid will still be added to the polypeptide chain and contribute properly to the protein. However, certain mutations can occur that result in a codon calling for an alternative amino acid. The ramifications of such a mutation depend on several factors, including location in the polypeptide chain, polarity (charge) differences, and structure changes.

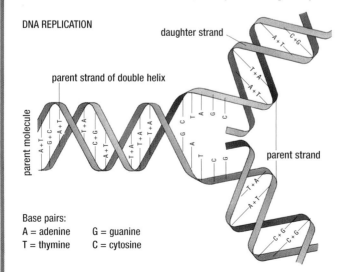

DNA REPLICATION

daughter strand

parent strand of double helix

parent molecule

parent strand

Base pairs:
A = adenine   G = guanine
T = thymine   C = cytosine

Before cell division occurs, each DNA molecule must replicate (copy itself) to ensure that the new daughter cells contain the correct amount of DNA. Before replication, a molecule of DNA occurs as a double helix comprising two sugar-phosphate "backbones" joined by paired bases (A and T; G and C). With the help of an enzyme, the parent molecule is partly "unzipped" by the breaking of base pairs. The resulting separate, single strands then pair up with free-floating bases to form new double helixes, each of which comprises an original (parent) strand and a newly built daughter strand.

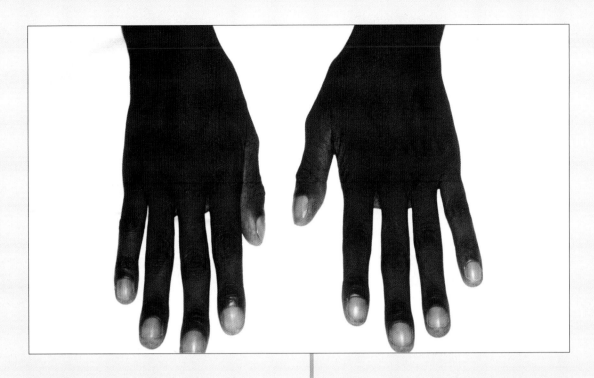

Mitosis. When a body cell replicates (copies itself), each strand of DNA acts as a template from which two new strands are formed to produce two new identical double DNA strands. These DNA strands coil up to form X-shaped chromosomes, each of which contains a double helping of DNA. The chromosomes line up in the middle of the cell, arranged on a network of threads that begins to pull the chromosomes apart. Half of each chromosome moves to the opposite side of the cell, which then divides into two. When a cell undergoes mitosis, the two resulting "daughter" cells contain exact copies of the original, or parent, cell's full set of DNA. So, each daughter cell has the full genome—46 chromosomes (23 pairs).

Meiosis. In this form of cell division, a parent cell divides in an ovary or testis in two stages to form four new sex cells (egg or sperm respectively). The parent cell contains 46 chromosomes, but since the DNA is only doubled at one of the two division stages, each of the four new cells contains only 23 chromosomes, half the normal amount. This process ensures that when an egg and sperm fuse at conception, the resulting fertilized cell contains the correct number of chromosomes—46. Twenty-three of those chromosomes have been inherited from the mother, and 23 from the father. Mitosis then takes over to complete development of the fertilized cell.

Marfan syndrome is a rare genetic disorder of connective tissue in which people grow tall and thin with long fingers. This genetic disorder, which leads to many physiological problems, is inherited in an autosomal dominant manner.

Genetic mutations

There are three possible sources for mutations. An inherited mutation is one that was passed down from one of the person's parents, or both of them, through meiosis. The mutation could be present in all of the parent's cells, potentially making him or her susceptible to the manifestations of the mutation, and transmittable via egg or sperm to the offspring.

The mutation could exist solely in the parent's ovaries or testes (gonadal mosaicism); although offspring would not be susceptible to manifestations of the mutation, they would have the potential to pass on the mutation to several offspring.

New spontaneous mutations can occur during cell division; however, the cell contains mechanisms to overcome these. Some mutations in sperm can be lethal and prevent their perpetuation into the next generation. Some mutations can be silent, that is, they do not alter the protein, or they may occur in genes that are inherited in an autosomal recessive manner. Finally, some mutations can be in areas of noncoded DNA, and hence are thought to be of no known

CRACKING CODES AND MAPPING GENOMES

In 1966, Marshall Nirenberg, H. Gobind Khorana, and colleagues, "cracked" the genetic code. They discovered the correlation between the four base pairs and 20 amino acids that are produced by the body as building blocks for proteins. In effect, scientists were then finally able to "read" the triplet code carried by DNA and the "mirror-image" code carried by mRNA. This "reading" was limited, however, to knowing the production of which amino acid is coded for by which codon. Figuring out which triplet codes formed particular genes took longer. That work was undertaken by the Human Genome Project, a project partially funded by the U.S. Government. In 2003, researchers on the Human Genome Project announced the complete sequencing ("reading" of the triplet code) of the human genome. The "human genome" refers to a single entity, since the genetic code is more than 99.9 percent identical from one human to the next. As a result of this work, it has been possible to map where genes occur on chromosomes. Genetic linkage maps provide the relative location of genes based on how frequently genes are inherited together. Physical gene maps place genes in relation to the presence of known sequences that can be considered chromosomal landmarks.

significance. Mutations can alter protein structure, function, or dosage; this can be benign, beneficial, or detrimental depending on the location in the genome. On inheritance, chromosomes can be missing or sometimes an extra chromosome is gained. During mitosis or meiosis, chromosomes can break off and are consequently missing. Conversely, an additional chromosome or a piece of a chromosome can be donated during meiosis. Having an extra chromosome in the twenty-first pair can result in Down syndrome. Sometimes chromosomal accidents can result in miscarriage because the defects are too severe. If the child survives and is born, the defect remains in the genes throughout his or her life.

Single gene disorders

Individual gene defects are common. Genes occur in paired forms called alleles, one allele on each chromosome of a pair. Mutations of genes on X chromosomes result in conditions called X-linked disorders. Mutations on other chromosomes result in autosomal disorders. Each cell has 22 pairs of autosomes, which are the non-sex chromosomes. Single gene disorders are classified according to the type of inheritance, which can be autosomal dominant, autosomal recessive, or X-linked. Another category also exists, that of multifactorial disorders, which are caused by a mixture of factors, such as the environment, genes, and lifestyle.

Autosomal dominant. Only one copy of a defective gene in parental alleles is sufficient for an individual to display features of a disease. Males and females are equally at risk of being affected since the gene lies on an autosome. If an affected person has offspring with an unaffected person, each child will have a 1 in 2 chance of inheriting the mutant (defective) allele (gene form), and inversely, a 1 in 2 chance of being unaffected after inheriting the normal allele.

If two affected individuals have offspring, each child will have a 1 in 2 chance of inheriting the mutated allele, a 1 in 4 chance of being homozygous (inheriting two identical alleles) for the normal allele, and a 1 in 4 chance of being homozygous for the mutant (this might lead to prenatal death).

When a pedigree is investigated, usually multiple generations are found to have affected individuals, which is called vertical inheritance. Examples of diseases inherited vertically through autosomal dominance include achondroplasia, neurofibromatosis, and Marfan syndrome.

Achondroplasia is characterized by small stature, large head, trident-shaped hands, and other bony problems of the spine and long bones. It occurs with a frequency of 1 in 15,000 to 20,000 live births. In about 90 percent of cases, the mutation is new in the family. In the rest of the cases it is associated with advanced paternal age. Mutations occur on the gene encoding for a cell receptor called fibroblast growth factor receptor 3. A homozygous (both alleles affected) form of achondroplasia can occur and is lethal secondary to lack of sufficient lung development caused by restriction in the growth of the rib cage.

PATTERNS OF INHERITANCE

In most genetic disorders, the defect is passed through the genes from parent to child. A child inherits one of each pair of genes from the mother and father; these genes may be dominant or recessive; dominant genes hide any effect from recessive genes. Single gene disorders are distinguished by their patterns of inheritance, which may be autosomal dominant, autosomal recessive, or X-linked.

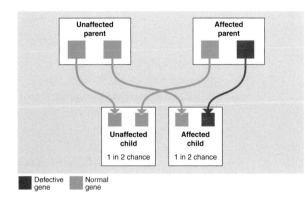

Autosomal dominant

Males and females are equally at risk because the defective gene is present on an autosome (not a sex chromosome).

Examples of disorders caused by this type of inheritance are: achondroplasia, Huntington's disease, and Marfan syndrome.

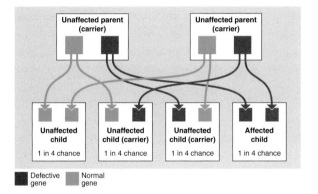

Autosomal recessive

Males and females have the same chance of being affected. A pair of defective genes is inherited, usually one from each parent.

Examples of disorders are Tay-Sachs disease, cystic fibrosis, and phenylketonuria.

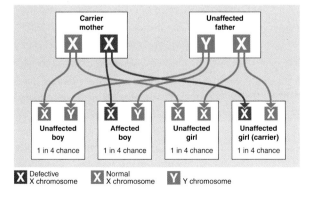

X-linked recessive

Males are most commonly affected since the defect cannot be masked by a second normal X chromosome. A boy who receives the gene will be affected; a girl will be a carrier.

Examples include hemophilia, muscular dystrophy, and fragile X syndrome.

Type 1 neurofibromatosis has a high penetrance (that is, the genetic mutation causes observable manifestations in a population), but there is wide variability in how the gene is expressed (observable manifestations vary). This disorder occurs with a frequency of 1 in 3,500 individuals. Findings on clinical examination include multiple fleshy benign lesions on the skin called neurofibromas, multiple irregularly shaped pigmented lesions of the skin known as café-au-lait spots, small benign tumors of the iris called Lisch nodules, and possible effects on the central nervous system, including tumors, seizures, and potential for malignant changes in the neurofibromas. Neurofibromas rarely develop in children less than 6 years of age, with a potential for increase in tumor size during puberty, pregnancy, and later in life. The majority of affected individuals have a benign life. Type 2, or acoustic, neurofibromatosis is also autosomal dominant and it is often more severe than type 1.

Marfan syndrome is characterized clinically by a tendency toward tall stature with long slim limbs, long fingers with joint laxity, lens problems, and dilation (widening) of the root of the aorta. The variability in expression of Marfan syndrome is sufficiently wide to make the diagnosis difficult with a new mutation. Mutations occur in the gene for fibrillin (a glycoprotein that is the major component of elastic tissues in the body), which is located on chromosome 15. Diagnosis is important because treatment with pharmacological agents to block or slow the heart rate will significantly reduce the rate of dilation of the aortic root and might lead to further complications.

Autosomal recessive. In an autosomal recessive disorder, patients are affected because they have inherited a pair of defective genes, usually one from each parent. The parents are usually carriers of the defective gene and are unaffected by the disorder. A mutation in both alleles of a gene is required for an individual to display features of a disease. Males and females have an equal chance of being affected because the gene lies on an autosome and not on a sex chromosome. An individual who has one mutation is called a carrier or a heterozygote (that is, the person has both a defective allele and a normal allele of a particular gene). A carrier does not display the classical features of the disease in question. If a

person does not display features of this disease, he or she can be homozygous for the normal allele or can be heterozygous for a mutation (and therefore a carrier). Affected individuals usually have unaffected parents but may have affected siblings, which is a form of horizontal inheritance.

If two carriers have a child, each child has a 1 in 4 chance of being a carrier and being unaffected, a 1 in 4 chance of having inherited the mutant allele from each parent and therefore being affected, and a 1 in 4 chance of having both normal alleles.

If an affected individual mates with an individual who has both normal alleles, every child will be a carrier. If a carrier mates with an individual who has both normal alleles every child has a 1 in 2 chance of being a carrier, and a 1 in 2 chance of having both normal alleles. Examples of autosomal recessive disorders include phenylketonuria, cystic fibrosis, and Tay-Sachs disease.

Phenylketonuria is a disorder in which an abnormal enzyme fails to convert the amino acid phenylalanine into tyrosine. The resulting buildup of phenylalanine, if untreated, leads to neurological problems. The problem is quickly corrected by a modified diet that excludes the amino acid.

Cystic fibrosis is a severe genetic disorder that is life threatening. It is characterized by a buildup of sticky mucus in the airways and intestines. This requires regular and intensive physiotherapy and treatment with antibiotics to attempt to keep the disease at bay. Cystic fibrosis occurs if both parents are carriers and their child inherits a faulty gene from each of them. If only one defective gene is inherited, the person will be a carrier with the potential to pass on the gene.

Tay-Sachs disease is an inherited metabolic disorder, in which a vital enzyme is deficient; its lack causes a buildup of a dangerous substance in the brain that is potentially life threatening. The disease was prevalent among Ashkenazi Jews but genetic counseling has helped to reduce its prevalence.

X-linked disorders. In X-linked disorders, there is a mutation on the X chromosome. Males are generally more severely affected than females because they do not have a second unaffected X chromosome to compensate for the mutation. The severity of the disease in females can range from asymptomatic to severe, as it is in males.

Females who have a mutation are said to be heterozygous, since they have a normal allele on their second X chromosome. Males who have a mutation are said to be hemizygous, since they only have one X chromosome so can only have one allele of the gene.

If a heterozygous female and an unaffected male have offspring, every male child they have has a 1 in 4 chance of being affected, and a 1 in 4 chance of being unaffected. Every female child has a 1 in 4 chance of being a heterozygote (carrier), and a 1 in 4 chance of being unaffected.

If an unaffected female mates with an affected hemizygous male every male child they have will be unaffected, because males can only inherit the Y chromosome from their father. Every female will be a heterozygote after inheriting one X chromosome from her mother and the only (mutated) X chromosome from her father.

If a heterozygous female mates with an affected hemizygous male every male child they have has a 1 in 2 chance of being an affected hemizygote, and a 1 in 2 chance of being unaffected. Every female child has a 1 in 2 chance of being a heterozygote, and a 1 in 2 chance of being affected as she may inherit a mutated X chromosome from either parent.

Some scientists classify X-linked diseases that render heterozygous females asymptomatic as "X-linked recessive" and those that render them symptomatic as "X-linked dominant." Examples of X-linked recessive diseases include hemophilia and Duchene muscular dystrophy. Hemophilia A, or Factor VIII deficiency, is characterized by easy bruising and bleeding into the joints and muscles. It affects 1 in 10,000 Caucasian males and is the most common type of hemophilia. Treatment is directed at replacement of missing blood factors, particularly during surgery or after trauma.

In Duchenne muscular dystrophy, because boys have only only X chromosome, if they inherit a copy of a defective gene from their unaffected mother, they will develop the full disorder. Around half the sons of carrier mothers will be affected; the other half will neither be carriers nor will they be affected. Because girls have two X chromosomes, they will not be affected by the disorder, but they will be carriers and could pass it on to their children. The symptoms of this type of muscular dystrophy are curvature of the spine,

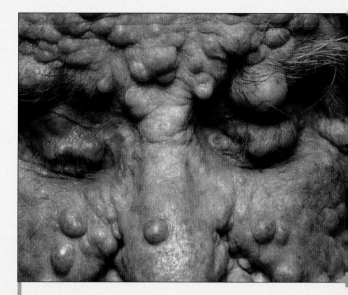

This woman has a severe form of neurofibromatosis, an autosomal dominant disorder in which benign (noncancerous) tumors called neurofibromas arise from nerves in the skin.

difficulty walking, and learning difficulties. Children with this disorder often succumb to heart problems or chest infections.

Another example of an X-linked dominant disease is Coffin-Lowry syndrome, in which there is severe mental deficiency. Clinical findings include a coarse-appearing face, short stature, and thick soft hands with tapering fingers. Abnormal curving of the spine can occur later in childhood.

Other X-linked disorders include color blindness, fragile X syndrome, and Christmas disease. Fragile X syndrome is an inherited abnormality on the X chromosome that results in learning difficulties for the person affected. It tends to mainly affect males, although females can develop the disorder also. Other symptoms are large ears, nose, and jaw, and men with the disorder tend to have large testes. Although the syndrome does not affect longevity, it does affect quality of life and if it runs in the family, couples contemplating pregnancy are advised to seek the advice of a genetic counselor before proceeding.

It is important to note that although females have two X chromosomes, only one of them is functional. One X chromosome is randomly inactivated in every cell of the body. It is presumed that 50 percent of the cells will inactivate the maternal X chromosome, and

50 percent will inactivate the paternal chromosome. However, for ill-defined reasons, skewing might take place, leading to overexpression of one or the other X chromosome in a female. Because of the randomization of inactivation, female carriers for X-linked diseases might display mild features of an X-linked disease.

Y-linked disorders. A mutation in a gene on the Y chromosome results in affected males and unaffected females since they do not have a Y chromosome. However, because the Y chromosome does not carry much genetic material in the same way that the X chromosome does, there are no major diseases that are linked to Y chromosome defects. The main function of the Y chromosome is to stimulate the development of the testes in a male embryo.

Genetic counseling

Genetic counseling is a communication process about the occurrence and the risk of recurrence of genetic disorders in a family. The aim of counseling should be to describe the genetic disease as fully as possible and discuss survival and prognosis along with the options available for diagnosis, treatment, and prevention. The accuracy of proper diagnosis, along with unbiased and nondirective counseling, concern for the individual, confidentiality, and trust are important features of genetic counseling.

In clinical genetics, geneticists do a careful family history noting the age, sex, and lineage of all members of the extended family to try to gain clues as to the possible genetic disorder and inheritance pattern if a disorder is present in a family. This pedigree, combined with a careful physical examination, laboratory evaluation, and possibly radiological studies, such as X-rays, computed tomography (CT), or magnetic resonance imaging (MRI), can aid in the diagnosis of genetic disorders. Not all features of the genetic disease can be found or are expressed in all individuals.

The pattern of findings in an individual or family can be compared to data available in massive databases compiling the known genetic conditions reported in humans. Sometimes a clear diagnosis cannot be made until later in life when other features start to express themselves.

Testing during pregnancy

Certain pregnancies fall into a higher risk group, including advanced maternal or paternal age, a prior affected child, a parent with a genetic disorder or who is known to be a carrier of a disorder, family history of a genetic disorder, consanguinity (having a child with a close relative), and environmental exposures. In addition, some ethnic groups have a higher incidence of certain genetic disorders, including sickle-cell anemia in African Americans and Tay-Sachs disease in Ashkenazi Jews.

There are many problems associated with trying to diagnose chromosomal changes and other genetic mutations during pregnancy, including the fact that there are so many genetic disorders. Many genetic diseases are first detectable during pregnancy as aneuploidy (deviation from the normal number of chromosomes). While many of these problems can be diagnosed through an invasive procedure such as amniocentesis, there is a risk of miscarriage attributable to the procedure. The risk of miscarriage as a result of amniocentesis in most centers is less than 0.5 percent. The loss rate for chorionic villus sampling (CVS) has been quoted as 1 to 2 per 100 procedures and for genetic amniocentesis to be 1 in 200 to 800. With a CVS sample, a portion of the placenta is obtained by a needle to check the fetal chromosome number; genetic amniocentesis utilizes fetal cells that have sloughed off into the amniotic fluid. Rare complications associated with these procedures include bleeding, infection, and fetal or maternal injury. It must be kept in mind that for many of the genetic conditions that can be diagnosed prenatally, there is no treatment available. Couples often cite the need for early diagnosis to prepare for caring for an affected child or the desire for pregnancy termination. Pregnancy termination is not legal in all countries; some countries place limits on how far along in the pregnancy abortion is considered legal.

Given the risk of these invasive techniques, many couples elect to undergo less risky screening evaluations for aneuploidy or for particular disorders such as cystic fibrosis. These tests do not reveal whether the child has the disease or problem, but rather whether the child is in a higher risk group to have this problem and whether the mother should have prenatal diagnosis.

Practitioners can screen the pregnancy in the first or second trimester for chromosome problems using ultrasound—the more defects noted, the higher the risk of aneuploidy—and also by using hormonal markers in the maternal blood. These hormone levels are compared to other women who have already delivered for which the outcome of their pregnancies is already known (for example, in cases of Down syndrome or spina bifida). Other tests to screen for problems such as cystic fibrosis check parental blood for the most common mutations associated with cystic fibrosis.

One diagnostic technique that is still in its early stages of development examines fetal cells in the mother's circulation for genetic abnormalities. Although fetal cells (particularly in the case of Down syndrome) and fetal DNA can be found in the maternal circulation, the low number of cells and the difficulty in differentiating between maternal and female fetal cells in the circulation currently limit the usefulness of this technique.

The persistence of certain white blood cell types such as lymphocytes across multiple different pregnancies is another limitation that needs careful evaluation.

Treatment

The goal of treating genetic diseases is to eliminate the effects of the disorder or at least lessen its effects to provide a better quality of life for the affected individual and her or his family.

Screening for genetic disease should occur at or before birth to try to catch problems before damage occurs. As some disorders can develop or worsen over time, it important to continue assessment for genetic disease throughout the life of each person. When an individual has a significant change in the chromosome content or number, no effective therapy is possible because of the large number of genes involved.

Multifactorial diseases or single gene disorders represent the main targets for therapy. The strategies utilized by researchers involve intervention at different levels of the problem: the mutant gene (transplantation or gene therapy), the mutant protein (protein replacement or enhancement of protein function), metabolic or biochemical dysfunction (dietary or pharmacological treatment), clinical phenotype (medical or surgical intervention), or the family (genetic counseling, carrier screening, and presymptomatic diagnosis).

If the genetic disease causes an effect on a specific organ or structure (for example, congenital heart defects, cleft lip and palate, and pyloric stenosis), surgical repair can cure or decrease the risk of other problems such as the infections associated with spina bifida. In some cases such as phenylketonuria (PKU), the mechanism by which elevations of the amino acid phenylalanine impair brain development and function is not well understood. Recent advances have discovered the function of abnormal proteins in diseases such as cystic fibrosis or certain types of muscular dystrophy. With these findings as a basis, research continues to formulate these findings into a possible therapy.

Single gene disorders represent an area of great hope and yet still even greater disappointment. Of the more than 370 disorders identified with

SUPPLEMENTS

Genetic factors are thought to play a role in the development of spina bifida, which appears to run in families. However, the risk of spina bifida and other neural tube defects in a child can be significantly reduced if the mother takes supplements of the B vitamin folic acid, or folate, in the months preceding pregnancy and the first few weeks of pregnancy. Folic acid is essential for the proper development of the nervous system early on in fetal growth. This supplemental vitamin may also help decrease the risk of congenital cardiac disease and cleft lip and palate.

Other disorders will cause problems unless medical treatment occurs before birth. In congenital adrenal hyperplasia, a rare genetic disorder, there is a defect in an enzyme that blocks the production of corticosteroid hormones (hydrocortisone and aldosterone) from the adrenal glands. The result is large amounts of male sex hormones (androgens), which can severely affect the unborn child. Maternal treatment in utero with the drug dexamethesone can prevent problems in genital development, and sometimes later problems such as premature puberty and infertility, if the drug is started at the proper time during pregnancy.

THE FUTURE OF GENETICS

Gene therapy involves the transfer of functional copies of a missing or defective gene to correct or reverse the effects of a genetic mutation. Scientists are able to introduce normal genes into cells through the use of recombinant DNA technology. The introduced gene can possibly compensate for a mutant gene by providing functional copies of genes (for example in phenylketonuria), to replace or inactivate a mutant gene's abnormal product (as in Huntington's disease), or to provide a pharmacological effect to counteract the effects of mutant cellular genes or pathogenesis (cancer).

Although the possibilities of this therapy are extremely exciting, it is fraught with significant technical and ethical difficulties. Any study carried out would be subject to an extremely rigorous review. Given the significant possibility to relieve human suffering, virtually all religious and government organizations have agreed that investigation of this form of therapy should be undertaken. A permanent genetic cure is not yet possible.

Some risks of gene therapy have already been demonstrated whereas others are thought to be possible and have a significant effect. Gene therapy requires a vector (carrier) to transport a gene into the cell. At least one patient has died from an adverse reaction to this vector or transferred gene. These vectors allow the incorporation of the transferred gene into the patient's DNA at a random location in the somatic or germ cell line. There is a risk that the process might turn on a cancer gene or inactivate a tumor suppressor gene. Since gene therapy trials are currently carried out only when no other therapy is available, these risks have been considered acceptable. If the vector is inserted into an essential gene, the procedure would result in the death of a single cell; however, cell death would be unlikely to occur in all transfected cells.

Genetic scientists have been trying to help victims of cystic fibrosis. The patient is given a mixture of healthy genes and an adenovirus, or modified virus that does not insert its own DNA into the host cell. The virus invades the cells of the lungs; at the same time, the virus carries the healthy genes into the cells. So far the technique looks promising, but more research is needed.

single gene defects, only 12 percent have completely effective therapies, 54 percent partially effective, and 34 percent with no apparent benefit with therapy.

For some diseases, the damage occurs before a diagnosis is made, which can be after or before birth. These possibilities underscore the importance of genetic counseling prior to attempting pregnancy in couples with a family history of genetic disorders.

Dietary restriction is the oldest treatment option for genetic disease, with more than 24 gene defects managed this way. While a change in diet can be effective, it requires strict and lifelong compliance with often very restrictive dietary options. Children with phenylketonuria are normal at birth; the mother clears excess phenylalanine through the placenta. After birth, levels of phenylalanine will accumulate unless there is strict dietary adherence.

Other methods of treating genetic disease include avoiding substances that can precipitate a problem; replacing missing components; and diversion, inhibition, or depletion of substances in the body. Another form of genetic therapy is modification of the somatic genome through transplantation, such as a bone marrow or liver transplant, for severe cases of cystic fibrosis.

Prevention

Couples with the risk of a specific devastating or lethal condition running through the family may try to select for a child without this specific condition. Preimplantation genetic diagnosis allows couples undergoing in vitro fertilization (IVF) to select embryos that are free of a specific genetic condition prior to transfer of the embryo to the uterus. Using techniques under a microscope, a single cell can be removed from the developing embryo at around the eight-cell stage to look for single gene mutations or an abnormal chromosome number. Affected or abnormal embryos are discarded, which raises ethical concerns about this procedure. There do not seem to be any documented problems for the developing embryo with this technique. Current techniques of preimplantation diagnosis do not allow selecting for multiple genetic conditions because of the limited number of cells that can be removed at this early stage in pregnancy.

Lama Eldahdah and Brian Brost

Giardiasis

Giardiasis is an infectious disease of the intestines caused by the microscopic parasite *Giardia lamblia*. Symptoms include diarrhea, stomach cramps, dehydration, and weight loss. In many less-developed countries, most children have had giardiasis by their third birthday.

More than 20,000 new cases of giardiasis are reported every year in the United States alone. The cause is a microscopic, single-celled parasite belonging to the genus *Giardia*. Scientists are still not certain about the classification of this organism, but there appear to be various species, each of which can infect several different kinds of animals. The main species that affects humans is called *Giardia lamblia*.

The symptoms that a *Giardia* infection produces, such as diarrhea, can also be caused by many other disorders. If giardiasis is suspected, examination of a fecal sample or a blood test will discover if the patient has produced specific protective antibodies (see IMMUNE SYSTEM DISORDERS).

Pathogenesis

Giardia can survive in the environment because the parasite is surrounded by a thick outer coat to form a cyst (an inactive, nonfeeding form). After a person or animal swallows the cysts present in contaminated food or water, the cysts break open when they reach the small intestine, releasing mature parasites that feed and multiply. The parasite does not attack intestinal cells directly. *Giardia* parasites, by attaching to and covering the inner intestinal surfaces, interfere with nutrient absorption and water transport and cause diarrhea, cramps, and sometimes dehydration. As the parasites pass through the small intestines to the large intestines, they form new cysts that pass out of the body. These new cysts, if they infect other people or animals who come in contact with contaminated food or water, start another cycle of infection.

Epidemiology, prevention, and treatments

People get giardiasis when they drink river, stream, or lake water contaminated with fecal matters from wild animals such as bears and beavers. Infection is also possible from drinking insufficiently processed municipal water. Outbreaks sometimes occur in day care centers and nursing homes when caregivers do not wash their hands after a bowel movement. Giardiasis does not spread by exposure to blood or other body fluids, but some people can be infected without apparent symptoms and may spread the infection.

Prevention is mainly a matter of personal hygiene habits such as washing hands after a bowel movement. River, stream, and lake water should be boiled or filtered before it is drunk. Eating uncooked food in countries where giardiasis occurs should be avoided. Nearly four thousand people per year in the United States have giardiasis severe enough to require hospitalization. Treatment is with drugs such as metronidazole, furazolidone, and nitrazoxanide. Patients take medication for 5 to 10 days. When diarrhea is severe, replacing lost fluids is also important.

Janet Yagoda Shagam

KEY FACTS

Description
Parasitic infection of the small intestine.

Cause
Infection with *Giardia lamblia*, a single-celled microscopic parasite.

Risk factors
Drinking untreated or undertreated water, or eating contaminated raw foods or inadequately cooked foods.

Symptoms
Diarrhea, abdominal cramps, and weight loss.

Diagnosis
Identifying parasites in feces of infected person, or immunological testing.

Treatments
Drugs, plus hydration treatment.

Pathogenesis
Parasites interfere with absorption of nutrients and also cause diarrhea.

Prevention
Good hygiene. Boiling or otherwise treating potentially contaminated water.

Epidemiology
More than 20,000 new cases each year in the United States.

See also
• Diarrhea and dysentery • Digestive system disorders • Gastroenteritis • Infections, animal-to-human • Infections, parasitic

Glaucoma

A serious eye disorder involving damage to the optic nerve, glaucoma is usually caused by a buildup of pressure within the eye. Because of age, glaucoma is the second most common cause of blindness worldwide after cataracts. As a population grows older, the prevalence of glaucoma rises. It is important to detect and treat the disease as early as possible because damage caused by glaucoma cannot be undone.

Glaucoma is sometimes called the "silent thief of sight" and may be well advanced before individuals become aware that their eyesight is becoming impaired. Typically, vision around the edges of sight (peripheral vision) is affected first. In the United States, an estimated 3 million people have glaucoma; 50 percent of these remain undiagnosed. Glaucoma is the leading cause of blindness in the United States for which treatment is available.

Risk factors

Everyone is potentially at risk. Advancing age is a major risk factor (glaucoma is six times more prevalent in individuals over 60 years), but the disease also occurs in babies and adolescents. It is the leading cause of blindness in African Americans, who are at much higher risk (and at a younger age) than Caucasians. A person's risk of developing the most common form of glaucoma (primary open angle glaucoma) increases if another family member already has it. Normal tension glaucoma (see below) is more common in people of ethnic Japanese origin.

Causes and pathogenesis

Glaucoma is usually caused by a buildup of pressure in the eye. The pressure increase begins in the eye's front chamber, which is filled with a watery liquid called aqueous humor. If too much of the liquid is produced and it cannot drain properly, increased intraocular pressure (IOP) results, which can damage the eye's nerve cells. The most common type of glaucoma is called primary open angle glaucoma (POAG), which develops gradually. In this type, the openings to the drainage tubes for aqueous humor are clear, with blockage occurring farther inside the drainage canals. By contrast, in angle closure glaucoma (also called narrow-angle or closed-angle glaucoma), the drainage openings suddenly become blocked, as with a blocked sink drain. IOP rises suddenly, sometimes just in one eye, resulting in attacks of headaches, nausea, eye pain, and blurred vision. Acute angle closure glaucoma is a

medical emergency: the pressure in the eye must be reduced rapidly to prevent permanent loss of vision. More rarely, people can be born with glaucoma or develop it during childhood or adolescence. Glaucoma can also arise from other causes, including eye injuries, infections, diabetes, cataracts, or use of steroid drugs.

KEY FACTS

Description
Partial or complete blindness involving damage to the eye's nerve cells, usually caused by increased pressure within the eye.

Causes
In most cases of glaucoma, overproduction or reduced drainage of aqueous humor is the primary cause.

Risk factors
Increasing age, race, family history, steroid use, diabetes, eye injury.

Symptoms
Depend on type of glaucoma, but can include apparent halos around light, headaches, nausea, blurred or reduced vision, or eye pain. Fifty percent of people with glaucoma show no symptoms until late stage.

Diagnosis
Various procedures, including checking pressure within eye, evaluating quality of vision, and checking damage to optic disk.

Treatments
Drugs or surgery (laser or conventional) aimed at reducing intraocular pressure (IOP).

Pathogenesis
Nerves transmitting information from eye to brain are damaged.

Prevention
Risk can be reduced with eye drops aimed at decreasing IOP, cholesterol-reducing drugs, and regular eye exams.

Epidemiology
Estimated 3 million people in the United States currently affected, 120,000 of whom are blind.

Increased pressure in the eye endangers vision by damaging the optic disk, the area (sometimes called the blind spot) where the cablelike axons that carry messages from the eye's nerve cells to the brain group together. Once their axons are damaged, the nerve cells of the eye die and cannot be replaced. Similar damage to the optic disk sometimes occurs for unknown reasons without increased IOP, in so-called normal tension glaucoma.

Diagnosis

Measuring IOP can be done in various ways. One method (applanation) is to direct a puff of air at the eye, measuring how much force is needed to dent the surface. For best results, the thickness of the cornea should be measured at the same time, because it varies between individuals and can distort readings. A doctor may also carry out a visual perimetry test, in which the extent of vision loss is mapped: Individuals are asked to look ahead and indicate when they detect a moving stimulus introduced into their peripheral vision. Gonioscopy is a technique that uses a mirrored contact lens to examine the angle the iris makes with the cornea, to confirm whether angle closure glaucoma or POAG is involved. Finally, an ophthalmoscope can be used to look into the eye to check whether there is any visible damage to the optic disk.

Treatments

Glaucoma cannot be cured, and dead retinal cells are irreplaceable. Most treatments are aimed at reducing intraocular pressure to prevent or reduce further damage.

Eyedrops or other drugs can be prescribed to lower production of aqueous humor or increase its outflow, or both. A disadvantage of these drugs is that they may have to be taken regularly for life. Laser surgery can be used to clear out the meshwork of drainage canals, inactivate part of the tissue that produces aqueous humor, or open a new hole in the iris. A technique called selective laser trabeculoplasty uses a low-energy laser to make very small disruptions to clogged drainage canals. Because it causes so little damage, the procedure can be used repeatedly.

Nonlaser microsurgery is also used, for example to make a tiny opening in sclera so liquid can drain out. Where necessary, a tiny tube can also be implanted in front of the iris to provide an alternate drainage route. Infection, irritation, bleeding, or scarring may be complications of surgery, although scarring can be minimized with drug treatment.

Alternate treatments like homeopathy, bilberry

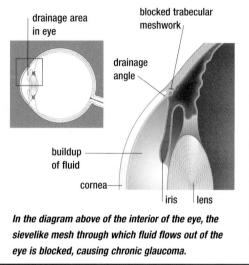

CHRONIC GLAUCOMA

In this condition, the fluid that is secreted into the anterior part of the eye, to retain the shape and feed the tissues, cannot flow away normally. A blockage in the drainage angle prevents the release of excess fluid, and the pressure in the eye builds up until there is a loss of vision, by which time the condition is advanced and chronic.

drainage area in eye

blocked trabecular meshwork

drainage angle

buildup of fluid

cornea

iris   lens

In the diagram above of the interior of the eye, the sievelike mesh through which fluid flows out of the eye is blocked, causing chronic glaucoma.

juice, yoga, and use of biofeedback techniques are used by some patients, but there is no clear evidence of their therapeutic value for glaucoma. Earlier tests of medicinal use of marijuana showed some effectiveness in reducing IOP, but safer and more effective drugs are now available. A vaccine that may slow glaucoma progression is currently being developed. Recent research indicates that cholesterol-reducing drugs (statins) may protect against glaucoma.

Prevention

Until recently, no preventive measures were known for glaucoma. However, investigators have now shown that drugs applied to the eye aimed at reducing IOP in individuals who were at risk for glaucoma reduced by 50 percent the chance of developing the disease. With such preventive measures available, screening to detect early symptoms of glaucoma is increasingly important. People can now buy a test kit to measure their IOP.

Sonal Jhaveri

See also
- Blindness • Cataract • Eye disorders
- Macular degeneration • Retinal disorders

Gonorrhea

Gonorrhea is a sexually transmitted disease caused by the bacterium *Neisseria gonorrhoeae*. The bacteria grow and multiply in the warm, moist areas of the reproductive tract, like the cervix, uterus, and fallopian tubes in women, and the urethra (urinary tube) in men and women. Other sites of infection include the eyes, rectum, throat, and mouth; rarely, infection spreads to the blood and joints.

Gonorrhea is the second most commonly reported infectious disease in the United States after chlamydia, another sexually transmitted disease, although it is believed that only about half of all gonorrhea cases are reported. More than 330,000 cases of gonorrhea were reported in the United States in 2004. This was the lowest recorded rate since 1941 when records began and, according to the Centers for Disease Control and Prevention (CDC), a 75 percent fall in rates since 1975, when the national gonorrhea control program began and gonorrhea rates were at their peak. However, while cases have been steadily decreasing, antibiotic resistance has been increasing.

Risk factors

Seventy-five percent of reported gonorrhea cases are in people under 30 years old, with the highest rates occurring in sexually active teenagers, young adults, and African Americans. The greater the number of sexual partners, the greater the risk.

Symptoms and signs

Most women have no symptoms, so many infections go undiagnosed. This can lead to pelvic inflammatory disease and cause chronic pelvic pain, infertility, and ectopic pregnancies. Left untreated in men, gonorrhea may cause epididymitis, a painful inflammation of the testicles that can result in infertility.

When symptoms are present in women, they include vaginal discharge, burning on urination, vaginal bleeding between periods, or only vague symptoms. In men there may be a thick fluid discharge from the penis 2 to 10 days after sexual contact, or as much as 30 days later. An infected mother can pass gonorrhea to the newborn as it passes through the birth canal; the result can be an eye, joint, or life-threatening blood infection.

Diagnosis and treatment

Microscopic examination of a swab sample taken from the infection site may show bacteria, and a urine test or culture can be sent for laboratory analysis. Gonorrhea is curable with antibiotics. In many cases, chlamydia and gonorrhea coexist, so a combination of antibiotics may be used. Sexual partners must be treated to prevent reinfection. Although antibiotics treat the infection, they do not reverse any damage such as scarred fallopian tubes.

Prevention

The best methods of prevention are to abstain from sex, or practice sex in a long-term monogamous relationship with an uninfected partner. Condoms reduce the risk of infection.

Ramona Jenkin

KEY FACTS

Description
A sexually transmitted disease (STD).

Cause
Infection with the bacterium *Neisseria gonorrhoeae*.

Risk factors
Highest rates of infection in sexually active teenagers, young adults, and African Americans.

Symptoms
There may be no symptoms. Men may have burning on urination and a penile discharge; women may have vaginal discharge and bleeding.

Diagnosis
Microscopic examination of a swab from the infection site; urine analysis.

Treatment
Antibiotics; treatment of sexual partners.

Pathogenesis
Gonorrhea increases the risk of contracting and transmitting HIV.

Prevention
Abstinence from sex. Latex condoms can reduce the risk.

Epidemiology
More than 330,000 infections reported in the United States each year.

See also
• AIDS • Chlamydial infections • Herpes infections • Sexually transmitted diseases

Gout

Gout is caused by the deposition of monosodium urate (MSU) crystals in or around joints, or both. It is the most common form of arthritis in men over 40 years old. Gout is less common in men under the age of 30 and in premenopausal women.

The primary abnormality in gout is an elevation in serum uric acid, which is called hyperuricaemia. Hyperuricaemia is defined as serum uric acid (SUA) level of more than 7 milligrams per deciliter (mg/dL). Uric acid is the end product of the degradation of chemicals called purines, and hyperuricaemia can result from overproduction of or reduced excretion of uric acid through the kidneys. When supersaturation levels are reached, MSU crystals form that deposit in joints and soft tissues, where they cause local mechanical pressure and acute or chronic inflammation.

Obesity, high blood pressure, poor kidney function, and use of diuretics are important risk factors. Dietary factors include increased consumption of alcohol, seafood, and red meat, which are all high in purines.

Symptoms and signs

In the early stages, gout is characterized by episodic attacks of joint inflammation, which are usually monoarticular (affecting one joint) and begin abruptly with intense pain, swelling, warmth, and redness of the affected joint. The metatarsophalangeal joint of the great toe is often the first joint involved. Symptoms generally settle over three to seven days, and between attacks the joints are normal. Such acute attacks may be triggered by trauma or consumption of alcohol or seafood. Over time, gouty attacks become more frequent and last longer. Some patients develop aggregates of MSU crystals in joints and soft tissues, called tophi. Recurrent attacks cause damage to bone and joint cartilage and lead to disability.

Diagnosis

A definitive diagnosis of gout requires demonstration of MSU crystals in joint synovial fluid or tophi. MSU crystals are typically needle-shaped and negatively birefringent (broken up) on polarizing light microscopy.

Acute attacks of gout are treated with medications that reduce joint inflammation such as nonsteroidal anti-inflammatories, corticosteroids, or colchicine. Such treatments have no effect on SUA concentrations. For MSU crystals in joints and soft tissues to dissolve and to prevent acute attacks, SUA levels have to be lowered. Urate-lowering therapies should be considered in patients who have hyperuricaemia and recurrent attacks of gout, tophi, or evidence of bone or cartilage damage. SUA can be reduced by lowering uric acid production or by increasing the excretion of uric acid via the kidneys. Allopurinol, a commonly used urate-lowering drug, inhibits xanthine oxidase, a critical enzyme in the production of uric acid, thereby reducing uric acid production. Dietary restriction of purines is also advised.

Lisa Stamp

KEY FACTS

Description
Acute arthritis, attacks of painful, swollen joints.

Causes
Deposition of monosodium urate crystals in joints and surrounding soft tissues.

Risk factors
High blood pressure, obesity, poor kidney function, diuretic use; dietary factors (alcohol, red meat, and seafood).

Diagnosis
Monosodium urate crystals in joint fluid or tophi.

Treatments
Acute attacks are treated with nonsteroidal anti-inflammatory agents, corticosteroids, or colchicine. Preventive treatments reduce uric acid production or increase excretion of uric acid.

Pathogenesis
Hyperuricaemia is due to overproduction or underexcretion of uric acid.

Prevention
Sustained reduction of serum uric acid less than 6 mg/dL through urate-lowering therapy and dietary restriction of purines.

Epidemiology
The most common form of arthritis in men older than 40 years. The incidence of gout is increasing.

See also
• Alcohol-related disorders • Bone and joint disorders • Kidney disorders • Metabolic disorders • Nutritional disorders • Obesity

Growth disorders

In growth disorders there is disturbance in one or more of the phases of growth during childhood, leading to increased or diminished height. Growth disorders have many causes, including malnutrition, hormonal and genetic abnormalities, and disorders of the digestive tract, bones, kidneys, lungs, and heart.

Before birth, the growth of the developing fetus is determined by factors that include genetics, the mother's health and standard of nutrition, and the functioning of the placenta (the organ that nourishes the fetus in the uterus). After birth, a child's rate of growth is influenced by genetic, hormonal, nutritional, and general health factors. Normal patterns of growth can be monitored at routine checkups by using charts that track height changes throughout childhood.

Growth phases
Growth occurs in three phases: the infantile phase, the childhood phase, and the pubertal phase. The infantile phase occurs during the first two years of life, when growth in height averages 12 to 14 inches (30 to 35 cm). The childhood phase occurs from the age of two until the start of puberty and is characterized by a constant steady height gain of 2 to 2½ inches (5 to 7 cm) per year. The pubertal phase occurs at the onset of puberty, the time of life when sexual development begins. Changes in hormones trigger a rapid increase in height called the pubertal growth spurt, with growth frequently reaching 3 to 5½ inches (8 to 14 cm) per year. In boys, peak growth velocity occurs near the age of 14, with achievement of final height occurring around 19 years of age; in girls, peak growth velocity is near the age of 12, with final height occurring around 16. In growth disorders there is disturbance in one or more of the phases of growth, leading to increased or diminished height.

Growth variations
Some variations in growth are considered normal. Such variations include constitutional growth delay, which occurs when children grow at a normal rate but are small for their age. These children reach puberty later than their peers, and their pubertal growth spurt

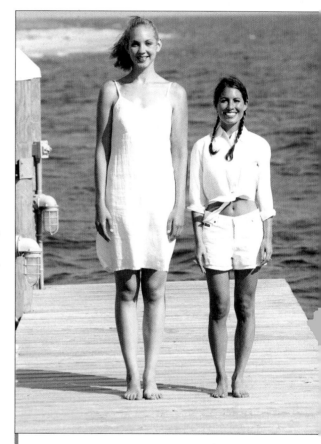

Though they are the same age, there is a big difference in the height of these girls. Many factors can lead to this variation: growth spurts at different times, a familial tendency to a certain height, delayed onset of puberty, or a growth disorder.

is delayed (puberty is considered late if it occurs after 13 in girls and 14 in boys). Frequently, children with constitutional growth delay continue to grow until a later age and have normal adult height. Also normal is short stature in children whose parents are shorter than average. Children with familial short stature enter puberty at a normal age and have normal adolescent growth spurts but have short adult height.

Causes and risk factors
Growth disorders have many different causes, including hormonal and genetic abnormalities, and diseases of the kidneys, heart, gastrointestinal tract, lungs, and bones. Worldwide the most common cause of growth disorders is malnutrition. Having adequate supplies

of calories and protein is of critical importance to maintaining growth and development, and if the diet contains insufficient nutrients, short stature is likely to occur.

Hormonal growth disorders are caused by an excess or a deficiency of a hormone. Growth hormone is made by the pituitary gland located at the base of the brain. Low production of this hormone can occur if the gland malfunctions, is damaged, or does not form properly. Tumors, infections, or injury to the pituitary or to adjacent areas can damage or destroy the gland. Radiation therapy used to treat other diseases may also damage the pituitary. Changes in genes that are critical for the development of the pituitary can lead to problems with the growth of the gland.

Rarely, pituitary tumors can produce too much growth hormone. If the tumor develops before puberty, the person grows abnormally and has a condition called gigantism. If the tumor develops once the long bones stop growing, the condition is called acromegaly. Typically, the hands, feet, jaw, and skull become enlarged, as well as some internal organs. Treatment for acromegaly may be the surgical removal of the tumor or drug treatment to try to shrink the tumor.

Thyroid hormone is also essential for normal growth. The thyroid, a gland located in the neck, makes thyroxine, a hormone critical for the growth and development of bones. If too little or too much thyroxine is produced, growth disorders can occur. Another hormone that affects growth is cortisol, which is produced by the paired adrenal glands located near the kidneys. If the adrenal glands produce too much cortisol, children usually have an increase in weight, although their height does not change. This overproduction of cortisol is called Cushing's disease. It is rare in children but may be related to treatment with glucocorticoids, which are steroid medications that act in a similar manner to cortisol.

Precocious puberty is a hormonal disorder that occurs when children enter the pubertal growth spurt early (before 8 years for girls and before 9 years in boys). Initially, most children with precocious puberty are taller than their classmates, but they may stop growing early and be shorter as adults. Growth may also be disturbed by delayed puberty, one cause of which is Turner's syndrome, a genetic disease that affects only girls and occurs in about 1 in 2,500 births. Girls with Turner's syndrome have an abnormal or missing X chromosome, and their ovaries are not properly formed. These children do not undergo puberty normally, which leads to very low levels of estrogen, a hormone that is important for growth in girls.

Down syndrome is another genetic disorder that affects growth. People with Down syndrome are generally shorter than their predicted height. Marfan syndrome is a genetic disease that is associated with a tall stature and very long arms and legs. Marfan, which is the result of defects in connective tissue, may also be associated with eye and heart diseases.

Disorders of the skeleton and cartilage may lead to growth disorders. In these conditions, the bones do not form normally, and children generally are shorter than expected.

Skeletal disorders can be genetic, for example X-linked hypophosphatemic rickets, in which children have bowing of the lower legs and short stature as a result of abnormal metabolism of the mineral phosphate and vitamin D. Vitamin D deficiency through

KEY FACTS

Description
Disrupted growth patterns leading to abnormally short or tall stature.

Causes
Malfunctioning, damaged, or absent pituitary gland; genetic disorders; malnutrition.

Risk factors
Tumors, infections, and injury to the pituitary gland; radiation therapy affecting the pituitary or nearby areas; genetic mutations that interrupt the formation of the pituitary; inadequate maternal diet or poor nutrition after birth.

Symptoms
Short stature with poor growth velocity; or abnormal height.

Diagnosis
Physical exam, laboratory testing, radiological testing, and growth hormone stimulation testing.

Treatments
Hormone replacement with growth hormone; correction of diet in cases of malnutrition.

Pathogenesis
Defects to or absence of the pituitary gland lead to deficiencies of hormones necessary for normal growth.

Prevention
Apart from growth disorders caused by malnutrition, most cases are not preventable.

Epidemiology
Growth disorders appear in an estimated 1 in 10,000 births.

poor nutrition can also cause rickets. Achondroplasia is a disorder of cartilage that is the most common form of disproportionate growth retardation. People with achondroplasia have an average-sized trunk but short limbs because of a progressive decrease in the growth velocity that begins in infancy.

Children with chronic diseases may also have growth disorders. Many different diseases, such as kidney disease, liver disease, sickle-cell anemia, diabetes mellitus, and cystic fibrosis, may slow growth; diseases of the intestines that impair the ability to absorb nutrients from the diet sometimes lead to poor growth. In addition, any disease that is severe, untreated, or poorly controlled can have a negative impact on growth. Severe stress is another possible cause of decreased growth.

Diagnosis

An abnormality in stature is determined by the comparison of a child's height to the average height, plotted on a growth curve, for a child of the same age and sex. If the measured height is not what would be predicted, it is important to evaluate other features of growth. One consideration is the growth velocity, which is based on the change in height estimated to occur in one year. For example, if height measurements are taken four months apart and a 1-inch (2.5 cm) increase in height occurs during that period, the growth velocity is 3 inches (7.5 cm) per year. In children with a suspected growth disorder, it is also important to assess a mid-parental height. For boys, a mid-parental height is calculated by adding 5 inches (13 cm) to the mother's height and averaging this height with the father's height. For girls, 5 inches (13 cm) are subtracted from the father's height, and this height is averaged with the mother's height. A target height can be predicted by (for a boy) adding $3\frac{1}{2}$ inches (8.5 cm) to or (for a girl) subtracting $3\frac{1}{2}$ inches (8.5 cm) from this calculated value. Target heights are considered normal for that family.

Body proportions should also be evaluated. This assessment includes a comparison between the height of the upper body and the height of the lower body, called an upper segment/lower segment ratio (US/LS). Another important measurement is the comparison between the arm span and the height. If either the arm span/height difference or the US/LS is abnormal, the growth disorder may be characterized as disproportionate growth.

Once it is determined that there is a disorder of growth, there should be a physical exam, and possibly laboratory and radiological tests, to look for a possible cause. Laboratory testing may be used to investigate hormone levels, kidney function, liver function, and chromosomes. Sometimes growth hormone stimulation is performed. In this test, a medication is given to see if the pituitary gland responds appropriately. If a person is suspected of having a pituitary problem, a magnetic resonance image (MRI) might be done. In children with delayed or accelerated growth, a bone age should be obtained. A bone age is an X-ray of the wrist that is done to determine if the skeletal age and the chronological age are the same. If the bone age is advanced, it suggests that there is less time available for growth. If the bone age is delayed, there may be more time for growth to occur. The bone age can be used to predict the final height the child will achieve as an adult, to see if it is expected to be normal for that family (within the target range).

Children with normal growth variants like constitutional growth delay or familial short stature are usually monitored with repeated physical exams and height measurements.

Treatments

There are many different causes of growth disorders, and the specific treatment depends on the cause. In growth hormone deficiency, growth hormone can be given as an injection. Growth hormone injections are also sometimes used to treat people with Turner syndrome and those with chronic kidney disease. If thyroid hormone levels are low, thyroid hormone can be replaced with an oral medication. In short stature linked to nutrition, supplying the proper nutrients leads to improved growth rates and frequently to normalization of height.

Epidemiology

Although acromegaly and gigantism are not strictly growth disorders, they are both caused by an abnormality of the growth process. In the United States only 40 to 60 people per million of the population suffer from acromegaly (which sometimes runs in families), and about 15,000 suffer from achondroplasia (dwarfism).

Mary Ruppe

See also
- Adrenal disorders • Down syndrome
- Hormonal disorders • Nutritional disorders
- Thyroid disorders • Turner's syndrome
- Vitamin deficiency

Guillain-Barré syndrome

Guillain-Barré syndrome is a form of polyneuritis, in which several peripheral nerves are inflamed. It was initially described by Guillain, Barré, and Strohl in 1916. Guillain-Barré syndrome (GBS) is characterized by loss of myelin covering the nerves, which results in symmetrical and progressive weakness in the limbs, loss of spinal reflexes, and sensory loss.

In two-thirds of patients affected, GBS follows an upper respiratory or gastrointestinal infection, surgery, or immunization. The preceding infection is most commonly intestinal, and it is caused by the bacteria *Campylobacter jejuni*. There may be an associated risk with immunocompromised states, but a clear relationship has yet to be defined.

Symptoms and diagnosis

GBS occurs in people of all ages and can begin with paresthesias (tingling) in the feet and progressive and symmetrical weakness in the legs, causing an ascending paralysis and loss of reflexes over hours to days, for up to four weeks. Diagnosis is made based on the patient's history and physical examination and cerebrospinal fluid analysis, which shows a high content of protein in proportion to inflammatory cells. Electromyography (nerve conduction studies) may be used to assist in diagnosis.

Treatments and prevention

Treatment is based on the severity of the illness and the muscle groups involved. Plasma exchange may be used early in the disease to remove autoantibodies, although alternative treatment is high-dose intravenous immune globulin (IVIG), which is thought to neutralize autoantibodies. These treatments are equally effective, and using IVIG and plasma exchange confers no additional benefit. If respiratory muscles are affected by the ascending weakness, mechanical ventilation may be needed, as well as support for unstable blood pressure and heart arrhythmias caused by involvement of the autonomic nerves. There are no prevention strategies.

Pathogenesis

GBS is thought to be caused by an immune response to an infection, whose molecular signature shares that of the myelin covering peripheral nerves (molecular mimicry). This process results in an autoimmune response causing breakdown of the myelin around peripheral nerves, leading to loss of nerve function and weakness. The illness should peak within four weeks of onset. Up to one-third of patients will need mechanical ventilation; if the person is over 60 years old with rapid progression of GBS, the prognosis is worse. Up to 70 percent of patients recover in the year following the illness.

Epidemiology

Mean annual incidence of GBS is 1.8 per 100,000 population. Men and women are equally affected. GBS has several variants; the most common form in North America and Europe is acute inflammatory demyelinating polyradiculopathy (AIDP). Other variants include acute motor axonal neuropathy (AMAN) and the Miller-Fisher syndrome (MFS).

Meredith Roderick and Robert Daroff

KEY FACTS

Description
A disease caused by progressive breakdown of the myelin in peripheral nerves.

Causes
Post infectious autoimmune response to a virus or often to a gastrointestinal infection.

Risk factors
No known risk factors

Symptoms
Progressive weakness and loss of reflexes.

Diagnosis
Cerebrospinal fluid examination and electromyography (recording of electrical activity in a muscle).

Pathogenesis
Autoimmune attack of the myelin of peripheral nerves.

Prevention
There are no specific preventative strategies.

Epidemiology
Mean annual incidence of 1.8 per 100,000 population with men and women equally affected.

See also
- Immune system disorders • Infections
- Infections, bacterial • Nervous system disorders • Paralysis

Gum disease

A potentially serious but preventable disorder, gum disease is a bacterial infection of the teeth and gums that can spread rapidly, causing severe inflammation, tooth loss, and loss of supporting bone. In serious cases, surgery is needed to restore bone in the jaw and prevent further tooth loss.

Gum disease, commonly called periodontal ("around the teeth") disease, involves the breakdown of gums as a result of the buildup of plaque (saliva, food, and bacteria) and tartar on the teeth's surface. It ranges from a mild disease causing moderate gum inflammation to a serious disorder in which bone becomes infected and breaks down. Periodontal disease comes in two forms: periodontitis and gingivitis.

Causes and risk factors

The mouth harbors bacteria which, with mucus and other particles, form an invisible, sticky substance called plaque that coats the teeth; if plaque builds up and hardens, it forms a sticky residue called tartar that is full of harmful bacteria. Tartar can cause gingivitis, a mild form of periodontal disease that causes inflamed and bleeding gums. If untreated, periodontitis can result; this is a serious disease in which the gums pull away from the teeth, forming pockets of infection. As the immune system reacts to fight the disease, both toxins in the bacteria and enzymes released by the body break down the connective tissue and bone that support the teeth. Apart from poor dental hygiene, periodontal disease is caused by stress; tobacco use; hormonal changes during pregnancy, puberty, menstruation, or menopause; diseases such as diabetes, cancer, and HIV; and the use of drugs that reduce saliva flow, which protects gums and teeth. Genetics may play a role since periodontal disease runs in some families.

Symptoms

Symptoms of gingivitis and periodontitis include red, swollen, sore gums that bleed during or after toothbrushing; bad breath; and a bad taste in the mouth. Periodontitis symptoms also include receding gums, the formation of pockets between the teeth and gums, shifting or loose teeth, and changes in the way the teeth fit together.

Diagnosis, treatments, and prevention

A dentist or periodontist checks for pockets among the teeth and gums, and X-rays are taken to determine if the surrounding bone has broken down.

Gingivitis is reversible with daily brushing and flossing and regular cleaning by a dentist or dental hygienist. Advanced gingivitis and periodontitis may be treated with a deep-cleaning method to remove bacteria and rough spots below the gum line; or with antibiotic medications, gels, mouth rinses, and in severe cases, surgery to restore bone. Peridontal disease can often be prevented by not using tobacco, brushing twice and flossing once daily, using toothpaste with fluoride, and drinking fluoridated water.

Lise Stevens

KEY FACTS

Description
Infection of the gums and tissues around the teeth.

Cause
Bacteria in plaque hardens on the teeth.

Risk factors
Crooked teeth, dental work such as bridges that no longer fit and broken fillings, tobacco use, hormonal changes, certain diseases, and some medications.

Symptoms
Frequent bad taste, bad breath, bleeding, red and tender gums, and loose, sensitive teeth.

Diagnosis
Examination of teeth by a dentist or periodontist; jawbone X-ray to detect breakdown of bone.

Treatments
Depending on seriousness: deep cleaning, antimicrobial treatment, bone or gum surgery, gum and bone grafts.

Pathogenesis
Bacteria in plaque break down the gums; teeth loosen; and underlying bone breaks down.

Prevention
Brushing and flossing teeth regularly, a healthy diet, stopping tobacco use, reducing stress.

Epidemiology
In the United States 80 percent of all adults have some degree of periodontal disease.

See also
- Dental and oral cavity disorders
- Diabetes • Tooth decay

Hay fever

The disorder hay fever is actually allergic rhinitis caused by grass, tree, and flower pollens in the air. The disorder usually has no connection with hay (mowed grasses), but the name probably developed because most sufferers are affected in the late summer and early fall of the year when hay is being baled. Ragweed, which is in bloom during the same season, has the most commonly identified offending pollen. However, the pollens of other plants may cause an allergic reaction similar to hay fever during other seasons.

Hay fever affects about 20 percent of people in the United States. It is the most common allergic condition. Molds in the air, dust mites, and animal dander or saliva are also frequent causes of allergic rhinitis, so susceptible people may develop symptoms that resemble those of hay fever from a variety of causes throughout the year.

Causes

When the body incorrectly identifies a protein as a potentially harmful invader, or allergen, it responds by producing antibodies to fight the perceived invader. These antibodies cause certain cells of the immune system to release chemicals such as histamine and leukotrienes in the upper respiratory tract, and these chemicals are responsible for producing the symptoms of allergic rhinitis. A type of antibody called immunoglobulin E (IgE) is particularly associated with respiratory allergies.

Exposure to allergens when the immune system is weakened, after an infection, or during pregnancy may increase the chance of an allergic response.

Symptoms

The characteristic symptoms of allergic rhinitis are a runny and sometimes itchy nose, nasal stuffiness, sneezing, watery, itchy eyes, and possibly an accompanying cough. Although very uncomfortable, these symptoms are considered mild reactions.

Because offending pollens are inhaled, symptoms are usually confined to the upper respiratory tract (nasal passages, throat, and voice box). Repeated exposure to inhaled allergens results in chronic inflammation of the lining of the upper air passages and swelling and redness of the protective lining (conjunctiva) of the eyes. Rarely, an extreme response to the offending allergen may result in a life-threatening inability to breathe, along with a severe drop in blood pressure, known as anaphylaxis, which requires immediate emergency treatment.

KEY FACTS

Description

An exaggerated immune response by the body to pollen, causing respiratory symptoms and discomfort.

Cause

Exposure to pollen, incorrectly identified by the body as an invader.

Risk factors

A family history of allergies.

Symptoms

Runny nose, sneezing, nasal stuffiness, and itchy, watery eyes, possibly accompanied by a cough.

Diagnosis

Evaluation of personal history along with intradermal (skin-prick) tests using dilute solutions of common allergens. Various other tests may be done to rule out the possibility of other causes of the symptoms.

Treatments

Medications to reduce the symptoms, such as antihistamines or antileukotrienes. Immunotherapy, or allergy injections, to reduce the body's response to particular, personal allergens identified by skin-prick tests.

Pathogenesis

Once an allergic response has been established, exposure thereafter to the offending pollen or substance (allergen) in the environment results in an inflammatory response, most often involving the upper respiratory tract. Without immunotherapy treatment the allergy is unlikely to disappear. However, children sometimes outgrow symptoms.

Prevention

Avoiding situations where the body would respond to a known allergen. Immunotherapy.

Epidemiology

Hay fever affects about 20 percent of people in the United States. It is the most common allergic condition. Allergies in general are the sixth leading cause of chronic illness in the United States.

ANAPHYLAXIS

Anaphylaxis is a sudden and severe, usually life-threatening, allergic reaction that requires immediate emergency treatment. Although the symptoms may start as the typical symptoms of a mild allergic reaction, within minutes they progress to severe difficulty in swallowing and breathing accompanied by a profound drop in blood pressure resulting in systemic (involving the entire body) shock. Hives (itchy welts), dizziness, and mental confusion may also occur with systemic involvement.

Immediate treatment with IV (intravenous) epinephrine (adrenaline), intravenous fluids, and oxygen is necessary if a fatal outcome is to be prevented. People who survive this type of attack, as well as their families, should be taught by their health care provider how, in the event of an emergency, to administer the necessary medication, usually an epinephrine formulation. They are advised to carry the emergency medication at all times.

Diagnosis

A thorough physical examination and review of an affected individual's personal and family medical history is the initial step for diagnosis. A family history of any type of allergy is significant because it suggests a tendency to be prone to allergy, although specific allergies are rarely inherited.

When allergy is suspected, a series of intradermal (skin-prick) tests using a tiny amount of very dilute solutions of specific common allergens is recommended. After injection of the allergen extract, the site is checked for possible development of redness and swelling. The amount of, or lack of, skin reaction determines the probability of allergy to the injected allergen.

If skin-prick testing is not possible, a RAST (radioallergosorbent blood test) may be done. A RAST test evaluates the amount of antibodies being produced by a person's immune system. In some cases, specific antibodies may indicate particular allergies, but skin tests are usually more accurate.

A complete blood count (CBC) and a differential white blood cell count may be ordered. An increase in the normal number of specific white blood cells (eosinophils and basophils) may suggest that the body is responding to an allergen. Occasionally, various other medical tests may be performed to rule out the possibility of other causes of the symptoms.

Treatments

Over-the-counter (OTC) and prescription antihistamines are the most widely used medications for relief of upper respiratory allergic symptoms. Drugs may be taken orally or as nasal sprays. Some antihistamines, such as diphenhydramine (Benadryl), may cause significant and potentially hazardous drowsiness.

Topical nasal anti-inflammatory steroids and cromolyn sodium may also be prescribed to treat allergic rhinitis, but cromolyn is most effective when taken before symptoms develop.

Decongestant sprays or pills may be used along with antihistamines to relieve nasal congestion, but should be avoided by people with high blood pressure, an enlarged prostate, or glaucoma.

Immunotherapy, or allergy desensitization injections—to reduce the body's response to particular, personal allergens identified by skin-prick tests—is the most effective method of controlling allergic rhinitis in the long term.

Drugs called antileukotrienes, frequently used for allergic asthma, may also be appropriate for treating hay fever, especially if the individual is troubled with large amount of mucous secretions.

Based on the presumption that an allergic attack may not develop if IgE is prevented from attaching to the cells that release the substances that cause allergic symptoms, new treatments using special injectable anti-IgE monoclonal antibodies are under development. However, IgE is not always present in allergic attacks.

Management and prognosis

Managing the environment to avoid exposure to the causative pollen is important in preventing symptomatic allergic rhinitis. Avoiding irritants such as smoke and strong chemical odors should also lessen discomfort.

Inadequately treated allergies may cause difficulty sleeping and fatigue, and possibly lead to more serious conditions such as asthma. The congestion often associated with upper respiratory symptoms may result in sinusitis or middle-ear infections. Without immunotherapy, an allergy is unlikely to disappear. However, children sometimes outgrow the characteristic symptoms.

Nance Seiple

See also
• Allergy and sensitivity • Asthma • Ear disorders • Respiratory system disorders • Sinusitis

Head injury

Head injury is a general term used to describe any trauma to the head, including injuries to the brain, scalp, and skull. Traumatic brain injury (TBI) is classified as either closed head injury or penetrating head injury. A closed head injury is any injury to the brain or structures within the skull not caused by a penetrating injury, like a gunshot wound. Brain injuries may be limited to a small area (focal) or may be more widespread (diffuse).

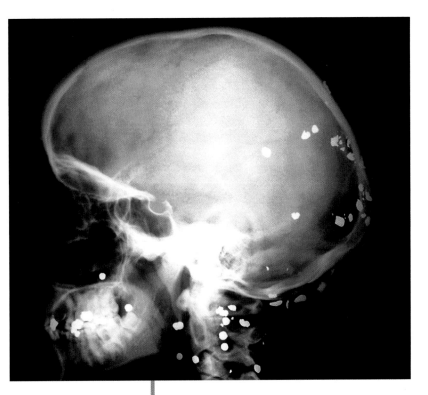

As a result of a hunting accident, this patient was hit by several shotgun pellets. On this colored X-ray of the side of the head, the pellets (white dots) are seen in the neck, around the teeth, and at the back of the skull.

Brain injuries are a common type of head injury. Primary brain injury refers to the initial structural injury to the brain as a direct result of the trauma. Secondary brain injury refers to any subsequent injury to the brain from lack of oxygen, low blood pressure, elevated pressure inside the skull, or as the result of physiological changes initiated by the original trauma. Mild traumatic brain injuries (TBIs) are commonly called concussions. A generally accepted description of concussion syndrome is a traumatically induced alteration in mental status with or without associated loss of consciousness. Injury to brain tissue can occur at the site of impact (coup), at the point opposite the impact (contrecoup), or due to rotational forces resulting in the shearing of axons (fiberlike processes of nerve cells). The direct force at the point of contact may not solely be responsible for the severity of injury if a significant shear effect occurs.

While not a life-threatening injury, concussions can cause both short-term and long-term problems. A mild concussion may involve no loss of consciousness or a very brief loss of consciousness. A severe concussion may involve prolonged loss of consciousness with a delayed return to normal function. Concussions do not include injuries in which there is bleeding under the skull or into the brain.

Diffuse axonal injury (DAI) reflects damage over a widespread area when compared to focal brain injury. Unlike direct brain trauma, DAI is the result of traumatic shearing forces that occur when the head is rapidly accelerated or decelerated, as may occur in auto accidents, falls, and assaults. It usually results from powerful twisting or rotational forces. Unlike concussion, DAI is associated with a high level of debilitation and is a frequent cause of persistent vegetative state.

A skull fracture is a break in the bone encasing the brain, which may or may not be associated with an injury to the brain itself. A linear skull fracture follows a relatively straight line. Depressed skull fractures, which cause dents in the skull bone, are common after forceful impact by blunt objects. Depressed fractures whose depth is equal to or greater than the thickness of the surrounding skull bone have a higher incidence of damage to the brain itself. A basilar skull fracture is a fracture of the bones that form the bottom of the skull and results from severe blunt force. A basilar skull fracture commonly connects to the sinus cavities, which may allow fluid or air entry into the interior of the skull, resulting in possible infection.

Intracranial hemorrhage is bleeding inside the skull, which may exert pressure on the brain. A subdural hematoma is bleeding of the veins between the brain and the dura mater (the brain's tough outer membrane). A subdural hematoma may be acute, developing suddenly after the injury, or chronic, slowly accumulating over a period of 12 days or longer after injury. An epidural hematoma is arterial bleeding between the dura mater and the skull bone, often from a blow to the temple area. Subarachnoid hemorrhage is bleeding into the subarachnoid space, the area between the arachnoid and the pia mater where cerebrospinal fluid flows. Intraparenchymal hemorrhage is bleeding into the brain tissue itself. Without intervention, any persistent increase in pressure on the brain as a result of bleeding will eventually lead to herniation, the pushing of the brain downward out of the skull. Herniation is not compatible with life.

Causes and risk factors

According to the Centers for Disease Control (CDC), the leading cause of TBI is falls (28 percent); rates are highest for children 0 to 4 years old and for adults over 75. Motor-vehicle injuries (20 percent) result in the greatest number of TBI-related hospitalizations. The rate of motor vehicle–related TBI is highest among adolescents 15 to 19 years old. Collisions with moving or stationary objects (19 percent) are the third leading cause of TBI. An estimated 300,000 sports- and recreation-related TBIs of mild to moderate severity occur in the United States each year. Firearm use is the leading cause of death related to TBI. Nearly two-thirds of firearm-related TBIs are suicidal in intent. All assaults comprise 11 percent, which includes child abuse. The male-to-female ratio for TBI is nearly 2:1, and TBI is much more common in persons younger than 35 years. Over half of all TBI incidents involve alcohol use.

Signs and symptoms

Signs and symptoms of head injuries vary with the type and severity of the injury. Some symptoms are evident immediately, while others may only surface days or weeks after the injury. Minor blunt head injuries may involve symptoms of being dazed or a brief loss of consciousness. Common symptoms include headache, confusion, dizziness, altered vision, fatigue, lethargy, altered sleep, mood changes, and trouble with memory, concentration, or thinking. Worsening symptoms indicate a more severe injury. With moderate or severe TBI there may be a loss of consciousness, personality changes, severe or worsening headache, repeated vomiting, inability to awaken, widening of one or both pupils, slurred speech, loss of coordination, increased confusion, and restlessness. Severe blunt head trauma involves a loss of consciousness lasting from several minutes to many days or

KEY FACTS

Description

Any closed or penetrating injury to the head, including bruises and cuts to the scalp, fractures of the skull, bleeding in and around the brain, bruising of the brain and the shearing of axons.

Causes

Falls; motor vehicle accidents; collisions; assaults; weapons.

Risk factors

Alcohol; male; age under 35.

Symptoms

Vary with type and severity. Being dazed; loss of consciousness; headache; dizziness; visual changes; vomiting; lethargy; seizures; cognitive, behavioral and psychological changes; strokelike symptoms; amnesia; coma.

Diagnosis

History; physical exam; X-ray; CT; MRI; angiography.

Treatment

Varies with type and severity. Wound care; observation; antibiotics; seizure medications; ICP monitoring; craniotomy surgery.

Pathogenesis

Varies with type and severity. No residual effects; chronic headaches and dizziness; permanent cognitive and behavioral changes; neurological deficits; coma. Effects over time are cumulative. Repeated TBIs over a short period of time can be catastrophic.

Prevention

Seatbelts; lock up weapons; never drive under the influence; helmets; improve safety of living areas for seniors and children.

Epidemiology

TBIs are responsible for significant death and disability, especially in adolescents and children. TBIs are responsible for over one million emergency room visits and cost $60 billion annually in the United States.

longer. The person may die or suffer from severe and sometimes permanent neurological deficits. Neurological deficits from head trauma include paralysis, seizures, difficulty speaking, seeing, hearing, walking, and understanding. Penetrating trauma may cause death, immediate severe symptoms, or only minor symptoms despite a potentially life-threatening injury. Contrary to Hollywood depictions, amnesia from TBI usually affects memories around and after the incident and not prior to it.

Diagnosis

The patient's medical history, description of the current symptoms, and a physical examination are all important in the diagnosis. In mild TBI, X-rays of the skull may be taken to look for a fracture in the skull bone. Skull fractures are not always associated with brain injury, and the absence of a fracture does not exclude a brain injury. The fracture itself will seldom need treatment, but an underlying brain injury may. In moderate to severe cases, a computed tomography (CT) scan should be obtained, which creates a series of cross-sectional X-ray images of the head; these images reveal bone fractures, hemorrhage, hematomas, contusions, brain swelling, and tumors. Magnetic resonance imaging (MRI) may be used after the initial assessment and treatment of the TBI patient. MRI uses magnetic fields to detect subtle changes in brain tissue content and can show more detail than X-rays or CT. In some cases of bleeding in or around the brain, angiography may be performed by injecting dye into the arteries to visualize the blood vessels and locate the area of bleeding. It is sometimes possible to stop the bleeding during angiography by injecting clot-forming agents. After major falls and car accidents, other imaging and laboratory tests may be performed to rule out other chest, abdominal, or bony injuries. Neck injuries are common in people with severe head trauma. Spine imaging is usually ordered before the head is moved if there is any neck pain or other symptoms of a neck injury.

The Glasgow coma scale (GCS) is used to describe the general level of consciousness of patients with TBI. The GCS is divided into 3 categories: eye opening (E), motor response (M), and verbal response (V). The score is the sum of all 3 categories, with a maximum score of 15 and a minimum score of 3. Mild head injuries are those with a GCS score of 13-15, and moderate head injuries are those with a GCS score of 9-12. A GCS score of 8 or less defines a severe head injury. These definitions should only be considered as a general guide to the level of injury.

Treatments

Treatment varies widely depending on the type and severity of injuries. Minor head injuries are often treated at home if someone is available to watch the person. Ice, bed rest, hydration, and a mild pain reliever may be prescribed. In the event of an open wound, cuts will be numbed, cleansed, and inspected for foreign matter. The wound usually is closed with skin staples, stitches, or special skin glue. An immunization to prevent tetanus is given if needed. People with serious closed head injuries are admitted to the hospital for observation and repeated studies. Seizure medication may be given, though seizures related to a head injury rarely recur. Antibiotics are usually not required in closed head injuries, while antibiotics are sometimes considered in cases of basilar skull fracture. An intracranial pressure (ICP) monitor probe may be surgically inserted into the brain. When there is a closed head injury with bleeding inside the skull, the doctor must consider the location of the bleeding, the severity of the symptoms, other injuries, and the progression of symptoms when determining the treatment plan. Craniotomy surgery may be needed to evacuate the blood and relieve the pressure.

Patients with severe TBI may need a breathing tube placed to protect the airway. Penetrating head injuries often require some sort of surgery, usually to remove foreign material or to stop bleeding. Visualization of the blood vessels (angiography) may also be needed.

Pathogenesis

The outcome of TBI is related to the initial level of injury. While the GCS score provides a description of the initial condition and helps predict death from the injury, it does not correlate tightly with other outcomes. For example, if a patient is older than 60 years, has an initial GCS score of less than 5, presence of an unresponsive dilated pupil, prolonged low blood pressure or low oxygen level, and presence of intracranial bleeding requiring surgery, a poor outcome is likely.

Prognosis varies and depends on the severity of the injury. Even minor head injuries can have long-term consequences (usually psychological or learning disabilities). Serious head injuries can result in anything from full recovery to death or a permanent coma. TBI can cause functional changes in thinking, sensation, language, and emotions. TBI can also cause epilepsy and increase the risk for conditions such as Alzheimer's disease, Parkinson's disease, and other brain disorders. Repeated mild TBIs occurring over an

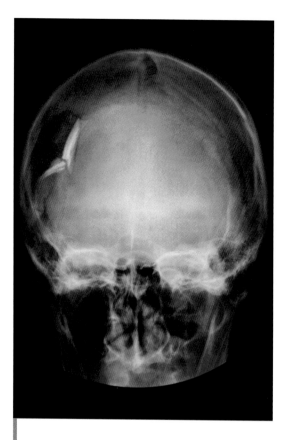

A colored X-ray shows a depressed fracture (red, upper left) in the back of a skull. This type of fracture is caused by a high-energy impact from a blunt object. Brain damage is a high risk for skull injuries such as this one.

extended period of time (months to years) can result in cumulative neurological and cognitive deficits. Repeated mild TBIs that occur within a short period of time (hours to weeks) can be catastrophic or fatal. The cause of the TBI also plays a role in determining the patient's outcome. Approximately 91 percent of firearm TBIs result in death, while only 11 percent of TBIs from falls result in death.

Prevention

There are many ways to reduce the chances of a traumatic brain injury. Firearms and bullets should be stored in a locked cabinet when not in use. Seat belts should be worn whenever driving or riding in a motor vehicle. Children should be buckled into the car using a child safety seat, booster seat, or seat belt. Driving should never occur while under the influence of alcohol or drugs. Helmets must be worn when appropriate, and children should also be asked to wear helmets when appropriate. Living areas can be made safer for

seniors by removing tripping hazards, using nonslip mats in washing areas, installing handrails in stairways and bathrooms, and improving lighting throughout the home. Living areas can be made safer for children by installing window guards and using safety gates. Shock-absorbing materials, such as hardwood mulch and sand, can be used under playground equipment to reduce the chance of injury in children.

Epidemiology

TBIs contribute to a substantial number of deaths and cases of permanent disability annually. Of the roughly 1.4 million who sustain a TBI each year in the United States, there are over 50,000 deaths and 450,000 hospitalizations. Greater than one million TBIs are treated and released from an emergency room each year. Among children age 14 years and under, TBI results in an estimated 2,685 deaths, 37,000 hospitalizations, and 435,000 visits to emergency rooms annually.

The mortality rate is high in severe TBI (33 percent) and low for moderate TBI (2.5 percent). About 75 percent of TBIs are concussions or mild TBI; the remaining injuries are divided equally between the moderate and severe categories. An estimated 15 percent of persons who sustain a mild brain injury continue to experience negative consequences one year after the injury.

The cost to society of TBI is staggering, from both an economic and an emotional standpoint. Almost all persons with severe head injury and nearly two-thirds of those with moderate head injury will be permanently disabled and will not return to their previous level of function. The CDC estimates that at least 5.3 million Americans currently have long-term or lifelong need for help to perform activities of daily living as a result of a TBI.

The financial cost is estimated at about $60 billion per year, which includes loss of potential income of the patient and relatives who may need to become caregivers, cost of acute care, and other medical expenses such as continual ambulatory and rehabilitation care. The impact is even greater when one considers that most severe head injuries occur in adolescents and young adults.

Medley O'Keefe Gatewood

See also
- Brain disorders • Diagnosis • Fracture
- Prevention • Shock • Trauma, accident, and injury

Health care

Health care is the prevention, treatment, and management of sickness and injury; the protection of people's health; and the maintenance of mental, physical, and spiritual well-being.

A widely accepted definition of health is the one used by the World Health Organization (WHO) in 1946. It states that "health is a state of complete physical, mental, and social well-being and not merely the absence of disease or infirmity." In 1978, the WHO modified the statement to include the following: [that health] "is a fundamental human right and that the attainment of the highest level of health is a most important worldwide social goal." The WHO definition is controversial, and it is considered by many as an altruistic goal for societies.

The Blum Model of Health suggests that there are four determinants of a person's health status: (1) genetics; (2) environmental factors; (3) lifestyle, and (4) use of health care services. In this model, the most important factor affecting a person's health status is the environment in which he or she lives, while the least important factor is the use of health care services (Blum, 1974). Additional research has shown the importance of lifestyle factors such as healthy diet, exercise, smoking cessation, and weight reduction as equally important factors in the maintenance of health status (Lalonde, 1974). Newer models of health that focus on wellness point out the importance of psychological and spiritual well-being in the promotion of health in the population.

Health care spending

The proportion of industrialized nations' production of goods and services (GDP, or gross domestic product) allocated to health care has increased dramatically in recent decades. Comparisons of international data show that the United States spends more on health care than its industrialized nation counterparts (Huber,1999). According to data compiled in 2000, the United States led the way in health care, spending at $4,631 per individual in the population, which is more than double the median of $1,983 per person (Anderson et al., 2003), which the Organisation for Economic Cooperation and Development (OECD) had suggested as a reasonable amount to spend.

Despite massive medical care expenditures, the Unites States lags behind its industrialized counterparts in major indicators of population health. For example, researchers have reported that people in the United States have lower life expectancy at birth and higher infant mortality.

These international differences are largely attributable to the greater degree of heterogeneity in the U.S. population, to various prominent risk factors such as violence, and to economic barriers to obtaining health care (Williams, 2001).

RELATED ARTICLES

In many emerging economies, low income per capita, lack of access to proper hygiene and sanitation, cultural mores, regional warfare and strife, and other socioeconomic factors have resulted in low health care spending per capita, low life expectancy, and high infant mortality rates within these populations. Over 24.5 million people were living with HIV in sub-Saharan Africa at the end of 2005, and an estimated 2.7 million new infections occurred that same year. AIDS is erasing decades of progress made in extending life expectancy. Millions of adults are dying young or in early middle age. Average life expectancy in sub-Saharan Africa is now 47 years. Studies indicate that it could have been 62 without AIDS (UNAIDS, 2006).

Providers and consumers of health care services

In order to maintain a state of health, individuals utilize services offered by medical and other health professionals. Health care services may be delivered in a variety of settings from a person's residence (home care) to a doctor's office (ambulatory care) to specialized facilities such as hospitals (acute care) or nursing homes (long-term care).

The use of technologies such as telemedicine (health care services provided over the Internet, with a video component) and Internet-based health care services is growing, particularly in rural areas and in emerging world economies that do not have well-developed transportation and communication systems.

The individuals and institutions producing health care services are called the providers of health care services, while the individuals using health care services are called the consumers of health care services. Providers of health care services include a variety of health care professionals such as doctors, dentists, nurses, therapists, chiropractors, specialized medical technicians, and allied health personnel, as well as a variety of institutions such as hospitals that provide care for acute health conditions, long-term care facilities that provide care for functional limitations, and end-of-life services, such as hospices.

Consumers of health care services include all members of a community such as children, families, working adults, individuals who have disabling or chronic health conditions, and the elderly.

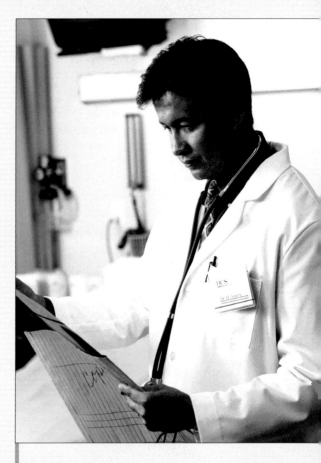

A hospital doctor examines a patient's records. Patients are admitted to the hospital for planned treatment for minor complaints, for major surgery, or they may be brought to the hospital as as the result of an emergency.

Public health systems

Governments may also provide health care services through a public health system. Public health services have their origins in the nineteenth century, when government officials assisted in the prevention of the spread of infectious diseases and in monitoring the quality of water and food supplies in urban areas. Now modern public health organizations ensure that the health of a community is protected, monitored and improved through the use of health education programs, programs to control communicable diseases (including vaccinations and health screenings), application of sanitary guidelines, and monitoring of environmental hazards. With the increasing incidence of natural disasters and threats of terrorism worldwide, the importance of global cooperation and sharing of public health information has grown beyond regional borders.

Public health has also been increasingly concerned with prevention programs aimed at health problems that disproportionately affect minority and economically disadvantaged groups. Programs such as Healthy People 2010 in the United States focus on reduction of health disparities and aim to eventually eliminate differences in provision within the population; similar initiatives exist in the European community. By focusing on issues of health promotion and disease prevention, public health activities provide a foundation for health care systems that may result in better quality services and lower health care costs.

How health care is used

In the acute care sector or curative side of health services, there are three levels of medical care that can be provided by practitioners.

The first level is primary care, which is the first contact that an individual would have with his or her physician. If additional services are required, such as X-rays or diagnostic tests, the individual would move to the second level of care.

The second level is called secondary care. These services can be provided at a local hospital or often within a physician's office.

The third level of care is called tertiary care, which typically involves use of medical services provided by a specialist, or the use of hospitals that specialize in services including cancer care, rehabilitation, and mental disorders.

These concepts, however, tend to apply to the use of health care services in highly industrialized economies that have well-developed health care delivery systems. In many emerging economies, the first contact for health care services is with nonmedically qualified personnel. Due to budgetary limitations, any contacts with medical personnel or a physician are rare to limited, and these medical extenders provide the bulk of basic health care services.

Health care services are used by individuals in a continuum of care over their lifetime, where the breadth of health care services ranges from preventive health care services to palliative and end-of-life care. There are typically seven stages in the continuum of health care services. These stages are: personal care (that is, the maintenance of one's well-being before illness occurs); primary care (direct access to a source of health care services from a family or primary care physician); specialty care (treating special health conditions with the services of an organ- or disease-specific medical practitioner); inpatient care (care in a primary care or specialty hospital); rehabilitative services such as physical, occupational, or speech therapy; long-term care (care that addresses functional or mental limitations delivered at a person's home, in a nursing home or other type of residence with continuous supervision; and hospice and palliative care (services appropriate at the end of life, which may include management of pain and other comforting services for the patient who is approaching death). Individuals may use health care services in the order indicated by the continuum, or may use them variably, depending on their stage of life, if they have a recurrent or chronic health condition that requires ongoing care by the medical community.

Within the continuum of health care services, there are a variety of important institutions. Hospitals are providers of acute care and specialty care, and their type and importance can vary in the global economy. While there are approximately 1.1 million hospital beds in the United States, the average length of a hospital stay is five days, in comparison with Japan, which has 1.6 million hospital beds with an average length of stay of 33 days (Japan Annual Report on Health and Welfare, 1999). Due to reduced reimbursement for inpatient health care services, there is increasing emphasis in the United States on ambulatory care (defined as "care for the walking"), which encompasses care in physicians' offices, outpatient or ambulatory care clinics that may have an affiliation with a hospital system, freestanding surgery centers, and emergency medical services. Long-term care services include a wide range of options, from residential settings (such as nursing homes providing skilled nursing care and residential care or assisted living facilities, or both, for 24-hour personal care services), to community-based services (such as adult day service centers and home health services provided by specialized agencies). Within many industrialized economies, there is greater emphasis on use of ambulatory care services as a result of rising health care costs and limited government financing resources. One of the greatest dilemmas facing OECD countries is the accelerating aging of the population and dramatic increases in consumption of health care services as a result of these changing demographics. In countries like Germany and Japan, long-term care services are reimbursed by special government-sponsored insurance systems, while in other countries, families are held financially responsible by their governments for provision of long-term care services.

With the aging of the world population, incidence of chronic illness increases. Chronic illness care is defined as treatment and care given to individuals whose health problems are long-term and recurring. Types of illness that fall into this category include asthma, diabetes, multiple sclerosis, lupus, Alzheimer's disease, and various types of mental illness. According to the National Chronic Care Consortium, more than 75 percent of all health care costs incurred are for people with chronic care conditions. The difficulty in providing care to chronically ill individuals is that they may need services provided in acute care as well as long-term care facilities. Rehabilitation facilities, nursing homes, and mental hospitals may be considered chronic care facilities.

With growing world publicity on problems with end-of-life care issues, many countries are expanding the use of hospice and palliative care services. The word *hospice* (from the same linguistic root as "hospitality") can be traced back to medieval times, when it referred to a place of shelter and rest for weary or ill travelers on a long journey. The name was first applied to specialized care for dying patients in 1967 by physician Cicely Saunders, who founded the first modern hospice, St. Christopher's Hospice, in a residential suburb of London. Saunders introduced the idea of specialized care for the dying to the United States during a 1963 visit to Yale University (National Hospice and Palliative Care Organization, 2006).

In the United States and United Kingdom, hospice provision focuses on caring, not curing, and, in most cases, care is provided in the patient's home. Hospice care also is provided in freestanding hospice centers, hospitals, nursing homes, and other long-term care facilities. Hospice services are available to patients of any age, religion, race, or illness. Hospice care is covered under Medicare, Medicaid, most private insurance plans, HMOs, and other managed care organizations. (NHPCO, 2006). There are an increasing number of health care organizations interested in providing hospice care and related services, and many have formed coalitions of service providers, government officials, educators, and legal or financial service professionals, or both, to promote education and training about these issues.

Palliative care extends the principles of hospice care to a broader population that could benefit from receiving this type of care earlier in their illness or disease process. No specific therapy is excluded from consideration. An individual's needs must be continually assessed, and treatment options should be explored and evaluated in the context of the individual's values and symptoms. Palliative care, ideally, would segue into hospice care as the illness progresses (NHPCO, 2006).

Associated with hospice and palliative care is the issue of advance directives (ADs). These are documents that indicate an individual's wishes for types of care provided at the end of his or her life. These documents may include items such as orders not to resuscitate (DNR) and orders not to intubate (DNI), as well as preferences for tube feeding, pain medication administration, and other types of life-sustaining treatments.

In the United States, the moral arguments supporting ADs are based primarily on the concept of respect for autonomy or on the patient's right to self-determination. The Patient Self-Determination Act of 1990 aims to encourage patients to take the initiative to ensure that their values are respected at the end of their life. Completion of formal documentation either in the form of ADs or durable powers of attorney are considered to be effective means in supporting patient autonomy and patient preferences regarding life-sustaining treatment. ADs and the use of a health care proxy have been recommended as a means to improve communication about the patient's preferences in making health care decisions (Akabayashi et al., 2003).

In the United States, states may have different sets of laws that address what is legally permissible for expression of end-of-life care wishes. In contrast, many countries such as Japan have more informal systems in which families and their wishes determine

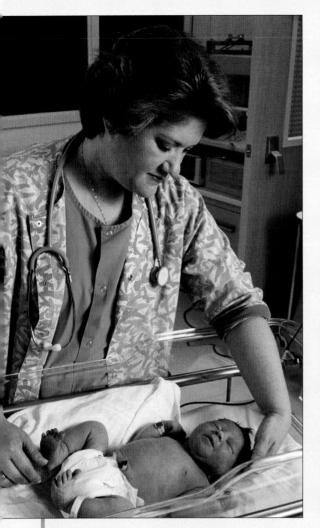

If a newborn baby needs special medical care, a hospital setting is usually the place that will provide the best outcome. Most pediatric providers will have immediate access to all the medical specialties.

the extent and quality of end-of-life care services for individuals.

Types of health care systems

The types of systems used to deliver health care services in world economies vary considerably. The United States utilizes a private, market-based system that combines use of services from private health care providers paid for by the use of private insurance policies, with services from government programs for special populations like the elderly (Medicare), indigent and poor (Medicaid), the military (Veterans Administration), and children (state-run Child Health Insurance Programs). There is no national health service or national health plan in the United States, resulting in a patchwork of medical service supply that frequently bases access to health care services on availability of health care insurance carried by the individual seeking care.

In contrast, many countries utilize a system of universal health care in which all residents have their health care services paid for by the government regardless of medical condition or financial resources. In these countries, the government controls the use of and payment for health care services in accordance with a national health plan. Services are frequently provided by a general practitioner who is trained in provision of a variety of health care services.

However, universal health care does not ensure that all types of health care services are given or paid for by the government, since countries have varying financial abilities to provide health care services.

Financing health care

Health care services may be reimbursed in a variety of ways, depending on the structure of a country's health care system. In the United States, there are three key sources for health care reimbursement.

First, there are government programs for targeted populations such as Medicare, which caters to individuals who are more than 65 years old and certain groups of disabled persons. There is also a means-tested program called Medicaid to provide for the poor and indigent, as well as programs for the military, veterans, and children.

Second, private health insurance policies, which are sometimes referred to as managed care plans, are typically offered at an individual's place of employment and may be jointly paid for by the employer and the employee.

Third, some people subscribe to private pay or out-of-pocket payments for health care needs.

Of the three sources of reimbursement, employer-sponsored health insurance is the most common form of reimbursement for health care services. Forms of this health insurance include indemnity plans, in which individuals can elect to consult any physician of their choice, and managed care plans, which provide services to individuals through a network of physicians that focus on management of patterns of health care service reimbursement.

In recent years, managed care plans have become the dominant type of health insurance coverage provided by employers, and three general types of plans have emerged.

The first plan is the health maintenance organization, in which an individual chooses a primary care physician from a network and consumes most of their health care services within that network

The second plan is a preferred provider organization, in which an individual can go to any physician that is in the network as well as physicians outside the network for reduced reimbursement levels.

The third plan is a point of service plan, a hybrid plan in which an individual must choose a primary care physician to access in-network services but has the opportunity to go to a provider out of the network for reduced reimbursement.

While managed care plans were promoted heavily during the 1990s in the United States as a way for employers to save on health care costs, these plans are experiencing problems in delivering continuous health care cost savings as the use of new, expensive technologies and increasingly expensive pharmaceutical drugs continues. While the tax burden on individuals in the United States to pay for government programs in this arrangement is smaller than in other industrialized countries, the cost of maintaining employer-sponsored insurance is much greater and may provide limited access to health care services.

Consumer-driven model

A new development in employer-provided health insurance in the United States is the emergence of consumer-driven models of insurance benefits. These benefits include health reimbursement accounts and health savings account plans that are accompanied with high deductible health insurance plans. In these insurance plans, employees are encouraged to educate themselves about the costs of items such as prescription drugs and other types of health care services in an attempt to encourage efficient use of health care services.

In contrast with managed care plans that have experienced significant cost increases, consumer-driven plans have typically experienced lower costs

Modern technology enables surgeons to carry out surgery with the aid of an endoscope and camera that projects a magnified image onto a monitor.

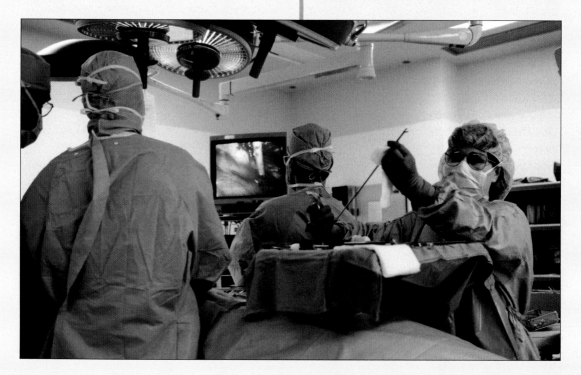

and lower cost increases, and there is evidence (Buntin et al., 2006) of modest favorable health selection (the enrollment of healthier beneficiaries into the plan).

Health care in other countries

In other global economies, the key source of reimbursement for health care services is a government plan paid for by tax revenues. There are varying models of government-provided health care services. One such model is the British National Health Service, which allocates tax revenues to primary health care trusts that commission health care services based on a fixed annual budget given to them by the Department of Health. Another example is the German health care system, which is similar to the U.S. health care system in that it utilizes third-party payors or sickness funds to contract with health care providers for services. In many countries, individuals seeking care not reimbursed in full by the government plan may supplement their coverage with specialized forms of private insurance policies. An important point to remember is that in the latter type of health care system, the tax burden on individuals to finance their health care system may be greater, but access to and coverage for health care services may also be more comprehensive.

Regulation of health care

The regulation of health care can vary, depending on whether a country has a mixed system of health care reimbursement, such as that in the United States, or a system in which the government is the primary source for reimbursement. In the United States, there are three levels of regulation for health care services.

First level. Federal laws and guidelines are in force that are broad and may cover issues including patient privacy and confidentiality of health information and access to emergency health care services.

Second level. State laws cover licensing of health care professionals and health care institutions, as well as collection of health care data and statistics.

Third level. There are local area laws and departments that may provide community-based health services and other types of health information and support services. The Congress of the United States as well as its judicial system may also be initiators, contributors, and modifiers of health care legislation. Health care organizations in the United States may also seek accreditation by independent agencies such as the Joint Commission on Accreditation of Health Care Organizations (JCAHO) and also from other entities to attract the best health care personnel to work in their facilities and provide quality services to consumers.

In other countries, health services may be regulated at a federal government level but may be distributed according to a system of regionalization in which various geographical areas provide health care services for their constituencies. Under this system, resources are allocated geographically and to population groups based on actual need as determined by careful health planning. Populations are enrolled in the plan and are usually assigned to a primary care physician, often using the gatekeeper mechanism (in which a patient can access a specialist only by referral from a physician). Local community hospitals are also allocated based on population size and health care needs. Local hospitals feed into regional and tertiary care hospitals, and physicians are allocated panels of patients with referrals, as needed, for specialty care. Ultimately, resources are strictly allocated so a community has only what it needs for its population, thereby reducing duplication, and strictly controlling resource allocation through budgeting and management of the patient (Williams, 2001).

Health care quality

The provision of quality health care services has become an important topic of discussion throughout the world. Health care quality is typically defined as quality of medical care provided, resulting in positive health outcomes for the recipient of care, but it may also include quality of services provided, which addresses issues that include the length of waiting time for an appointment and the professional demeanor of the health care provider.

Traditional measures of health care quality include quality assurance, which is the process of measuring the quality of care provided in a health care setting on a retrospective basis. In this model, quality of health care is measured by looking at structure (what are the services provided), process (what is done to the patient and its appropriateness), and outcome (the results of the care process) (Donabedian, 1980, 1985). It requires the availability of data from ongoing and reliable sources, such as medical records and claims forms, and may look at items such as appropriateness of hospital admissions and length of stay (Williams, 2001). In contrast, many health care organizations have moved to the use of continuous quality improvement, in which the process of providing medical care is examined with the goal of identifying opportunities for change in the health care services delivery process to improve the quality of care that the patient receives.

Other measures of care that are used in this process are benchmark data developed by government agencies as well as not-for-profit organizations that allow health care organizations to compare their administrative, clinical, and financial performance relative to their peers.

In many countries, government agencies and some private companies have developed quality indicators from data on health care services collected by health care providers and institutions participating in their programs. In the United States, Medicare has developed sets of quality indicators published on their Web site that look at care outcomes for hospitals, nursing homes, home care, and dialysis centers that accept payments for services rendered to Medicare recipients. Other nongovernmental agencies, such as JCAHO, that accredit hospital organizations require that quality indicator data be regularly collected and submitted to them for analysis as a condition of their accreditation. Frequently, these data sets are available to the public so that health care institutions and providers may be evaluated and consumers can use the data to make decisions on where to obtain their health care services.

Information technology

Countries are increasingly turning to information technology to improve the quality of health care services. It is believed that with the integration of sophisticated information systems to capture patient data accurately and comprehensively, fewer mistakes will be made and information can be shared simultaneously between departments to increase the efficiency of decision-making and discharge of patients. In many parts of the world, providers are encouraging the use of an electronic medical record to store all health care information about patients that can be shared between health care institutions to avoid medical errors in the provision of patient care. Although the cost of adopting this electronic medical record is significant, most European primary care physicians are utilizing these technologies. It is estimated that less than 10 percent of their U.S. physician counterparts have made a commitment to the use of these instruments.

The future of health care

The ideal health care system would provide access to high-quality and appropriate health services for all individuals. Resources would be used efficiently. Ideally, administrative complexity and paperwork burdens for consumers and providers would be reduced, and technological innovation would be brought to the bedside rapidly upon confirmation of its efficiency and safety. Physicians would make their decisions based on the best interests of the patient. Feedback mechanisms would monitor resource use and continually improve the system.

Finally, health care policy decisions would be made based on social and health care goals rather than economics and politics (Williams, 2001).

Global views of health care

Increasing globalization of world economies, changes in the global political and economic environment, expanded use of technology in the provision of health care services, and a more sophisticated health care consumer are all factors that will have an impact on health care systems in the future. Most countries acknowledge the importance of communication and sharing of information about advances in health care service provision, as well as improving the health status of countries with fewer resources to address their health care needs. As health care providers increasingly consult with each other across global borders, they will also need to be aware of a more educated health care consumer who will readily use technology to obtain a personalized approach to health care services. Hopefully these initiatives will result in greater access to health care services as well as increased quality of care and good outcomes provided for all consumers globally.

Mary Helen McSweeney

Heart attack

Heart attack, also called myocardial infarction, is sudden death of heart muscle. Heart attack is a major cause of death worldwide. The risk for coronary artery disease (CAD) and heart attack is increased by smoking, high blood pressure, high cholesterol, diabetes, and lack of proper exercise.

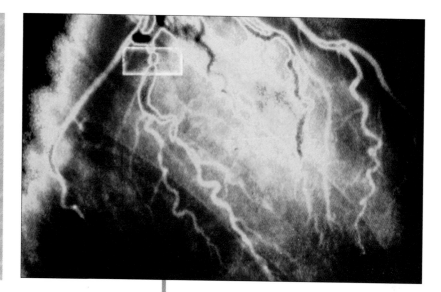

A heart attack, or myocardial infarction (MI), is caused by blockage of one or more of the blood vessels (coronary arteries) that supply the heart. Symptoms may include chest pressure and sweating, or, in about 15 percent of cases, there are no symptoms, in which case it is referred to as a silent heart attack.

Damage to the heart from a heart attack is directly proportional to the muscle mass involved. It may be small enough to be insignificant or it may be massive enough to cause sudden death. It can also cause long-term problems with heart failure and disability. Heart attack is a major cause of death and disability, but attention to proper diet and exercise, as well as control of blood pressure, cholesterol, diabetes, and smoking, may reduce the risk of heart attack.

Causes, risk factors, and pathogenesis

A heart attack is an acute manifestation of CAD. In persons with CAD, plaques composed of fat, cholesterol, calcium, platelets, fibrin, and other materials from the bloodstream build up in the coronary arteries that supply blood to the heart muscle. Plaques may be located in peripheral arteries feeding just a small part of the heart muscle, or in the main arteries responsible for blood flow to large areas of the heart muscle. While these plaques may remain stable or grow gradually in persons with relatively stable CAD, a heart attack occurs if one or more of the plaques ruptures. When a plaque in an artery ruptures, blood flow to the area of the heart supplied by that artery may be

This colored angiogram shows that a coronary artery, which supplies the heart muscle with blood, is narrowed. The box (upper left) highlights the area of narrowing, or stenosis, which is caused by deposits of fatty material on the artery walls, usually as a result of high blood cholesterol levels. This condition can lead to atherosclerosis of the coronary arteries, which in turn impedes blood flow to the heart.

blocked in one of two ways: pieces of the plaque (emboli) may flow downstream until they lodge in a smaller segment of the artery, or a clot (thrombus) may develop at the site where the remnant of the plaque is exposed to the bloodstream. Such blockage of one or more coronary arteries prevents the affected area of the heart from receiving nutrients and oxygen, leading to injury or death of the involved heart muscle tissue.

When an area of heart muscle in the ventricle is injured or dies as a result of blockage of an artery, several problems develop soon after. The injured area of the ventricle may generate electrical impulses that are either too fast (ventricular tachycardia) or too irregular (ventricular fibrillation) to allow for proper, coordinated pumping of the heart muscle. Ventricular fibrillation leads to sudden collapse and can lead to sudden death, and ventricular tachycardia can lead either to acute heart failure and pulmonary edema, or sudden death.

If a patient survives an acute heart attack but has permanent damage to part of the heart muscle, the heart may be able to fully recover most of its pumping function, but if a large enough area of the heart muscle is damaged or dies and is replaced by scar tissue, the heart will be unable to pump normally and will eventually develop chronic heart failure.

Risk factors

Risk factors for a heart attack are the same as those for CAD in general. Some risk factors, such as tobacco

---

KEY FACTS

Description

Sudden blockage of one or more arteries in the heart, causing injury or death of heart muscle.

Causes

Clots in the arteries that supply blood to the heart causing inadequate blood flow (ischemia) to all or part of the heart.

Risk factors

Tobacco smoking, high cholesterol, high blood pressure, physical inactivity, obesity, diabetes, age, male gender, family history and heredity, heavy use of alcohol, and cocaine use.

Symptoms

Anginal chest pain (squeezing chest discomfort or chest heaviness radiating to one or both arms or to the back), sometimes accompanied by nausea, vomiting, or sweating.

Diagnosis

Based on history of anginal symptoms, specific abnormalities on ECG consistent with ischemia of heart muscle, blood tests when history and ECG are not diagnostic.

Treatments

Oxygen, aspirin, heparin, and interventions to open blocked coronary arteries including fibrinolytic medications, angioplasty, or coronary artery stenting.

Pathogenesis

Rupture of plaques in the coronary arteries, which can lead to clots in the coronary arteries, death or injury of heart muscle due to ischemia, and either sudden death from abnormal heart rhythms or long-term heart problems including heart failure as a result of impaired pumping by a weakened heart.

Prevention

A healthy diet, regular exercise, avoiding smoking, control of high cholesterol levels, and regulating high blood pressure are all important preventive measures.

Epidemiology

Heart attack is a leading cause of death and disability worldwide. It is more common among people who are of lower socioeconomic status, older, male, and have risk factors for CAD.

---

smoking, high cholesterol, high blood pressure, physical inactivity, obesity, and diabetes, are modifiable and can be controlled or managed to reduce a person's chance of having a heart attack.

Other risk factors, such as age, male gender, and family history and heredity, cannot be changed. Heavy use of alcohol or use of cocaine may also increase a person's risk for CAD or heart attack.

Symptoms

The most typical symptom of heart attack is new or worsening central chest pain. The pain is often described as squeezing, heaviness, or pressure and may radiate to one or both arms or to the back. It may also be accompanied by nausea, vomiting, or sweating. Less typical symptoms of heart attack include discomfort radiating to the jaw, neck, or ear, and new-onset shortness of breath. Anyone with new-onset chest pain or pressure should be evaluated promptly at an emergency room.

Diagnosis

The first diagnostic step in determining if someone is having a heart attack is a brief physical examination. The initial evaluation focuses on the patient's airway, breathing, and circulation (ABCs). The heart is evaluated for murmurs or gallops, and the lungs are evaluated for crackles or rales that may signal pulmonary edema from acute heart failure. It is also important to evaluate for signs of stroke and for signs or symptoms of shock or hypoperfusion (low blood pressure) such as cool, clammy skin, or a pale or ashen appearance.

The most important diagnostic test in evaluating for heart attack is the 12-lead electrocardiogram (ECG). Electrical activity from the heart produces a trace with peaks called P, QRS, and T, which represent the waves. ST segment connects the QRS and T waves on the trace. Findings on ECG that most strongly suggest a heart attack are ST segment elevation, Q waves, or a new conduction defect such as a left bundle branch block (LBBB). New T wave inversion also suggests a heart attack (see box, page 407). An ECG showing ST segment elevation indicates the patient may be suffering from a heart attack affecting a large portion of heart muscle and may benefit from reperfusion (restoration of blood flow) therapy to open the blocked blood vessel or vessels. This is called an "ST-elevation myocardial infarction" (STEMI), and these patients are at highest risk of death or long-term complications from heart attack. An ECG that shows ST segment depression or no ST segment changes in a

ECG: FINDINGS THAT SUGGEST ISCHEMIA

Ischemia (lack of blood flow) or damage to the heart muscle will produce certain, typical changes on the ECG. A Q wave is an abnormally large "downstroke" at the beginning of the QRS complex, signifying heart muscle tissue that has been permanently damaged or is dead. A block of the right or left bundle conducting systems due to ischemic damage can lead to a prolonged QRS (points on a wave) complex. Acute injury to the heart, such as when a coronary blood vessel feeding the heart is first blocked off with a clot, leads to elevation of the ST segment (the portion of the ECG between the end of the QRS complex and the beginning of the T wave). Chronic ischemia (lack of blood flow that prevents heart muscle from getting enough blood but does not kill that area of muscle) will produce ST-segment depression, or cause the T wave to invert.

patient with chest pain suggests unstable angina or a "non–ST-elevation myocardial infarction" (NSTEMI), due to partial blockages of blood flow or partial damage to an area of heart muscle.

However, absence of ECG changes does not completely exclude heart attack, since up to 6 percent of patients with chest pain and a normal ECG may actually have had a heart attack or unstable angina.

Blood tests can be used to help clarify whether a patient is having a heart attack if the ECG does not definitively show a STEMI. Blood is drawn to measure levels of specific enzymes that are released from damaged heart tissue. Enzymes that are commonly measured are creatine kinase (CK), its MB subform (CKMB), and troponin T (TnT) and troponin I (TnI). Because CK and CKMB are present in both heart and skeletal muscle, elevated levels of total CK or CKMB are relatively nonspecific for heart attack, but CKMB is still the blood test most commonly used when evaluating for heart attack. Cardiac troponins T and I are much more specific indicators of heart damage. Individuals with chest pain and a low-risk history, a normal or near-normal ECG, and normal troponins can safely be further evaluated as outpatients. Overall, CKMB is the most efficient blood test for early diagnosis of heart attack within 6 hours of the beginning of symptoms, while TnT and TnI are much more efficient for late diagnosis of heart attack.

In short, when a patient presents with symptoms of heart attack, the history and ECG are used to decide whether the patient's symptoms are due to: heart attack from STEMI, unstable angina or heart attack from NSTEMI, or noncardiac problems, or CAD that is not causing acute damage to the heart.

Treatments

Any patient suspected of having a heart attack is usually started promptly on oxygen (to prevent death of heart muscle), given by a mask or through small tubes placed in the nose, and is given an aspirin to chew, as aspirin can help prevent blood clots. Heparin (a medication to prevent further blood clotting) is also important and is given either intravenously, or as an injection in the skin. A beta blocker, statin medication, and probably an ACE inhibitor may also be considered. A patient with severe anginal chest pain must be relieved of severe chest pain by powerful analgesics.

ST-segment elevation is diagnosed with STEMI based on history and ECG alone, and typically has complete blockage of one or more coronary arteries. This requires urgent treatment to reopen the blocked blood vessels, in order to minimize damage to the heart muscle and to prevent further complications.

One approach that can be used is to give a medication to break down the blood clot (a "fibrinolytic" medication). Another approach is using angioplasty (in which a catheter is inserted into an artery in the leg and threaded up to the heart) to find the blocked blood vessel or vessels, and to restore blood flow either by opening the blockage with a balloon on the tip of the angioplasty catheter, or by placing a stent in the vessel to keep it open.

A patient who has anginal chest pain and ischemic ECG changes, but no ST-segment elevation, may be having unstable angina or a NSTEMI due to a partially occluding blood clot in a coronary artery. Fibrinolytics are not given in this situation.

Important steps in evaluation of the patient include obtaining ECGs every few hours to look for the development of more severe ischemic changes, obtaining blood tests for heart enzymes such as CKMB, TnI, or TnT, and also evaluating for other nonischemic causes of chest pain. A patient with anginal chest pain and a normal or nondiagnostic ECG is unlikely to be having a heart attack, although CAD cannot be entirely excluded based only on the immediate emergency room evaluation. Evaluation focuses on CAD risk factors and considers further testing to clarify whether there is underlying CAD that has not yet been diagnosed. Exercise or chemical stress testing may be used to further evaluate a patient who has anginal chest pain and is at high risk for CAD but is not suffering acutely from heart attack. Stress tests can help determine the cause of chest pain or other symptoms.

After initial stabilization and treatment, any patient who has had a heart attack or is suspected to have CAD should be assessed for long-term cardiac risk. Advice to avoid smoking is one of the most important preventive measures. Blood pressure and cholesterol levels should be measured, and treated if they are high. Any patient with diabetes requires monitoring, since diabetes greatly increases the risk of CAD and heart attack. Close monitoring of rhythm disturbances and prompt treatment can avert disastrous arrhythmia.

Pathogenesis

If someone has never had a heart attack before and has prompt treatment, the outlook is promising. If there are no complications, the likelihood of another heart attack is reduced. However, the outlook also depends on the extent of damage to heart muscle. Rupture of plaques in the coronary arteries can lead to clots in the coronary arteries, death, or injury of heart muscle due to ischemia. Sudden death can occur if someone has abnormal heart rhythms or long-term heart problems, including heart failure, as a result of impaired pumping by a weakened heart.

Prevention

The prevention of heart attacks depends on controlling modifiable risk factors for CAD: eliminating smoking is essential, and blood pressure, cholesterol, and weight can be improved with a healthy diet and regular exercise. Only moderate amounts of alcohol should be taken, in the region of one to two small glasses of beer or wine a day. Smoking increases the risk of CAD; stopping smoking is the most important step in reducing heart attack risk.

A program of regular exercise and a healthy diet are also important for reducing the risk of CAD and heart attack. All persons should try to get at least 30 minutes of aerobic exercise on most days of the week, such as walking, bicycling, jogging, or swimming. A healthy diet should include at least five servings of fresh fruits and vegetables daily, plus plenty of fiber, and should avoid saturated fats.

A blood pressure above 140/90 is considered high, and for most people the goal is to keep the blood pressure below 140/90. Persons with diabetes or chronic kidney disease should try to keep their blood pressure below 130/80, since they are at much higher risk of heart attack.

An LDL (low-density lipoprotein or "bad") cholesterol level of 160 milligrams per deciliter (mg/dL) or less is acceptable for persons at low risk of CAD or heart attack. Persons at moderate risk of CAD or heart attack should try to keep the LDL cholesterol less than 130 mg/dL. Anyone at high risk of CAD or heart attack due to the presence of multiple risk factors, and anyone with diabetes, should try to keep the LDL cholesterol less than 100 mg/dL. Persons who have previously had a heart attack should also try to keep the LDL cholesterol less than 100 mg/dL.

For persons at risk of heart attack, medications may be needed if exercise and healthy eating are not enough to control high blood pressure or high cholesterol. High blood pressure may be treated with thiazide diuretics, beta-blocker medications, and angiotensin converting enzyme inhibitor or angiotensin receptor blocker medications. High cholesterol is most commonly treated with "statin" medications, although fibric acid derivatives and other medications are sometimes used instead. For men over age 50, taking one aspirin each day may also reduce the risk of CAD or heart attack. All persons with a previous heart attack should take an aspirin each day to prevent further heart damage.

Epidemiology

CAD is one of the most common causes of death worldwide. In 1990, CAD caused 6.3 million deaths worldwide, and in 2003 the rate of death from CAD in the U.S. population was 162 in 100,000. Unstable angina and NSTEMI account for 2.5 million hospitalizations per year. Each year about 900,000 people in the United States suffer a heart attack, and 225,000 of those die. One-half of deaths from heart attack occur within an hour of symptoms (sudden cardiac death). Rates of heart attack are higher among older individuals, are higher in men than in women, and are higher among people of lower socioeconomic status. Heart attack from CAD is a leading cause of death and disability around the world.

Bill Cayley Jr.

See also

• Arteries, disorders of • Cardiovascular disorders • Diabetes • Heart disorders • Obesity • Smoking-related disorders • Substance abuse and addiction

Heart disorders

The heart continually pumps blood throughout the body. Blood delivers oxygen and nutrition to the body's many organs and removes waste products for elimination. Normal heart function is essential to the body's health. Disorders affecting the heart's ability to pump normally may be a result of structural problems present from birth, valve disorders that develop later in life, or coronary artery disease, which blocks the blood vessels supplying the heart muscle.

The heart is located in the center of the chest and is about the size of a clenched fist. There are four muscular chambers, four valves, and a system of specialized muscle tissues that generate and conduct electrical impulses to coordinate the heart's pumping action. The heart is surrounded by a protective lining called the pericardium (*peri* means "around" and *cardia* means "heart"), which is filled with a small amount of fluid to allow for frictionless pumping. The right side of the heart consists of the small, thin-walled right atrium, the larger right ventricle, the tricuspid valve (named for its three cusps or leaflets) between the right atrium and right ventricle, and the pulmonary valve, where blood exits the right ventricle. Blood flows to the heart through the superior vena cava (from the upper part of the body) and the inferior vena cava (from the lower part of the body). After entering the right atrium, blood flows through the tricuspid valve into the right ventricle. Most of the blood flowing into the right ventricle travels through the atrium passively, pushed by the blood pressure in

the circulatory system, and contraction of the right atrium helps complete the filling of the right ventricle. After being filled, the right ventricle contracts to push blood through the pulmonary valve into the pulmonary artery and on toward the lungs. The tricuspid valve between the right atrium and right ventricle prevents blood from flowing backward into the right atrium. It is anchored to the inside of the right ventricle by chordae tendinae (tendinous or fibrous cords), which attach to papillary muscles on the inside wall of the ventricle and prevent the tricuspid valve from being pushed open backward by the pressure of the right ventricular contraction. After contraction, the right ventricle relaxes to allow filling for the next heartbeat. The pulmonary valve prevents blood from flowing backward into the heart from the pulmonary artery when the pressure in the right ventricle drops as it relaxes.

The left side of the heart functions similarly to the right side, although the left ventricle is much larger and more muscular since it pumps blood to supply the whole body. Blood flows from the lungs through the four pulmonary veins into the left atrium. From the left atrium, blood flows through the mitral valve (named for its resemblance to a bishop's miter, or hat) into the left ventricle. Once again, most of the blood flowing into the ventricle does so passively; the left atrial contraction completes the filling of the left ventricle. Contraction of the left ventricle pushes blood out through the aortic valve and into the aorta, the main artery of the cardio-vascular system. The two cusps (or leaflets) of the mitral valve prevent backward blood flow into the left atrium when the left ventricle contracts, and are

RELATED ARTICLES

anchored to the inside of the left ventricle by chordae tendinae (fibrous cords) attached to papillary muscles. When the left ventricle relaxes and begins filling for the next heartbeat, the three cusps of the aortic valve prevent blood from flowing backward into the ventricle from the aorta. A helpful measure of left ventricular function is the ejection fraction, which is the percentage of the heart's total blood volume that is pumped out in each cardiac cycle. A normal ejection fraction is about 50 percent.

Each heartbeat, or cardiac cycle, consists of two phases: systole, when both ventricles contract at the same time to pump blood out to the lungs and the body, and diastole, when the ventricles relax to allow inflow of blood through the atria. Coordinated systolic contraction and diastolic relaxation of the heart are important for normal cardiac function. On physical examination with a stethoscope, the two parts of the cardiac cycle are audible as a quiet "lub" (from the mitral and tricuspid valves as they are pushed shut by ventricular contraction at the beginning of systole) and a louder "dub" (from the aortic and pulmonic valves as they close with cardiac relaxation at the beginning of diastole).

The cardiac conducting system is made of specialized muscle fibers that regulate the rate and rhythm of each cardiac cycle. The sinus node is the heart's natural pacemaker. It is located in the wall of the right atrium and in healthy adults generates about 70 impulses every minute, though this rate may be increased or decreased, depending on the body's needs. From the sinus node, conducting tissue runs through the walls of the atria to the atrioventricular node (AV node), then divides into a right ventricular bundle supplying the right ventricle, and a left ventricular bundle which further divides into anterior and posterior branches supplying the ventricle's anterior and posterior walls. Thus, the electrical impulse for each heartbeat originates in the sinus node, which stimulates coordinated contraction of the atria and sends the impulse toward the AV node. The AV node slows each impulse slightly, then passes the impulse on to the right ventricular bundle and to the branches of the left ventricular bundle, causing coordinated contraction of the ventricles. The AV nodal delay of approximately 0.2 seconds allows coordination between the atria and ventricles, so that there is complete filling of the ventricles just before ventricular contraction pumps blood toward the rest of the body.

The heart does not receive any nutrition or oxygen from blood passing through the atria or ventricles, but depends on its own system of arteries and veins for supplying oxygen and nutrients and removing waste products from the heart muscle. The left coronary artery (left main coronary artery) originates at the aorta, travels a short distance down the anterior surface of the heart, then divides into the left anterior descending (LAD) artery, which nourishes much of the left ventricular muscle, and the left circumflex artery, which travels to the posterior part of the heart and nourishes the left atrium and much of the atrial conducting system. The right coronary artery also originates at the aorta, then travels around the right side of the heart, nourishing the right atrium and ventricle, and joining with the left circumflex artery to nourish the conducting system.

Congenital heart disorders

Congenital heart disorders refer to abnormalities of the heart that are present from birth. These may range from asymptomatic abnormalities that may only be discovered later in life, to severe abnormalities of heart structure and function that threaten the life of a newborn. Some form of congenital heart disease affects nearly 1 in 1,000 newborn children.

A common defect is an atrial septal defect, which is an opening occurring in the septum (wall) between the left and right atrium. Since blood pressure is higher in the left atrium than in the right, any opening between the atria can allow for shunting of blood from the left atrium to the right. Over time, this puts increased strain on the right atrium, the right ventricle, and the pulmonary circulation. Shunting due to an atrial septal defect can lead eventually to overload and enlargement of the right atrium and ventricle, dysrhythmias, ventricular dysfunction, and damage to the blood vessels in the lungs. Patients with significant shunting may live only about 45 years; thus surgical correction before age 4 is recommended.

Ventricular septal defects are openings in the septum between the left and right ventricles. These are much more common than atrial septal defects but are much less likely to cause symptoms. The only sign of a ventricular septal defect may be a slight heart murmur. If a defect is large enough to cause significant shunting, this will likely be apparent by the age of 6 weeks. If left unrepaired, a ventricular shunt can also cause overload,

HEART STRUCTURE

The heart is a hollow muscular organ, which is situated just to the left of the center of the chest. It acts as a pump, transferring deoxygenated blood from the body to the lungs, where blood is reoxygenated, then pumped to all parts of the body.

The heart is divided into four chambers: two upper chambers (atria), and two lower chambers (ventricles). The septum, a muscular wall, divides the two sides of the heart. Four valves ensure that blood flows in only one direction.

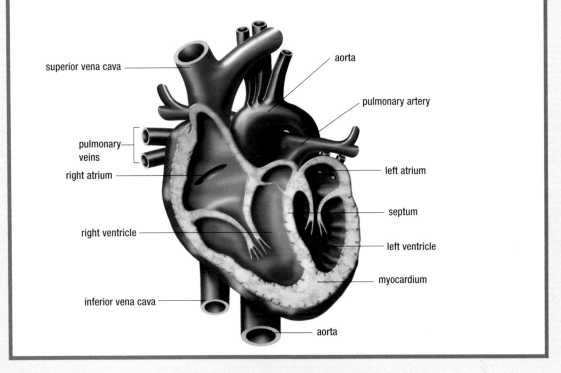

- superior vena cava
- aorta
- pulmonary artery
- pulmonary veins
- right atrium
- left atrium
- septum
- right ventricle
- left ventricle
- myocardium
- inferior vena cava
- aorta

enlargement, and dysfunction of the right ventricle. Significant ventricular septal defects are usually closed surgically or by a device placed through a catheter threaded up into the heart from an artery in the leg.

Atrioventricular canal refers to a combination of defects in the atrial and ventricular septa (walls), and can lead to left-to-right shunting with high pressures in the right side of the heart and to heart failure. Surgical repair is usually done around the age of 3 to 6 months.

Tetralogy of Fallot is a combination of four defects that usually occur together: a ventricular septal defect, obstruction of the pulmonary artery, in which the aorta lies over the ventricular septal defect, and abnormal thickening of the right ventricular muscle. This complex disorder requires surgical correction early in life. Other congenital heart disorders include transposition of the great arteries (reversal of the aorta and the pulmonary artery), tricuspid atresia (inadequate development of

the tricuspid valve), Ebstein's anomaly (the tricuspid valve has only one or two leaflets), pulmonary atresia (inadequate development of the pulmonary valve), hypoplastic left heart syndrome (inadequate development of the left ventricle), truncus arteriosus (a large ventricular septal defect with a single vessel leading out to the pulmonary artery and the aorta), double-outlet right ventricle, and total anomalous pulmonary venous connection.

Because of the complexity of congenital heart disorders and the surgical procedures that may be required to treat them, babies or children with congenital heart disorders require care at advanced medical centers. As these individuals grow into teenage and adult life, continued specialty care is important, as is coordination between the individual's primary care doctors and the heart specialists.

Valve disorders and endocarditis

All four of the heart's valves can suffer damage that causes either stenosis (tightness or incomplete opening that prevents proper blood flow through the valve) or insufficiency (leakage of a valve or incomplete closure that allows blood to flow backward through the valve). Valve insufficiency may also be associated with prolapse (most commonly found in the mitral valve), in which there is an abnormality of the valve leaflets that allows them to be pushed backward. Both valvular stenosis and valvular insufficiency can impair the heart's ability to properly pump blood, either by preventing adequate forward flow of blood (stenosis) or by allowing too much blood to leak backward during pumping (insufficiency).

The most common finding on physical examination associated with a valve disorder is a heart murmur, an extra hum or "whoosh" or other sound occurring between the normal "lub-dub" of each cardiac cycle. However, not all valve disorders cause murmurs, and not all murmurs indicate a valve disorder. Most patients who have a concerning heart murmur are evaluated with an electrocardiogram (ECG), a chest X-ray, and an echocardiogram. The most common valve disorders are aortic stenosis, aortic regurgitation, mitral stenosis, and mitral prolapse and regurgitation.

Aortic stenosis occurs when the valve's normal area of around ½ square inch (3–4 sq. cm) is reduced due to calcifications or degeneration due to aging. Early aortic stenosis may not produce any symptoms, but severe stenosis may impair blood flow enough to cause chest pain, lightheadedness on exertion, or shortness of breath. A valve area less than a fraction of a square centimeter is critical stenosis. Individuals with mild stenosis have a normal life expectancy, but once symptoms develop, life expectancy drops to about two to three years unless the valve is repaired. Aortic stenosis can only be corrected by open-heart surgical valve replacement and newer techniques of valve repair.

Aortic insufficiency, often caused by aging, is backward leaking of blood from the aorta to the ventricle during diastole, may be caused by damage to the valve from endocarditis, rheumatic fever, connective tissue disease, aortic dissection, or syphilis. Symptoms of aortic insufficiency include fatigue and a declining functional capacity. While medications may help delay the need for correction of aortic insufficiency for two to three years, surgery provides the only cure. Patients with aortic insufficiency also need to take antibiotics for certain medical procedures to prevent endocarditis (an infection of the heart valve by bacteria in the bloodstream).

Mitral valve stenosis is generally caused by damage to the valve from rheumatic fever, and it can take 20 to 40 years to become clinically apparent. Symptoms include shortness of breath on exertion or lying down, and swelling of the feet and legs. Additionally, the resistance to blood flow through the mitral valve causes increased stress on the left atrium and can eventually lead to atrial fibrillation. Medical management of mitral valve stenosis includes diuretics for fluid retention, management of atrial fibrillation, and antibiotics for certain medical procedures to prevent endocarditis. Correction of mitral valve stenosis in patients with mild disease is carried out using a balloon threaded through a catheter into the valve, which is then expanded to reopen the stenotic valve, while other patients require open-heart surgery to reopen the valve. Patients with severe disease may require surgical replacement of the damaged valve.

Mitral valve prolapse occurs when one or both of the mitral valve leaflets protrude into the left atrium during systole. About 10 to 20 percent of the population in developed countries is affected by mitral valve prolapse, but there is no increased risk of stroke, atrial fibrillation, or sudden death. Mitral valve insufficiency, with leakage of blood during systole, can be caused by endocarditis, rheumatic fever, or worsening of mitral valve prolapse. Chronic overload on the left atrium can lead to left atrial dilation, congestion of the lungs, and atrial fibrillation. Mitral valve prolapse usually causes no symptoms, but severe mitral insufficiency can cause shortness of breath and leg swelling. Mitral valve prolapse needs no specific medical management, but patients with mitral valve insufficiency need antibiotics for certain medical procedures to prevent endocarditis. Severe mitral valve insufficiency is treated with open-heart surgical valve repair or replacement.

Endocarditis is an infection of the inside of the heart, usually occurring in the valves, the chordae tendinae, or if there is a hole allowing leakage between chambers. Risk factors for endocarditis include valvular heart disease (congenital or acquired), diabetes, injection drug use, HIV infection, poor dental hygiene, and having an artificial heart valve. The bacteria causing infection are usually streptococci, staphylococci, or enterococci. Patients with endocarditis may be acutely ill with high fevers, or get sick more slowly with chronic low-grade fevers. Other symptoms may include stroke, heart failure, pneumonia, skin infections, joint infections, or general fatigue and weakness. Endocarditis is diagnosed by culturing the patient's blood for bacteria, and using an echocardiogram to look for vegetations on the heart valves (growths of bacteria and inflammatory cells). Endocarditis is treated with long-term intravenous antibiotics (it was fatal in the era before antibiotic use). To prevent endocarditis, individuals with artificial heart valves, prior endocarditis, heart valve disease, structural heart disease, or mitral valve insufficiency should take antibiotics before dental, respiratory tract, gastrointestinal tract, or urogenitary tract procedures that might allow bacteria to enter the bloodstream.

Heart failure

Heart failure refers to any condition in which the heart is unable to pump blood at a sufficient rate and volume to meet the body's metabolic needs. Typical symptoms include shortness of breath, fatigue, and swelling or fluid retention. Heart failure can be acute, that is, a sudden reduction of the heart's ability to pump efficiently. Chronic heart failure, on the other hand, is a long-term inefficiency of the heart, leading to poor circulation and edema. Causes of heart failure can be grouped as low-output, high-output, or fluid-overload heart failure.

Low-output heart failure occurs when the heart is unable to pump adequately due to systolic dysfunction, diastolic dysfunction, valvular disease, or dysrythmias (abnormal heart rhythms). Systolic dysfunction (when the heart cannot squeeze strongly enough) is generally defined as an ejection fraction of less than 40 percent. The most common cause of heart failure is cardiomyopathy (damage to the heart muscle) secondary to coronary artery disease. Other causes of systolic dysfunction include inflammation due to viral or bacterial infections or inflammatory diseases, or certain medications. Diastolic dysfunction (when the heart cannot relax enough to fill completely) may be associated with an elevated ejection fraction (60 percent or higher). Causes of diastolic dysfunction

include left ventricular hypertrophy (thickening of the ventricular muscle) due to chronic overload from hypertension, aortic stenosis, chronic lung disease, or tamponade of the left ventricle (when the pericardium fills with fluid, compresses the heart, and prevents the ventricle from expanding). Valvular heart disease can also cause low-output failure. Severe aortic stenosis may block outflow of blood from the heart so much that there is inadequate blood flow to meet the body's needs, and mitral insufficiency may allow enough backward leakage of blood during each cycle that there is inadequate pressure to force blood to flow forward out of the aortic valve. Dysrhythmias such as atrial fibrillation, ventricular tachycardia, or heart block may also cause low-output failure if they disrupt normal coordinated pumping of the heart chambers enough to prevent effective pumping action.

High-output heart failure occurs when excessive metabolic demands from the body cannot be met by the heart's normal pumping function, such as in mitral valve disease. Also, extreme hyperthyroidism causes a dramatic increase in the body's need for nutrition and energy, which may lead to demand for more circulating blood volume than the heart can deliver. Severe anemia may reduce the blood's ability to carry oxygen so much that the demands on the heart to circulate the remaining blood, with its reduced oxygen-carrying capacity, may also be more than the heart can deliver. Pregnancy is a third condition in which demand from the body for nutrients and oxygen to supply both mother and baby may outstrip the heart's normal pumping capacity.

Fluid-overload heart failure occurs when the volume of blood in the bloodstream is increased beyond what the heart can adequately pump. This generally can only occur during kidney failure (when the kidneys cannot properly eliminate excess fluid volume from the bloodstream) or when a patient receives more fluid through intravenous (IV) lines than the heart and kidneys can handle.

Treatment of heart failure involves addressing symptoms, causes, and long-term care of the heart. When heart failure is identified, symptoms are often relieved by use of diuretics and sometimes by digoxin. Diuretics are medications that cause the kidneys to draw extra fluid out of the bloodstream, thus reducing the volume of blood that must be pumped. Digoxin is a medication (derived from the foxglove plant and first used for heart failure in the 1700s) that slightly increases the pumping strength of the heart. It is also important to identify and treat any reversible causes of heart failure such as coronary artery disease (CAD), dysrhythmias, valve disease, anemia, or fluid overload. A low-salt diet is necessary. Long-term care of patients with heart failure involves treatment of any chronic heart disease, plus use of beta-blocker, angiotensin-converting enzyme inhibitor, or angiotensin receptor blocker medications, which have been shown to reduce symptoms and risk of dying for patients with heart failure.

Conduction system and rhythm disorders

Disorders of the heart's conducting system can lead to irregular or abnormal heart rhythms. They may be insignificant and asymptomatic, or may be life threatening. Abnormal heart rhythms include atrial fibrillation, abnormal tachycardias (heart beats faster than normal) or bradycardias (heart beats slower than normal), and ventricular fibrillation.

Atrial fibrillation occurs when damage to the atria (due to chronic pressure overload, heart attack, or other conditions) causes pulses to generate randomly from multiple sites throughout the atria, rather than coming regularly from just the sinus node. This causes the atria to fibrillate (quiver irregularly) rather than pump regularly. The AV node may allow these fast, random pulses through to the ventricles at a rate that is faster than, slower than, or about the same as the 60 to 100 beats per minute of a normal heart rate. Patients with atrial fibrillation may be asymptomatic or experience only mild palpitations if their heart continues beating at a normal rate, but if the ventricular rate is too fast, medications may be needed to slow the heart rate to a more normal speed, and if the rate is too slow, a pacemaker may be needed to ensure an adequate heart rate. Additionally, the lack of regular atrial pumping allows blood to pool in the left atrium and form clots. Patients with atrial fibrillation are usually given the anticoagulant medication warfarin to reduce the risk of such clots dislodging and flowing to the brain, which could cause a stroke.

Tachycardia refers to any condition in which the heart is beating faster than the normal rate of 60 to 100 beats per minute. Sinus tachycardia, a heart rate greater than 100, driven by the sinus node, usually

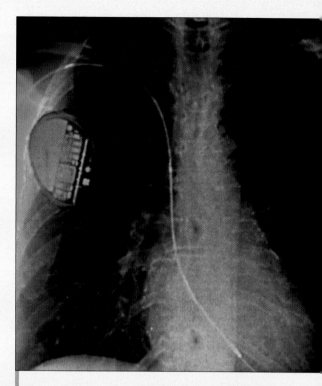

This colored X-ray shows a pacemaker or cardiac stimulator, which uses electrical impulses to help maintain a regular heartbeat. Pacemakers vary; some will stimulate the heart all the time, others only when the heart rate makes it necessary.

represents the heart's normal response to stress on the body. Tachycardia may also be caused by the congenital presence of abnormal conducting circuits in the heart, or by damage to the heart's normal conducting system. The tachycardic pulses may originate in the atria, the AV node, or the ventricle. The nature of the tachycardia may be diagnosed by ECG, and tachycardias are usually treated medically to control the heart rate, or with the use of medications or controlled electric shocks to reset the conducting system in an effort to reestablish normal conduction (also called cardioversion).

Bradycardia refers to any condition in which the heart is beating slower than the normal rate of 60 to 100 beats per minute. Healthy individuals and conditioned athletes can have a resting heart rate as low as 40, but an abnormal bradycardia occurs when the heart rate will not increase enough to meet the body's demands for blood flow. Abnormal bradycardia may be due to a medical condition or a medication overdose but can also be the result of damage to the heart's conducting system. Bradycardias due to conducting system damage usually require a pacemaker for correction.

Coronary artery disease and angina

Coronary artery disease refers to blockage of the arteries feeding the heart by plaques composed of fat, cholesterol, calcium, platelets, fibrin, and other materials from the bloodstream. Buildup of plaque is called atherosclerosis, and over time it can gradually decrease blood flow to the heart muscle. Plaques may be located in small, peripheral arteries feeding just a small part of the heart muscle, or in the main arteries responsible for blood flow to large areas of the heart muscle. As plaque builds up, the areas of the heart muscle supplied by the affected blood vessel may first function normally. However, as the blockage increases and blood flow in the affected artery decreases, the muscle supplied by the affected artery may become starved of oxygen and nutrients, suffer damage, or die. Depending on the location and severity of blockages, an individual with coronary artery disease may have no symptoms, may have vague chest discomfort, may have angina (chest pain that is brought on with exertion and relieved with rest), or may experience a heart attack if there is significant damage to a large enough portion of the heart.

Many different risk factors can increase a person's chance of developing coronary artery disease. Some risk factors cannot be changed: increasing age, male gender, and family history and heredity. Some risk factors for coronary artery disease can be controlled, managed, or modified: tobacco smoking, high cholesterol, high blood pressure, physical inactivity, obesity, and diabetes. Stress and alcohol use are two other factors that may contribute to heart disease. To prevent heart disease, it is important for individuals to understand their risk, and it is important for all individuals to control their modifiable risk factors for heart disease (risk factors that can be changed): smoking should be avoided, and a healthy diet and regular exercise are important to control blood pressure, cholesterol, and weight.

For persons at low risk of coronary artery disease, low-density lipoprotein (LDL, or "bad") cholesterol level of 160 milligrams per deciliter (mg/dL) or less is acceptable, while those at moderate risk of coronary artery disease should try to keep the LDL cholesterol less than 130 mg/dL, and those at high risk of heart disease should try to keep the LDL cholesterol less than 100 mg/dL. Blood pressure should be kept below 140/90 for most people, while those with diabetes or chronic kidney disease should try to keep their blood pressure below 130/80. Persons with diabetes are at high risk of coronary artery disease, and should be particularly careful to control their cholesterol levels and their blood pressure, in addition to controlling blood sugar levels.

Persons with coronary artery disease may be treated medically or surgically. Medical treatment of coronary artery disease consists primarily of aggressive management of risk factors. "Statin" medications are used to reduce cholesterol levels so that the LDL cholesterol level is below 100 mg/dL; beta-blocker medications are used to reduce stress on the heart by reducing blood pressure and heart rate; angiotensin-converting enzyme inhibitor or angiotensin receptor blocker medications are used to prevent long-term damage to the heart muscle; and aspirin or another anti-platelet medication is used to reduce blood clotting and help prevent blockage of arteries. Additionally, healthy diet and adequate physical activity are important.

Surgical treatment of coronary artery disease may involve angioplasty with stenting, or coronary artery bypass grafting (CABG) to allow blood to flow around blocked arteries. Angioplasty is used if there are blockages in one or two of the main arteries in the heart. A catheter is inserted into the femoral artery (a main artery in the leg), threaded up into the heart and then into the blocked coronary artery, and a stent (a small tube) is placed in the blocked portion of the artery to reopen it and allow continued blood flow. The doctor performing the procedure guides the catheter and the stent using X-ray pictures, as is done with angiography. CABG is used to treat severe blockages or blockages of multiple main vessels. CABG involves surgically opening the chest and using a blood vessel taken from another part of the body (usually the saphenous vein from the leg) to create alternate paths around blocked coronary arteries. Patients who are treated surgically for CAD are also prescribed medications for aggressive medical management, and should follow a healthy diet and get adequate physical activity.

Diagnosis

The most basic and widely used test for evaluating the heart is the electrocardiogram (ECG). Using electrical leads attached to a patient's limbs and chest, an ECG monitor records on graph paper the electrical impulses generated each time the conducting system causes the heart to beat. The electrical impulses from each part of the cardiac cycle generate characteristic patterns, or waves, on the ECG tracing, and the size, timing, and relationship of the waves provide a snapshot of the heart's electrical function. The initial impulse from the sinus node that starts each cardiac cycle and causes the atria to contract is recorded as a small "P" wave, the "QRS" complex is a set of larger downward and upward waves generated when the ventricles contract, and the "T" wave is a smaller round wave produced when the conduction system resets itself for the next cycle. The standard ECG tracing is a "12-lead ECG," since multiple leads attached to the patient's body are used to "look" at the heart from 12 different angles. Thus, the size and direction of the P wave, the QRS wave complex, and the T wave differ from lead to lead, but their rate and pattern should be consistent throughout all 12 leads. Problems with heart function due to insufficient blood flow, abnormal heart muscle function, or abnormal heart rate or rhythm will produce characteristic changes in the pattern and timing of the ECG tracing.

A chest X-ray can provide information about heart function. On a standard chest X-ray, the width of the heart is typically less than half the width of the rib cage. Cardiomegaly (enlarged heart) is diagnosed if the width of the heart on chest X-ray is more than half the width of the rib cage, and may be due to systolic dysfunction or heart failure, or less commonly due to ventricular hypertrophy. Increased vascular markings in the lung fields can suggest pulmonary edema, which may be due to heart failure. Significant pleural effusions (collections of fluid around the lungs, often due to infection, fluid overload, or inflammation) may also suggest heart failure or fluid overload. A chest X-ray is limited by the fact that it can only show a silhouette of the heart, and nothing of the internal structure or function of the heart.

Echocardiography uses ultrasound waves to create images of the heart's internal structures, and can provide two-dimensional images of the heart's structure and function. Echocardiography allows evaluation of the size of each atrium and ventricle, and can assess whether the heart muscle is contracting in a normal organized pattern with each beat or is disorganized or simply not contracting. Echocardiography can also show the size, shape, and function of each heart valve, and can help determine the pressures in each heart chamber and whether valves are functioning properly by measuring the speed of blood flow across each valve. Lastly, echocardiography can help assess whether or not there is an effusion (fluid collection) in the pericardial sac around the heart that might indicate inflammation of the heart muscle, or that could cause tamponade and impair heart function.

Angiography is used to evaluate the anatomy of individual coronary arteries and determine whether there are plaques from coronary artery disease that could be responsible for a heart attack or anginal chest pain. An angiogram is performed by inserting a catheter through a small skin incision into one of the femoral arteries, then threading it up through the femoral artery and the aorta into the heart. The catheter is then inserted into the opening of each coronary artery one at a time, and as X-ray dye is injected into each coronary artery, continual X-ray pictures are taken that show the pattern of blood flow through the artery. The result is an X-ray "motion picture" of the heart as it pumps, demonstrating the location of any plaques and their effect on the flow of blood through arteries. Angiography is used to guide decisions about whether to treat symptomatic coronary artery disease with medical therapy, stenting, or CABG.

Stress testing allows evaluation of the heart by measuring its response to increased workload in a monitored setting. During stress testing, exercise or medications are used to increase the heart rate and the cardiac workload. The effect is assessed based on the patient's symptoms, changes observed on continuous ECG monitoring, and sometimes using radioactive (nuclear) contrast to assess bloodflow in the heart. Stress testing can be used to help diagnose the cause of chest pain or other symptoms that are suspicious for heart disease, and it can be used to reevaluate patients with known coronary artery disease to determine their exercise capacity or determine if their coronary artery disease is worsening.

Bill Cayley

Hemochromatosis

One of the most common genetic disorders in the United States, hemochromatosis involves mutations in many different genes, all of which cause the body to be overloaded with iron. The excess iron builds up in various organs, including the heart, liver, and pancreas, leading to serious tissue damage and life-threatening illness.

Iron is an essential nutrient that enables red blood cells to transport oxygen around the body. Normally, only about 10 percent of iron is absorbed from food. A deficiency of iron is fairly common, especially in women, and can cause anemia.

People with hemochromatosis have the opposite problem; they absorb much higher levels of iron than normal. Iron gradually accumulates to toxic levels and is moved into various tissues and organs, which can lead to life-threatening damage. It is not clear exactly how high iron levels damage tissue, but it is probably because of an increase in the production of highly destructive molecules called free radicals.

Causes and risk factors

Hemochromatosis is a genetic disorder that can result because of mutations in at least five different iron metabolism genes. Some of these genes produce proteins responsible for absorbing iron; others are involved in iron transport or storage. Whichever genes are affected, the outcome is always the same: the body becomes overloaded with iron. In most cases, the disease is inherited as an autosomal recessive disorder, meaning that both parents must carry a disease gene for offspring to inherit the disorder. Type 1 hemochromatosis affects about 1 million people in the United States. It is one of the most common genetic disorders, and families of northern European descent are at highest risk; the estimated carrier rate is 1 in 9 people. A rare form, type 4 hemochromatosis, is autosomal dominant. In this case, a single copy of the faulty gene is sufficient to cause disease. Another rare form of the disease, called neonatal hemochromatosis (NH), affects newborns and is usually fatal. Although the inheritance pattern of NH is uncertain, the risk of having a second child with the disorder is 80 percent in women who have had one NH baby.

Gender is an important factor in hemochromatosis. Women, who lose iron through menstruation, typically do not experience symptoms of hemochromatosis until after menopause. Men are five times more likely to develop hemochromatosis than women.

Symptoms

Hemochromatosis type 1 can go undiagnosed for many years, mainly because it has low penetrance (percentage of people with the mutation who show signs of the disease) and because its symptoms mimic so many other disorders. The most common symptoms are joint pain, abdominal pain, heart disease, and fatigue. Some people may also show darkened or

KEY FACTS

Description

A genetic disorder that results in iron overload.

Cause

A mutation in the genes involved in the absorption, transport, or storage of iron in the body.

Risk factors

People with a family history of the disease are at greatest risk. Males are at higher risk of developing symptoms early in life.

Symptoms

Joint pain, darkened skin color, fatigue, abdominal pain, or heart disease.

Diagnosis

Blood tests and a family history.

Treatments

Drawing blood every few months is usually sufficient to maintain normal iron levels.

Pathogenesis

Early diagnosis and treatment needed. Iron overload may eventually damage many organs, leading to complications such as diabetes, liver disease, heart disease, and arthritis.

Prevention

Screening is recommended for any adults with a family history of the disease, so early treatment can prevent serious organ damage.

Epidemiology

The highest rates of the disease are in people of northern European descent. In the United States, roughly 1 person in 10 is a carrier for the disease. About 0.5 percent of people in the United States are susceptible to developing the disease.

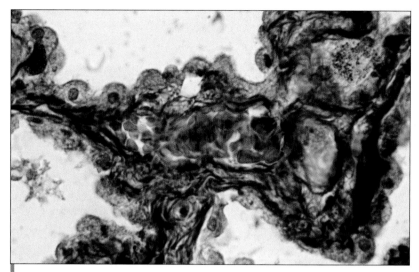

A light micrograph of a section through brain tissue shows a brown area; this patch is as a result of hemochromatosis, an excessive buildup of iron in the body.

(perform phlebotomies) until iron levels are restored to normal. It can take up to a year of weekly blood draws to return patients to a healthy iron level. After that, blood is drawn every two to four months. Blood donation may be an option; since 1999, the FDA announced that blood from patients with hemochromatosis was safe to use.

Diet is another key component used in treating hemochromatosis. The aim is to limit the consumption and absorption of iron. Eating foods that contain antioxidants (chemicals that neutralize harmful free radicals) may also be of benefit. Alcohol and large amounts of vitamin C increase absorption of iron and should be avoided. Vitamin C supplements (less than 500 milligrams per day) should be taken between meals. Reducing the amount of red meat in the diet and increasing the amount of fruits, nuts, and vegetables is recommended. Most important, anyone with hemochromatosis should never eat or touch raw shellfish. Shellfish often harbor a bacterium that can be fatal to people with iron overload.

bronzed skin tones. The vast majority of patients are not diagnosed until adulthood. In men, symptoms are most likely to appear between the ages of 30 and 50. The disease does not usually become apparent in women until they are past the age of 50.

If hemochromatosis progresses unchecked, iron overload can damage essential organs such as the heart, liver, and pancreas. Liver failure can result from scarring of the tissues (cirrhosis), and untreated hemochromatosis increases a person's risk of liver cancer. Damage to the pancreas can cause diabetes. Hemochromatosis may even affect bones and joints, leading to a type of arthritis.

Diagnosis

Laboratory tests determine the amount of iron in the blood and the level of iron in the liver. In each case, the tests measure the iron bound to iron-transporting proteins (ferritin and transferrin). If iron levels are abnormally high, genetic tests can be used to look for mutations in the most common hemochromatosis gene. These tests cannot identify mutations in the other genes linked to the disorder.

Treatments

The most important way to avoid life-threatening complications from hemochromatosis is to diagnose and treat the disorder early. Once the disease has affected organs, the damage is difficult to reverse. Treatment is simple and safe. Physicians draw blood

Prevention

Screening for hemochromatosis is controversial, because no definitive and inexpensive test is available. Blood tests can provide misleading results, and not all people with iron overload develop complications, so a positive screening test could have the effect of making it more difficult for a healthy person to get life or health insurance. On the other hand, if there is a family history of the disease, it is important to be diagnosed before symptoms develop to reduce the risk of organ damage. The American College of Physicians has reviewed the possibility of establishing routine screening for hemochromatosis, but lack of information about the risks and benefits means that screening is unlikely to be available in the near future.

Chris Curran

See also
• Diabetes • Genetic disorders • Metabolic disorders • Nervous system disorders

Hemophilia

Hemophilias are disorders of coagulation characterized by ineffective blood clotting. Hemophilia results from an inherited inability to produce sufficient amounts of one of these clotting factors. The ability of blood to clot or coagulate, that is, to turn from liquid to solid, at the site of damage to a blood vessel restricts blood loss following injury and is the initial step of wound repair.

Blood clotting is necessarily finely regulated through a large number of interacting clotting and anti-clotting plasma proteins, since excessive clotting results in vessel obstruction (thrombosis), ineffective clotting in blood loss. Deficiencies of almost all factors have been described. However, more than 95 percent concern factors VIII (Hemophilia A) and IX (Hemophilia B). Absence of factor VIII stabilizing factor (von Willebrand factor), as occurs in a rare subtype of von Willebrand's disease (type 3), causes severe depletion of factor VIII and may thus manifest with a hemophilia-like phenotype. Depending on the remaining amount of coagulation factor, mild, moderate and severe forms of hemophilia are distinguished; two-thirds of cases are severe.

In hemophilia, as a result of the clotting factor deficiency, blood does not coagulate efficiently. Severe and prolonged external and internal bleeds ensue, often without any significant trauma. Any organ can be affected by such bleeds. Blood loss can be significant, even fatal, if untreated. In addition, bleeding into organs causes damage to the organs. The joints are commonly affected, and accumulated blood leads to destruction of cartilage and joint deformation. Bleeds into the head can be rapidly fatal.

Although relatively rare, hemophilia enjoys a certain public notoriety because of its prevalence among European royalty. Queen Victoria of the United Kingdom (1819–1901) acquired and spread a de-novo mutation in her factor VIII gene, which she passed on to at least three of her children, whose own children in turn spread it through several of Europe's royal families, including those of Russia, Germany, and Spain.

Causes

Hemophilias are inherited diseases caused by mutations in any of the clotting factor genes, which lead to deficiency of that factor. Hemophilia A and B are inherited in an X-chromosomal recessive pattern, since the genes for factors VIII and IX are located on the X chromosome. This pattern of inheritance implies that for males, who have only one X chromosome, inheritance of one defective gene is sufficient to cause (almost) complete absence of this coagulation factor and thus disease. In males, the mutation may either be

KEY FACTS

Description

Hemophilias are disorders of blood clotting, manifesting as prolonged bleeding without (adequate) trauma.

Causes

Inherited deficiency of a blood clotting factor.

Risk factors

The most common types of hemophilia are inherited in an X-chromosomal recessive pattern. De-novo mutations also occur. Because of this pattern of inheritance, most hemophiliacs are male.

Symptoms

Easy bruising or bleeding, spontaneously or after minor trauma, which can affect all organs. Without prompt treatment, patients may bleed to death. Disability frequently results from repeated joint bleeds.

Diagnosis

Suspected from the clinical presentation, a blood sample is required to establish abnormal blood clotting and identify the deficient clotting factor.

Treatments

Replacement of the missing clotting factor through injection into the bloodstream is the mainstay of therapy.

Pathogenesis

A tightly regulated cascade of different interacting protein molecules (clotting factors) regulate the ability of blood to turn from liquid to solid within seconds of an injury at the site of that injury. Severe deficiency in any of the clotting factors leads to impaired clotting.

Prevention

Genetic counseling, abstention of carriers from reproduction.

Epidemiology

The two more common forms of hemophilia, A and B, occur in all races with a frequency of 1 in 5,000 and 1 in 25,000 males, respectively. Females are rarely affected.

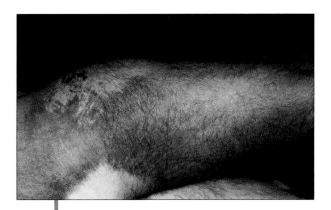

A 55-year-old hemophiliac has a large hematoma (bruise) on his leg after a fall. Because of a deficiency in clotting factors, wounds or injuries bleed into muscles and joints.

Diagnosis

The diagnosis of hemophilia may be suspected from a family or personal history of abnormal bleeding, and is established by blood tests. Absence of a relevant family history does not rule out hemophilia, since approximately 30 percent of mutations are newly acquired. After confirmation of abnormal blood clotting, in subsequent tests the individual clotting factors are quantified. Based on the residual quantity of coagulation factor, mild, moderate, and severe forms of the illness are distinguished. Patients with severe hemophilia have less than 1 percent of normal factor activity. After making the diagnosis, family genetics are frequently studied to identify carriers.

Treatments

There is currently no cure for hemophilia. The principle of hemophilia therapy is to prevent or aggressively treat bleeding. The mainstay of treatment is replacement of the deficient clotting factor by injection into the bloodstream. Lifestyle adaptations, such as avoidance of extreme or contact sports, are also generally recommended. Parental over-protection is a common problem, possibly more so than in many other chronic diseases, because mothers may feel guilty for passing on the causative "bad gene" to their sons. The need for factor injection into the bloodstream, which necessitates frequent needlesticks, adversely affects the quality of life of hemophiliacs, particularly of children, but this discomfort compares favorably with the severe disability and early death occurring in people who are not being treated with substitute clotting factors. Most patients with hemophilia learn to inject themselves and become quite expert at handling their condition in everyday life. The overall clinical management as well as treatment of emergencies belongs in the hands of specialized comprehensive care clinics, if possible. All hemophiliacs should wear emergency bracelets. Joint bleeds are addressed with high-dose factor substitution, rest or immobilization, or both, and external cooling. Head injuries are also treated with high-dose factor substitution. Imaging studies to rule out intracranial bleeds may be indicated.

Most clotting factors used for substitution today are produced in genetically modified cell lines. This has minimized the risk of blood-borne viral infections, such as HIV and hepatitis, associated with older factor preparations that were generated from human volunteer donors. Generally, individuals with less severe forms of hemophilia require factor substitution

inherited from the mother or newly acquired. Hemophilia in females is rare. In contrast to their brothers, who do not inherit a paternal X chromosome and will therefore generally be normal at the hemophilia locus, on average half the daughters of an affected father will carry the hemophilia gene and can pass it on to future generations. Half their sons will again be affected, and half their daughters will be carriers like themselves. In contrast to hemophilias A and B, and with the exception of factor XI deficiency, which follows autosomal dominant inheritance, all the other, rarer hemophilias, as well as type 3 von Willebrand's disease, are inherited in an autosomal recessive mode, that is, two faulty genes are needed to cause abnormality.

Risk factors and symptoms

Since the X-chromosomal hemophilias A and B together make up more than 95 percent of all hemophilias, most hemophiliacs are male. The frequency of factor XI deficiency is very high (around 8 percent) among Ashkenazi Jews, but it is very rare in the general population.

Hemophilia manifests as internal or external bleeding without or with minor trauma. Repetitive and prolonged nosebleeds are as much part of the picture as protracted bleeding from small wounds, bleeding after dental procedures, and bleeds into muscles or joints or any other organ in the body. A frequent cause of disability is ankle or knee joint destruction as a consequence of repeated bleeds. A particularly grave complication is spontaneous bleeding into the brain, which can cause irreversible neurological damage or even death.

INHERITANCE OF HEMOPHILIA

Hemophilia is a result of an inherited faulty gene on the X chromosome, which is inherited in a recessive way. A woman cannot develop the disease but can pass the abnormal gene to her children. Each child has a 1 in 2 chance of inheriting the gene; only boys will be affected by it.

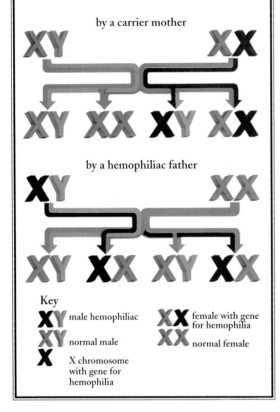

by a carrier mother

by a hemophiliac father

Key

XY male hemophiliac

XY normal male

X X chromosome with gene for hemophilia

XX female with gene for hemophilia

XX normal female

provided. Irrespective of future results from clinical studies, financial considerations—prophylactic treatment of a hemophiliac costs more than $50,000 per year—will likely remain a major obstacle to the general acceptance of this treatment. Over time a considerable number of patients develop inhibitory antibodies against the injected factor, which may make normal factor replacement ineffective. For such patients, alternative clotting agents are available. These include porcine factor VIII, activated prothrombin complex concentrate, or activated factor VII.

Several considerations, including the fact that as little as 3 to 4 percent normal activity is sufficient for near-normal function, identify hemophilia as a presumably ideal target for somatic gene therapy. Transgenic animals as sources of factor, that is, animals that are genetically engineered to produce human clotting factor, are also the subject of research.

Pathogenesis

A tightly regulated hierarchical cascade of different interacting protein molecules (clotting factors), which is activated by substances released by injured tissue, regulates the ability of blood to turn from liquid to solid within seconds of an injury. Normally, the clotting reaction is normally restricted to the site of injury. Severe deficiency in any of the clotting factors, due to genetic mutations, prevents solidification of blood, leading to easy and prolonged bleeding. Replacement of the missing factor itself or of one of its products further along the cascade allows for coagulation to occur normally.

Prevention and epidemiology

Genetic testing can identify carriers, but global screening in the absence of a relevant family history is not rational, given the low frequency of hemophilia. Abstention of known female carriers from reproduction may be recommended, but will only reduce the number of patients by two-thirds, since one-third of mutations are newly acquired by mother or child.

The two more common forms of hemophilia, A and B, occur in all races with a frequency of 1 in 5,000 and 1 in 25,000 males, respectively. Females are infrequently affected. All other forms of hemophilia are rare.

Halvard Boenig

only after injuries (most hemophiliacs keep factor concentrate in their refrigerator for self-injection) or during surgery. For around two-thirds of hemophilia patients whose disease is classified as "severe," with less than 1 percent residual factor activity, prophylactic factor repletion has been proposed as a better alternative to the on-demand regimen, to prevent pathological bleeding. Since injected clotting factors circulate for very short times, particularly in children, this necessitates frequent injection, such as thrice weekly for factor VIII or twice weekly for factor IX. Such treatment would be initiated after the first year of life and ideally continued lifelong. Many clinicians and the World Health Organization recommendations advocate this prophylactic approach, although a recent Cochrane review concludes that insufficient evidence for prophylactic factor substitution has been

See also
• Anemia • Blood disorders • Bone and joint disorders • Genetic disorders • Hepatitis infections • Von Willebrand's disease

Hepatitis infections

Infectious hepatitis is the inflammation of the liver, usually caused by one of the five hepatitis viruses: A, B, C, D, and E. In the United States viral hepatitis is most commonly due to hepatitis A virus (HAV), hepatitis B virus (HBV), and hepatitis C virus (HCV). Chronic hepatitis, especially from infection with hepatitis C virus, can lead to long-term damage of the liver (cirrhosis) and liver cancer. Vaccines are available to prevent infection with hepatitis A and B viruses.

According to the National Institutes of Health (NIH), viral hepatitis is the leading cause of liver disease in the United States and the world. The mode of transmission and the length and severity of the disease vary in the different types of viral hepatitis, but all five viruses can cause an episode of acute hepatitis. Virus types B, C, and D sometimes can cause chronic lifelong infections that can lead to cirrhosis of the liver and liver cancer.

Symptoms

Symptoms of hepatitis can include fatigue, fever, jaundice (yellowing of the skin and eyes due to bile pigments normally processed in the liver), loss of appetite, vomiting, diarrhea, dark urine, light-colored stools, and headache. In some types of hepatitis there may be no symptoms.

Diagnosis and prevention

Blood tests can be carried out to detect the presence of the virus or of antibodies and antigens that have built up in response to the virus. In some cases a liver biopsy may be done to determine whether there is hepatitis-related damage to the liver, including cirrhosis and liver cancer. There may also be imaging tests that can help assess damage. These include ultrasound, computed tomography (CT), and magnetic resonance imaging (MRI). Vaccines are available to prevent hepatitis A and hepatitis B; as yet no vaccines have been developed to prevent the other types of viral hepatitis.

Hepatitis A

Hepatitis A is caused by infection with the hepatitis A virus (HAV). In the United States, HAV is spread pri-

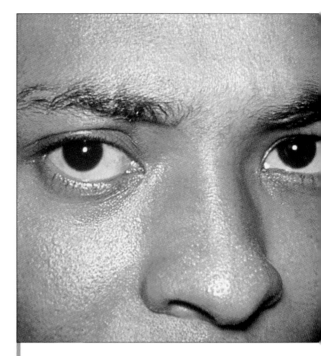

The young man above has infection with hepatitis A virus, which causes jaundice: yellowing of the conjunctiva—the white of the eyes—and facial skin due to bile pigments that are normally broken down by the liver.

marily through the fecal-oral route, whereby the virus from the stool of an infected person is swallowed by another person. This type of transmission can happen when the virus is on surfaces or hands and there is inadequate hygiene and hand washing, or from sexual contact. Localized outbreaks can occur from eating food contaminated with HAV that is uncooked, undercooked, or prepared by HAV-infected food handlers. In developing areas of the world where the water supply may be contaminated with sewage or inadequately treated, drinking water and ice, as well as food, may be contaminated. On rare occasions HAV has been transmitted through blood or blood products taken from infected donors.

Symptoms in people with HAV infection can range from none or mild to severe, and fatal cases are rare. When symptoms are present, they usually last for less than two months. In about 10 percent of people there will be relapses, which can last for as long as nine months. Often children infected with HAV have no symptoms, so they can play a large role in HAV transmission. Hepatitis A is not a long-term illness, and a single episode gives lifelong immunity against the disease. Diagnosis is made with a blood test for the hepatitis A virus.

Rates of hepatitis A in the United States have steadily declined in the last decade, from more than 31,000 reported cases in 1995 to under 6,000 cases in 2004, which is largely due to the introduction of the hepatitis A vaccine in 1995. This vaccine is the best method of prevention for hepatitis A and now is routinely recommended by the Centers for Disease Control and Prevention (CDC) for children age one to 18 years and for all people traveling to risk areas. The risk of infection when traveling outside the United States depends on the sanitary conditions and the rate of infection in the area of travel, as well as the length of the trip and the amount of time spent in rural areas where conditions may be particularly poor. While traveling in risk areas, boiling or cooking food and drinks to 185°F (85°C) for at least one minute inactivates the virus. According to the CDC, hepatitis A is the most common cause of vaccine-preventable infection acquired during travel.

In addition to the hepatitis A vaccine, hygienic measures such as hand washing after using the toilet, changing a baby's diaper, and before preparing food help prevent the spread of HAV. When a person who has not been vaccinated is exposed to the virus, a sterile injection of concentrated antibodies, called immune globulin (IG), can give some protection depending on when the exposure occurred.

Hepatitis B

Hepatitis B is spread through blood or body fluids and is a sexually transmitted virus and a global public health problem. The World Health Organization (WHO) estimates that more than 2 billion people worldwide have been infected with the hepatitis B virus (HBV), and more than 350 million have chronic lifelong infection. These people are at an increased risk of contracting cirrhosis of the liver and liver cancer, two serious disorders that kill about one million people each year.

In the United States it is estimated that more than 1.2 million people have chronic hepatitis B infection, although reported new cases have steadily declined in the United States in the last 20 years, from more than 26,000 in 1985 to 6,000 in 2004. Estimates of the number of new HBV infections have also declined, from about 260,000 each year in the 1980s to about 60,000 in 2004. The highest rate of decline occurred

in children and adolescents, which was a result of the introduction of the hepatitis B vaccine in 1982. Since 2004 more than 90 percent of children aged 19 to 35 months and more than 50 percent of all 13- to 15-year olds have been fully vaccinated with three

KEY FACTS

Description

Inflammation of the liver due to infectious agents that cause acute (short-term) health problems or chronic (long-term) effects.

Causes

The most common cause is infection with one of the five hepatitis viruses: A, B, C, D, or E. In the United States hepatitis viruses A, B, and C are the most common.

Risk factors

For hepatitis virus types A and E, transmission is via the fecal-oral route, which involves fecal contamination of food and water; for hepatitis virus types B, C, and D, spread is through blood or body fluids from an infected person. An infected mother can pass the infection to her baby in the uterus.

Symptoms and signs

These range from none to severe, including fever, flulike illness, jaundice (yellowing of skin and eyes), abdominal pain, nausea, vomiting, poor appetite, and dark urine.

Diagnosis

Blood tests to detect the specific type of hepatitis; liver function tests; biopsy.

Treatment

Depends on infectious agent and ranges from none to a shot of a drug called immune globulin, which increases antibodies against the virus; antiviral drugs are given for hepatitis types B and C.

Pathogenesis

All five viruses can cause acute hepatitis, in which liver cells become inflamed. Hepatitis virus types B, C, and D can cause chronic hepatitis and may result in cirrhosis and liver cancer.

Prevention

Vaccines are available for types A and B. For types B, C, and D, avoid contact with blood or bodily fluids of an infected person; to avoid types A and E, use clean water and practice hand washing, safe food handling and preparation, and general personal hygiene.

Epidemiology

Rates of reported cases have been declining for hepatitis A, B, and C in the last decade. Type E is rare in the United States, and type D only occurs in people with type B.

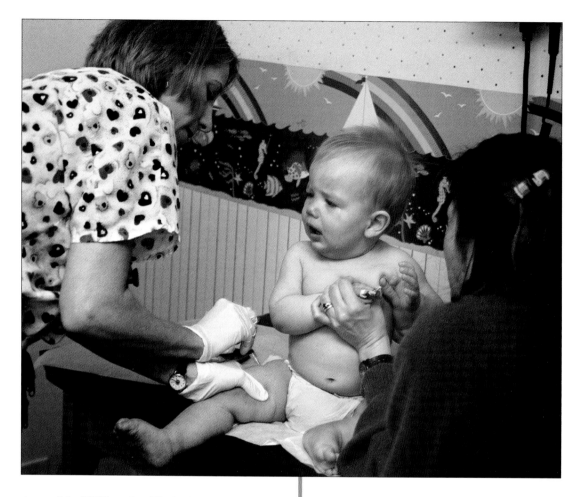

doses of the HBV vaccine. The highest rate of hepatitis B is in the 20- to 49-year age group.

HBV is transmitted through contact with the blood or body fluids of infected people in the same way that the human immunodeficiency virus (HIV), the virus that causes AIDS, is spread—although HBV is about 100 times more infectious. Risk factors include sex with HBV-infected partners; sex with multiple partners; sex with a partner with a diagnosed sexually transmitted disease; men who have sex with men; intravenous drug use; everyday household contact with an infected person; infants born to infected mothers; patients who have hemodialysis for kidney failure; and hospital workers.

Most infants and children with hepatitis B never develop symptoms or signs, and most newly infected adults recover fully from hepatitis B, even though symptoms can be severe. However, when an acute episode does occur, it progresses to a chronic, long-term infection in 30 to 90 percent of infants and children and 6 to 10 percent of adolescents and adults.

In recent years the incidence of hepatitis A and B infections in children has dropped greatly in the United States, due to the introduction of routine vaccination against hepatitis A in 1995 and hepatitis B in 1982.

There are several diagnostic blood tests for hepatitis B. These include a test to check liver function; a test for antigens that indicate current infection; and a test for antibodies that indicates recovery from a prior infection or response to the vaccine. If chronic infection is suspected, a liver biopsy may be performed to establish the extent of the disease. Blood and screening tests may also be carried out to detect the early stages of liver cancer, which can be a complication of chronic infection.

In the United States and many other developed countries, it is now routinely recommended that children and teenagers be vaccinated, as well as people in high-risk groups and people traveling to areas of the world where there is a high rate of HBV. It is also recommended that all pregnant women be screened for HBV. Treatment for chronic hepatitis B includes antiviral drugs. In severe cases a liver transplant may be carried out.

Hepatitis C

The WHO estimates that around 180 million people, or three percent of the world's population, are infected with hepatitis C virus (HCV), and 130 million are chronic carriers at risk of going on to developing cirrhosis of the liver and liver cancer. Each year more than 3 million people are infected with HCV, for which there is no vaccine.

In the United States it is estimated that more than 4 million people, which is about 1.6 percent of the population, have been infected with HCV, and of these more than 3 million have chronic infection. Although the estimated number of new infections each year has decreased from about 240,000 in the 1980s to 26,000 in 2004, HCV infection is sometimes called "a viral time bomb," as about 80 percent of newly infected people have no symptoms and if symptoms do occur they are usually mild. Chronic HCV infection, which progresses slowly over the years, develops in about 75 to 85 percent of infected people with the most common symptom being general fatigue. HCV infection occurs in about one-quarter of all people infected with HIV. This combination can cause higher levels of HCV in the blood and a more rapid progression to liver disease, so all HIV infected people should be screened for HCV.

Like HBV infection, hepatitis C infection is transmitted through virus-contaminated blood. The biggest risk factor is the use of intravenous drugs, which accounts for about 90 percent of cases. Cases associated with blood transfusion or organ transplant occurred before 1992 when screening for HCV began. Although the virus can be sexually transmitted, this is much less common than it is for HBV. A pregnant mother with HCV can pass the virus to her baby, usually while it is in the uterus. Sixty to 70 percent of people with chronic HCV infection develop chronic liver disease, and 1 to 5 percent of people with chronic liver disease die from cirrhosis or liver cancer. According to the CDC, chronic HCV infection is the leading cause of liver transplants in the United States.

HBV is diagnosed by blood tests to check the liver function, and to look for the virus and antibodies to the virus. Unlike many other infections, the presence of antibodies in the blood does not mean that the infection has cleared. Chronic infection is usually treated with a form of an antiviral medication called interferon for several months or longer in combination with another drug. In some people, this helps clear the virus from the liver. Imaging scans may be taken, and a liver biopsy, in which a sample of liver is removed and analyzed, may be carried out to check the progression of the disease.

Hepatitis D

Hepatitis D virus (HDV) is a defective virus that only occurs in people who already have HBV. The WHO estimates that there are more than 10 million people worldwide infected with HDV, although it is thought that the rate of infection in the United States is low. The risk factors and modes of transmission for HDV are the same as for HBV, although the virus is spread more easily by needle transmission and is less likely to be passed on by way of sexual contact, and transmission from a mother to her baby is rare.

When HBV and HDV infect a person simultaneously, it is called coinfection; when HDV infects a person who already has chronic HBV infection, it is called superinfection. In coinfection there is a greater chance of severe acute hepatitis and liver failure and a lower risk of chronic HBV infection. In superinfection there is a greater chance of developing chronic HDV infection, which can progress to chronic liver disease and cirrhosis. Hepatitis B vaccine can prevent coinfection, and chronic HDV infection can be treated with antiviral drugs and, if needed, a liver transplant.

Hepatitis E

Hepatitis E virus (HEV) is transmitted by the fecal-oral route through virus-contaminated drinking water or food. Person-to-person transmission is uncommon. HEV infection usually affects young adults and does not cause chronic infection, but can cause a life-threatening form of hepatitis in pregnant women in their third trimester, with death in about 20 percent of cases. Reported cases of hepatitis E in the United States are rare, with outbreaks more common in developing countries with poor sanitation. There is no vaccine for hepatitis E, and the best way to prevent infection is with a clean water supply, avoiding potentially contaminated water, ice, and food, and practicing good hygiene.

Ramona Jenkin

See also
AIDS • Cancer, liver • Cirrhosis of the liver • Infections, viral • Liver and spleen disorders • Prevention • Sexually transmitted diseases

Hernia

The word *hernia* is a Latin term that refers to tissue or an organ in the body pushing through a weak area. In reference to modern medicine, "hernia" is often caused by a weakness of the abdominal wall that allows abdominal contents to protrude from their normal positions outward. This protrusion relates to a visible or otherwise noticeable bulge beyond the point of herniation.

There are many types and causes of hernias, but certain regions of the abdomen are weaker than others and more likely to cause hernias. Hernias result from either a failure of the abdominal wall to close properly during development as a fetus, or more commonly, weakening and enlargement of a defect in the abdominal wall musculature. However, hernias can also occur elsewhere in the body. Examples include hiatus hernia (in which part of the stomach pushes upward through the diaphragm) and hernias in invertebral disks (slipped disk), in the brain as a result of compression by a hematoma, and in the eyelids.

Inguinal hernias

The most common location for hernias to form is in the area of the inguinal canal, leading to what is commonly referred to as a "groin hernia." Other common areas for hernias to develop are at the base of the umbilicus and within the scar tissue of a prior surgical incision.

Visible or painful bulges at the juncture of the lower abdomen and the top of the scrotum in men are typical symptoms in patients who have developed an inguinal hernia. Although identical hernias can also occur in women, they are more common in men as a result of a larger abdominal wall defect present in men that allows passage of the spermatic cord from the abdomen to the testicle. The spermatic cord contains a testicular artery and veins that supply the testicle, as well as the vas deferens, which allows passage of mature spermatozoa from the testicle to the seminal vesicles and prostate within the pelvic cavity. Since the spermatic cord that passes through the inguinal canal is larger in men than the round ligament that passes through the inguinal canal in women, men are more likely than women to develop hernias.

The inguinal canal is a complex anatomical area in the lower abdomen situated between muscular layers of the abdominal wall. The integrity of the anterior abdominal wall is maintained principally by three separate muscle layers. The outermost muscle layer is the external abdominal oblique muscle, the middle layer is

the internal abdominal oblique muscle, and the innermost layer is the transversus abdominus muscle. Toward the midline of the abdominal wall, the connective tissues associated with these three muscles, or fascia, fuse into a two-layered sheath containing the rectus abdominus muscle that connects the lower rib cage to the pubic bone. In the lower abdomen a window, known as the internal inguinal ring, below the transversus abdominus and internal abdominal oblique muscles allows passage of the spermatic cord

KEY FACTS

Description
Weaknesses or ruptures of the abdominal wall that allow abdominal contents to protrude.

Causes
Hernias develop at sites of natural defects and weaknesses in the abdominal muscles, which enlarge further when repetitively stressed.

Risk factors
The male gender, chronic coughing, straining, and heavy lifting.

Symptoms
Vague discomfort associated with a bulge in the inguinal region or in the scrotum.

Diagnosis
Physical examination.

Treatments
Surgery.

Pathogenesis
Anatomical weaknesses in the abdominal muscles allow passage of structures to and from the testicle. Repetitive activities increase intra-abdominal pressure, and enlargement of these defects allows hernias to form.

Prevention
Proper lifting techniques may reduce the risk.

Epidemiology
In the United States, 700,000 hernias are repaired annually. Hernias are the most common cause of bowel obstructions in the world.

STRANGULATED HERNIA

Hernias can be pushed back and kept in place with a surgical truss until surgical intervention eliminates the danger of strangulation.

This strangulated hernia has caused part of the intestine (orange) to burst through the abdominal wall. If the neck of the hernia is tight, arterial blood can pass through, but venous blood cannot get back out. Swelling may cause the blood supply to be cut off, leading to a danger of gangrene. Only surgery can prevent this outcome.

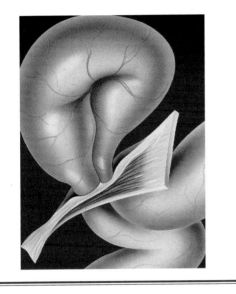

(or round ligament in females) out of the abdomen and into the inguinal canal.

Chronic increases in abdominal pressure, from persistent coughing, straining, or heavy lifting, pushes abdominal contents, such as the small bowel or colon, through the naturally occurring defects of the inguinal canal that enlarge with time and allow hernias to form. In other cases, the inguinal floor represents an area of relative weakness of the abdominal wall. This may become disrupted and allow herniation of abdominal contents through a defect that does not occur naturally. In either case, the protrusion of bowel or other abdominal contents in the inguinal region is perceived by the patient as a noticeable, and sometimes painful, bulge.

Surgical treatment

Inguinal hernias are defects for which the only available treatment is a surgical operation. Numerous approaches to hernia repair have been employed in the past, and they continue to evolve. All types of repair involve strengthening the floor of the inguinal canal and tightening the internal inguinal ring. These procedures ei-

ther pull the lower abdominal wall muscles down toward the pelvic bone or reinforce the area with a sheet of synthetic material.

Umbilical hernia

Another common location for hernias is at the base of the umbilicus. In contrast to most inguinal hernias, which develop later in life, umbilical hernias are frequently present at birth and fail to close spontaneously. During development, the entire small bowel protrudes through a large abdominal wall defect that is centered at the umbilicus. As development progresses and the fetus grows, the bowel returns to the abdominal cavity and the abdominal wall closes. The last area to close is at the base of the umbilicus. When this area fails to close completely, a hernia is present. Treatment of an umbilical hernia depends on the age of the patient. Children younger than five will be observed because the hernia may close spontaneously in the early years of life. After the age of five, however, the likelihood of a spontaneous closure diminishes, and surgical repair with sutures or synthetic material is recommended.

Incisional hernia

A third common area for hernias to occur in the abdominal wall is through a prior incision. After six weeks of healing, muscle layers of an incision approach their maximal strength, which is about 80 percent as strong as the muscle layers prior to the incision. The resulting weakness represents an area of potential herniation as subsequent increases in abdominal pressure, from straining, heavy lifting, or chronic coughing may encourage scar tissue to reopen. As with other types of hernias, an incisional hernia is identified by the presence of a bulge under the incision, particularly when the patient is straining. Surgical repair is recommended.

Incarceration

With hernias the bowel can protrude through the abdominal wall defect and become stuck or incarcerated. Hernias that can be pushed back into the abdomen, or reduced, are not threatening, but hernias that cannot be reduced are surgical emergencies. The blood supply of incarcerated bowel may be restricted, resulting in death of the bowel, which is life threatening and must be urgently treated surgically if the patient is to survive.

Chadrick Denlinger

See also
- Digestive system disorders • Muscle system disorders

Herpes infections

Herpes is a common and usually mild but contagious infection caused by herpes simplex viruses (HSV). HSV can cause repeated outbreaks of blisters and sores on the skin in the area of the genitals or mouth. Unlike many other viral infections, HSV sets up a lifelong hidden presence in the body with recurring outbreaks in or near the area of the original infection when the virus is reactivated.

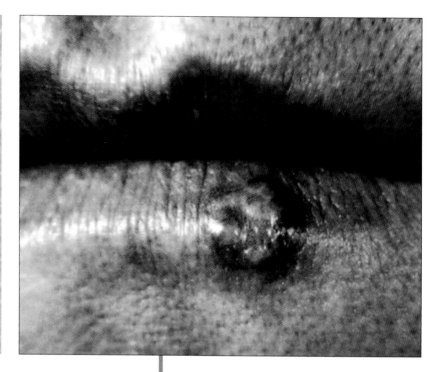

The herpes simplex virus causes painful blisters, usually affecting the mouth and nose, although they can also appear on the cheeks or chin. An attack usually clears up after about 7 to 10 days, but herpes can recur at any time.

According to the National Institutes of Health (NIH), most people in the United States have been infected with oral herpes by the age of 20. Oral herpes is commonly contracted at a young age, by a kiss from a person with oral herpes or from other physical contact, such as in a day care setting, or by sharing utensils, razors, and towels. The Centers for Disease Control and Prevention (CDC) estimates that at least 45 million people in the United States have genital herpes infection, a sexually transmitted disease that is most common in women.

Causes and risk factors

There are two viruses that can cause what is commonly known as herpes: herpes simplex virus type 1 (HSV-1) and herpes simplex virus type 2 (HSV-2). Generally, oral herpes infections, cold sores or fever blisters in the mouth area, are caused by HSV-1. HSV-2 more frequently causes sores in the genital area (genital herpes), although HSV-1 is thought to cause as much as 30 percent of all first-time genital herpes episodes. Another type, HSV-6, tends to affect infants and may be a factor in causing chronic fatigue syndrome.

The risk of contracting genital herpes increases with an increased number of sexual partners, sexual activity starting before age 17, a history of sexually transmitted diseases, HIV infection, multiple sexual partners, and a partner diagnosed with genital HSV infection.

Another virus in the herpes family is varicella-zoster virus, which causes chicken pox. After chicken pox infection, the varicella-zoster virus hides in nerve cells and can be reactivated later in life to cause what is commonly called shingles, a painful outbreak of blisters on the skin. Epstein-Barr virus, which causes mononucleosis, or glandular fever, also belongs to the herpes family.

Symptoms and signs

In genital herpes, symptoms vary greatly from none to severe painful blisters, with fever and flulike symptoms and swollen glands in the groin area. Blisters containing the contagious virus turn into painful ulcers and deep sores in the buttocks, rectum, penis, scrotum, vagina, or cervix, and can make urination painful. Lymph nodes in the groin may swell. However, according to the NIH, more than 80 percent of people in the United States who have genital herpes are not aware of their infection because they have mild symptoms or no symptoms, and may unknowingly infect sexual partners.

In young children a first episode of oral HSV can result in painful blisters and sores inside the mouth on the hard palate (roof of the mouth) and the gums, and lymph nodes in the neck may swell. The child may have a fever and feel ill, but usually recovers in 7 to 14 days. However, as in genital herpes, many people with oral herpes never have symptoms, and the NIH estimates that only 20 to 40 percent of people with oral herpes have recurrent outbreaks as adults. The classic symptom is a single blister or cluster of blisters on the lips or mouth, but they can appear on the nose, cheeks, or chin. A mild infection can appear as a crack or chapped lips or may be mistaken for a bug bite. There may be tingling or pain in the area before the sore breaks out, during which time the virus is already contagious. After blisters form, they crust over and may become itchy as they heal; they usually recur in the same location.

The most noticeable symptoms of herpes infection are usually found in people who have only recently been infected because they do not yet have an immune response to the virus. In recurrent episodes the body's immune response recognizes the virus and responds to it, so the symptoms are usually much milder.

Diagnosis and treatments

A clinical examination can be useful if a typical outbreak with blisters is present, but this is not usually the case. Furthermore, other sexually transmitted infections cause sores in the genital area that can look similar to herpes sores. Viral cultures, in which a swab is taken from a blister or sore and a culture is grown in a laboratory to identify the virus, become less sensitive as the sores heal, but if successful they can distinguish between HSV-1 and HSV-2. Special blood tests can measure the presence of the different HSV antibodies that form in the first few weeks after the first infection, which can be helpful, especially if the viral culture was taken too late and is negative. Since almost all HSV-2 is sexually transmitted, a positive HSV-2 antibody blood test strongly indicates a genital infection. Even though about 30 percent of all new genital outbreaks may be due to HSV-1, recurrent episodes of genital herpes are more likely to be due to HSV-2.

There is no cure for herpes. Cold sores usually heal without treatment in 7 to 10 days. Special medica-

tions, called antivirals, can shorten the duration of an outbreak of genital herpes. When antiviral medication is used to prevent frequent outbreaks, the treatment is called suppressive therapy, although this does not kill the virus or change the frequency or severity of outbreaks once the medication is stopped. Using special

KEY FACTS

Description
Lifelong infection caused by two viruses (HSV-1 and HSV-2) that can cause recurrent episodes of blisters on the mouth, face, genitals, or both.

Cause
Infection with the herpes simplex virus.

Risk factors
Skin-to-skin contact, kissing, and sexual contact. For genital herpes infection the risk increases with an increased number of sexual partners, sexual activity starting before age 17, a history of sexually transmitted diseases, HIV infection, multiple sex partners, and a partner diagnosed with genital herpes simplex virus infection.

Symptoms
Most people are unaware that they are infected with herpes simplex virus, as many have no symptoms. Some have outbreaks with recurrent blisters, painful sores, and flulike symptoms. The blisters are located in the genitals or mouth area.

Diagnosis
Clinical examination; viral culture; antibody blood test.

Treatment
No cure. Antiviral medication during breakouts, or suppressive therapy. Local treatment to ease discomfort of sores.

Pathogenesis
After the first infection, herpes simplex virus sets up a lifelong presence in the body by traveling into and remaining in nerve tissue, and later reactivating, causing an outbreak. It can "shed" and infect others even when there are no symptoms.

Prevention
Avoid skin-to-skin contact if blisters or other symptoms are present. Abstinence from sex; long-term monogamous sexual relationship with uninfected partner. To prevent infection in newborns it is necessary to ensure there is no active genital infection in the mother during delivery, or a Caesarean delivery may be necessary.

Epidemiology
At least 45 million people in the United States are thought to have genital herpes infection, and it is estimated that more than half of all adults in the United States have oral herpes infection.

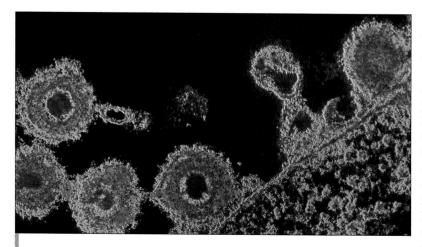

This colored transmission electron micrograph shows a recently discovered strain (HSV-6) of the herpes simplex virus, which may cause chronic fatigue syndrome.

mild soaps to keep the infected area clean, or using ice or warmth, may decrease pain. Rarely, herpes infections can be severe enough to need hospitalization.

Pathogenesis and transmission

HSV enters the body through skin or the soft mucous membranes and multiplies in the skin in the infected area. When the infection heals, the virus leaves the skin and travels along the sensory nerve to its root and remains in the ganglia, a bundle of nerve cells that supply the area of skin where the infection took place. The herpes virus sets up a lifelong presence in the nerve, lying dormant (asleep) and hidden for a period of time. When it is reactivated, the virus travels through the nerve and back to the skin site of the original infection, where it can cause blisters and sores, or it "sheds" (is released through the skin) without symptoms. Reactivation of the virus may be triggered by fever, menstruation, emotional stress, or a suppressed immune system, but often the trigger is unknown.

Genital herpes is easily spread through sexual contact, which can be genital-to-genital or oral-to-genital, either during an outbreak, during or just before an outbreak, or even when there are no blisters, sores, or symptoms, but the virus sheds.

Oral herpes can be transmitted through kissing, oral-genital contact, or other skin-to-skin contact involving the area of the sores, even before they break out. HSV can also be transmitted to other parts of the body, to a finger, for example, when it touches the infected genital area. The finger can then touch and infect other parts of the body like the eye, causing a severe infection.

Usually herpes infection is not dangerous in healthy people. Some people may have severe or prolonged symptoms, or the infection may be in the eye; in these cases a doctor should be consulted. In people with immune system problems herpes symptoms can be more severe. Having genital herpes makes it easier to transmit or acquire HIV, the virus that causes AIDS.

Active genital herpes infection in pregnant women at the time of birth increases the risk of transmission to the newborn as it passes through the birth canal. The risk is higher for women who have a first episode of genital herpes during pregnancy than for women with a history of genital herpes.

Usually, babies of mothers who have active genital herpes are delivered by Caesarean section to reduce the transmission risk. Herpes infection in newborns can be very serious and is almost always treated with antiviral medications.

Prevention

Herpes is a widespread and contagious infection. Prevention may be difficult, especially since most people with HSV-1 and HSV-2 are unaware that they are infected and, even for those who are aware, there may be periods of shedding even when they have no symptoms. The surest way to avoid sexual transmission of genital herpes is to abstain from sex, or to be engaged in a long-term monogamous sexual relationship with an uninfected partner.

People with outbreaks or symptoms should not engage in sex with uninfected partners. Condoms do not always cover the genital areas that may be infected or areas that harbor the infection, so they may not prevent transmission, even with correct and regular use. Daily suppressive antiviral medication can help reduce transmission to sexual partners.

Ramona Jenkin

See also
- Chickenpox and shingles • Infections
- Infections, viral • Prevention • Sexually transmitted diseases

Hodgkin's disease

Hodgkin's disease, or Hodgkin's lymphoma, was first recognized in 1832 by Thomas Hodgkin. Hodgkin's disease is a kind of cancer that originates in lymphatic systems, which are part of the body's immune system.

Hodgkin's disease, in most cases, originates in lymph nodes, especially those in the upper body, such as the chest, the neck, and under the arms.

There are two main types of Hodgkin's disease: the classical type and nodular predominant type. The exact causes of Hodgkin's disease are not yet known, and no major risk factors for the disease have been discovered. However, a few factors, including age, sex, infections, and certain medical conditions such as low immunity, seem to be linked to the disease.

According to the National Cancer Institute (NCI), Hodgkin's disease occurs more often in males than females, and it often occurs in early adulthood (between 15 and 34) and late adulthood (after 55).

According to research done by the American Cancer Society (ACS), people who have had infectious mononucleosis, which is an infection caused by the Epstein-Barr virus, tend to have a higher chance of contracting Hodgkin's disease. People with lower immunity also tend to have higher rates of contracting Hodgkin's disease.

According to the ACS, death rates of Hodgkin's disease have decreased by more than 60 percent since the 1970s. Chemotherapy, radiation therapy, and surgery are, currently, the three main types of treatment for patients with Hodgkin's disease. Chemotherapy uses chemical drugs to stop the growth of cancer cells by killing the cancer cells or by stopping them from dividing. Chemotherapy can be administered orally or by injection, and it can also be placed directly in the areas where cancer cells are found. Radiation therapy uses high energy X-rays to kill the cancer cells. Radiation therapy is either external or internal. External therapy uses a machine outside the body to kill cancer cells, whereas internal therapy uses needles or wires inserted inside the body to kill the cancer cells. Chemotherapy and radiation therapy are often combined in the treatment of Hodgkin's disease. Cancer cells and tissues can also be removed surgically. However, all the treatments for Hodgkin's disease, especially radiation therapy, have significant adverse effects.

Although Hodgkin's disease can strike both adults and children, the treatment for each can be different. For children who are still growing, radiation therapy is generally used with great caution because the radiation could affect bone and muscle growth. Because children tend to tolerate chemotherapy better than adults, doctors often prefer chemotherapy to radiation therapy to treat childhood Hodgkin's disease.

Clinical studies of new types of treatment for Hodgkin's disease, such as high-dose chemotherapy and radiation therapy with stem cell transplant, are ongoing. Because the causes are unknown and the main risk factors are not yet clear, it is currently very difficult to prevent Hodgkin's disease.

Y. Wang

KEY FACTS

Description
A type of cancer originating in lymphatic tissues.

Causes
The exact causes are unknown.

Risk factors
Age, sex, infection, and some medical conditions.

Symptoms
Enlarged lymph nodes, trouble breathing, fever, night sweats, itchy skin, and weight loss.

Diagnosis
Physical exam, biopsy, thoracentesis, chest X-ray, and CT scan.

Treatments
Chemotherapy, radiation therapy, and surgery.

Pathogenesis
Hodgkin's disease can form almost anywhere and can spread through the lymphatic vessels.

Prevention
Because the causes and risk factors of Hodgkin's diseases are not clear, it is very difficult to prevent the disease.

Epidemiology
Hodgkin's disease can strike adults and children. It often occurs between 15 and 34 years of age and late adulthood (older than 55 years of age). About 10 to 15 percent of cases are found in children 16 years old or younger.

See also
- Cancer • Immune system disorders
- Lymphoma

Hormonal disorders

Hormones play a critical role in maintaining the physiological balance of all the systems of the body. A hormone is a chemical messenger that circulates in the bloodstream and can move from one organ to another, that is, hormones are released from cells in one organ for delivery to distant cells of another organ. The target or destination cells receive hormonal signals through receptors, interpret the signals, and respond through a variety of biochemical changes. Hormones are responsible for a wide range of biological activities involving growth, development, reproduction, sexual characteristics, regulation of body fluids, and energy use and storage. The endocrine system consists of hormones and their associated glands and organs; the study of this system is called endocrinology.

Hormonal disorders occur when there is an imbalance in the endocrine system. Often hormone or endocrine disorders are caused by abnormal quantities or by the quality of the hormones. Quantitatively, there may be too much, too little, or no hormone at all, while qualitatively, the hormone may be biochemically abnormal. In addition, if there is a problem at the level of the receptor (for example, the receptor does not bind its corresponding hormone, a receptor does not communicate hormone signals to the cell, or a receptor binds too many similar hormones), a hormone disorder can develop. Hormone disorders can affect people of all ages, from newborns to the elderly. For example, children who have stunted growth may have a growth hormone disorder, while elderly individuals who cannot regulate their blood sugar may have an insulin hormone disorder. Thus, hormone disorders are not age or gender specific.

Glands and organs of the endocrine system

In the endocrine system, both glands and organs secrete and receive hormones. A gland is an organ that specifically produces hormones, and an organ is a group of tissues that perform a specific function or group of functions. The major glands of the endocrine system are the hypothalamus, the pituitary gland, the thyroid gland, the parathyroid glands, the islets of the pancreas, the adrenal glands, the testes in men, and the ovaries in women. In addition, during pregnancy, the placenta functions as an endocrine gland. Each of these glands produces one or more specific hormones. The major organs of the endocrine system are spread throughout the body and include the liver, kidney, stomach, pancreas, small intestine, skin, testes, ovaries, and placenta. Through this system, hormones can communicate with glands and organs all over the body and can have a powerful effect on the body. Therefore, when an imbalance causes a hormonal disorder, the impact is similarly potent.

Signs and symptoms

Symptoms of hormone disorders depend upon the affected tissue. However, general symptoms may include weight loss or weight gain, increased fatigue, darkening or thickening of the skin, increase or decrease in body hair, change in libido or sexual functioning, changes in mood or personality, and increased thirst, hunger, or urination. Specific symptoms may indicate the type of hormone disorder that is present. For example, frequent urination accompanied by abnormal thirst may be the first signs that the regulation of blood sugar in the body is abnormal. If facial features become coarse, and the hands and feet enlarge, this may indicate a dysfunction of growth hormone. Decreased energy, slow heart rate, dry skin, and feeling cold all the time may be symptoms of a dysfunction in the thyroid

RELATED ARTICLES

Adrenal disorders vol. 1, p. 18	**Metabolic disorders** vol. 2, p. 570
Diabetes vol. 1, p. 257	**Pancreatic disorders** vol. 3, p. 656
Growth disorders vol. 2, p. 386	**Parathyroid disorders** vol. 3, p. 661
Immune system disorders vol. 2, p. 443	**Thyroid disorders** vol. 3, p. 847

HORMONES AND THE ENDOCRINE SYSTEM

The endocrine system is a group of glands concerned with the secretion of hormones into the bloodstream. Those hormones regulate many of the important mechanisms in the body. The pituitary secretes stimulating hormones that regulate many of the glands. If too much or too little hormone is produced by a particular gland, a feedback mechanism comes into operation. High or low levels of hormone are regulated by an area of the brain called the hypothalamus, which produces its own hormones to influence the pituitary to modify its output of stimulating hormones and thus restore the balance. The pituitary influences the thyroid, the adrenals, and the gonads. The pituitary gland produces prolactin, oxytocin, antidiuretic hormone, and growth hormone.

The pituitary plays a major part in the endocrine system. In addition to producing several pituitary hormones, it stimulates other glands to produce hormones.

COLOR CODE
Purple: pituitary hormones influencing body directly
Red: pituitary hormones influencing other glands
Yellow, orange, and brown: hormone production controlled by pituitary
Gray, green, blue: hormones produced independently

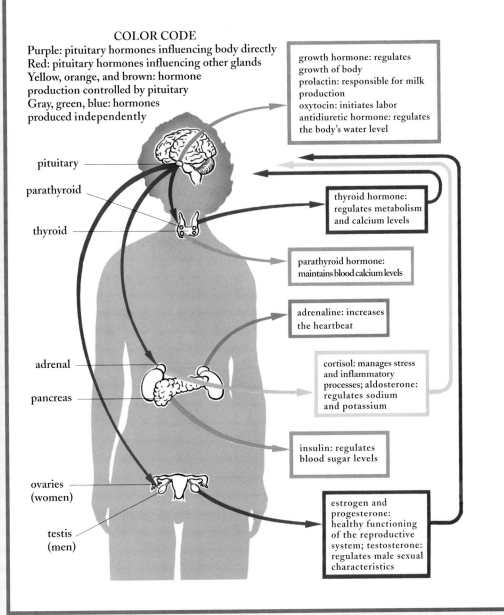

growth hormone: regulates growth of body
prolactin: responsible for milk production
oxytocin: initiates labor
antidiuretic hormone: regulates the body's water level

pituitary

parathyroid

thyroid

thyroid hormone: regulates metabolism and calcium levels

parathyroid hormone: maintains blood calcium levels

adrenaline: increases the heartbeat

adrenal

pancreas

cortisol: manages stress and inflammatory processes; aldosterone: regulates sodium and potassium

insulin: regulates blood sugar levels

ovaries (women)

testis (men)

estrogen and progesterone: healthy functioning of the reproductive system; testosterone: regulates male sexual characteristics system. Hormone replacement therapy will control the symptoms of most endocrine disorders, but most treatments must be continued throughout life. Specifics of each disorder will be discussed at length below.

Biology of hormone action and disorders

In general, hormones are secreted in response to behavioral or biological changes. For example, a behavioral trigger of the endocrine system occurs when a meal is eaten and the hormone insulin is released to metabolize sugar from food. A biological change occurs during puberty when the endocrine system is triggered to release sex hormones for growth and development. All hormones exert their effects through their receptors. Hormones are released into the bloodstream, where they circulate until they find their respective receptors. Target organs have specific receptors on either the surface of cells or inside the cells. Hormones bind to their receptors causing changes in growth, development, and metabolism. There are two kinds of hormones that work through different kinds of receptors: protein hormones and steroid hormones.

Protein hormones, sometimes known as peptide hormones, bind to receptors on the surface of cells. Binding causes receptors to undergo conformational changes that charge different enzymes to become active. Enzymes catalyze (stimulate) a variety of biochemical reactions in the cell, and most enzymes shuttle between states that are catalytically active versus inactive, or "on" versus "off." Binding of hormone to receptor turns enzymes on by using a system of second messengers (the hormone is the first messenger). The second messengers then trigger a series of molecular interactions that alter the physiological state of the cell responding to the original message of the hormone. After a hormone has bound to its receptor, it must be destroyed so that it does not overstimulate the system. In many cases, the receptor and hormone are internalized into the cell, where they are destroyed. Another term used to describe this entire process is *signal transduction*. This process can be illustrated by describing the action of glucagon. Glucagon is an important hormone in carbohydrate metabolism. It binds to its receptor on the surface of liver cells and activates adenylate cyclase, a common second messenger. Through a series of other

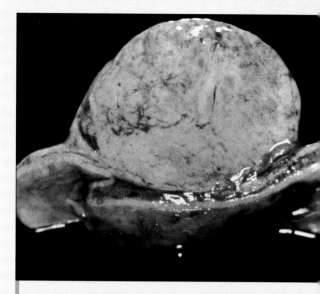

A benign adenoma has distorted this adrenal gland. That type of growth may lead to under- or overproduction of the hormone cortisol, which is produced by the adrenal gland.

biochemical reactions, multiple enzymes are activated and the cell has been changed. The result is the release of glucose so that the body has energy. Because protein hormones cause activation of several enzymes, a seemingly small change induced by hormone-receptor binding can lead to widespread consequences within the cell.

Receptors for steroid hormones are located inside the cell. Because steroids are lipids, they readily diffuse through the membranes of the cell to find their receptors in the cytosol (fluid around the nucleus) or the nucleus. Like protein hormones, steroid hormones change their receptors. The new hormone-receptor complex is changed in a way that allows them to bind with DNA at specific sites. By binding with these elements, the hormone-receptor complex becomes a transcription factor that controls whether a gene is transcribed (synthesizes RNA) or inhibited. For example, multiple hormones from the thyroid bind to their receptors in a variety of brain cells. Thyroid hormones diffuse through the plasma membrane, find their receptors, and bind to thyroid response elements in DNA to stimulate or inhibit transcription of genes that regulate the metabolism of the entire body.

Depending on the hormones and receptors, there are a number of variations on the themes described above. These variations account for many hormone disorders. Hormone disorders are the result of too much, too little, or no hormone at all. The amount of receptors available for binding can create an imbalance in a system and lead to illness. If a receptor is in some way dysfunctional, the binding of hormone may not have any impact. Also, if a steroid hormone is unable to disengage from its receptor at the level of DNA transcription, continual stimulation can lead to cancers and hormone disorders.

As mentioned earlier, hormone disorders can originate from various points within a particular part of the endocrine system and depend upon the affected tissues. Major types of hormonal disorders include diabetes, acromegaly, thyroid hormone disorders, and Cushing's syndrome.

Diabetes mellitus

Diabetes mellitus is a disease in which the body does not produce or properly use insulin. The hormone insulin is required to convert sugar, starches, and other food into energy needed for daily life. Insulin is secreted by the pancreas, which is a large gland behind the stomach. Diabetes is thus a hormonal disorder originating in the pancreas, but the disease has a wide impact on the whole body.

The imbalance of insulin results in varying or persistent hyperglycemia (high blood sugar levels). The most common kinds of diabetes mellitus are type 1, type 2, gestational diabetes, and pre-diabetes. In diabetes mellitus type 1, previously called juvenile onset diabetes or insulin-dependent diabetes mellitus (IDDM), insulin production is decreased or completely absent so that it has to be injected into the body. In this case, acquiring insulin from an external source is required for life. In diabetes type 2, previously known as adult onset diabetes, obesity related diabetes, or non-insulin-dependent diabetes mellitus (NIDDM), body tissue becomes resistant to insulin action. There is insulin in the body, but insulin receptors fail to communicate insulin signals to cells. Gestational diabetes is a form of insulin resistance (similar to type 2 diabetes) that occurs during pregnancy. It is thought that hormones from the placenta block insulin receptors, making it hard for the mother's body to metabolize sugars. Thus, more insulin or low-sugar diets are required. Most newly defined is pre-diabetes,

a condition that is a precursor to either type 1 or type 2 diabetes.

Approximately 7 percent of the population, or 20.8 million children and adults, in the United States are estimated to have diabetes. While it is probable that 14.6 million have been diagnosed with diabetes, it is thought that 6.2 million people are unaware that they have the disease. The number of individuals with diabetes doubles every 15 years. Statisticians list diabetes mellitus among the top 10 causes of death in the United States.

These major types of diabetes have similar symptoms, including frequent urination, excessive thirst, extreme hunger, unusual weight loss, increased fatigue, drowsiness, irritability, and blurry vision. High levels of blood sugar lead to excess sugar spilling into the urine; in turn, high urine sugar causes the kidneys to excrete additional water to dilute the large amount of sugar, leading to frequent urination, which brings on excessive thirst. Because calories are lost in the urine, a diabetic person loses weight, causing the person to feel hungry most of the time. In type 2 diabetes, however, enough insulin is present to avoid a loss of weight until the condition becomes severe.

The cause of the imbalance in insulin or its receptor is currently unknown. It is clear that this hormonal disorder is the result of too much, too little, or no insulin at all. At times, it may not be a function of the quantity of insulin, but rather in the quality of the receptor. When the receptor cannot communicate the signal of insulin to the cell, the result is diabetes. Risk factors include both genetics and environmental factors. Risk factors for developing diabetes include family history of type 2 diabetes, obesity, lack of exercise, racial or ethnic background, or both, and previous history of gestational diabetes for women.

All types of diabetes are diagnosed by measuring sugar levels in blood using a fasting plasma glucose test (FPG) or an oral glucose tolerance test (OGTT). With the FPG test, a fasting blood glucose level between 100 and 125 milligrams per deciliter (mg/dl) signals pre-diabetes. A person with a fasting blood glucose level of 126 mg/dl or higher has diabetes. In the OGTT test, a person's blood glucose level is measured after a fast and two hours after drinking a glucose-rich beverage. If the two-hour blood glucose level is between 140 and 199 mg/dl, the person tested has pre-diabetes. If the two-hour blood glucose level is at 200 mg/dl or higher, the person tested has diabetes.

Treatment of diabetes involves diet, exercise, education, and, for most people, medication. If a person with diabetes keeps blood sugar levels tightly controlled, complications—such as heart and blood vessel disease, blindness, kidney failure, and foot ulcers—are less likely to develop. The goal of diabetes treatment, therefore, is to keep blood sugar levels within the normal range as much as possible.

People with type 1 diabetes can eat a normal diet as long as they balance food with insulin. People with type 2 diabetes need to be more careful about what they eat, especially if they need to lose weight. Alcohol should be consumed with caution since it may cause a low blood sugar. Daily exercise is encouraged to help insulin metabolize glucose. When necessary, as in the case of type 1 diabetes, insulin is given by multiple injections each day or by continuous infusion using an insulin pump. In other cases, such as type 2 diabetes, insulin-stimulating tablets may be taken before or after meals to regulate blood sugar levels. Sometimes, when there is too much insulin in the body, the result is hypoglycemia (low blood sugar). Symptoms of hypoglycemia such as hunger, nervousness and shakiness, perspiration, dizziness, sleepiness, confusion, and weakness are relieved within minutes of consuming sugar in any form, such as candy or glucose tablets, or of drinking a sweet drink, such as a glass of fruit juice.

Acromegaly

Acromegaly is a hormonal disorder in which the pituitary gland located in the brain overproduces growth hormone (GH). The pituitary gland, located at the base of the brain, is sometimes called the master gland because of its huge influence on the other body organs. It controls the activity of many other endocrine glands, such as the thyroid, ovaries, and adrenals. Acromegaly has a prevalence of 40 to 60 cases per million and an incidence of 3 to 4 new cases per million annually. There are an estimated 10,880 people with acromegaly in the United States.

People with acromegaly have enlarged skeletal extremities; their hands and feet are large, and facial features are exaggerated as the jaw lengthens and the nose and brow ridge grow thicker. The skin thickens, and most internal organs enlarge. The onset of acromegaly is gradual, leading to long-term complications. Overgrowth of bone and cartilage often leads to arthritis. When tissue thickens, it may trap nerves, causing pain such as that of carpal tunnel syndrome, characterized by numbness and weakness of the hands. Other symptoms of acromegaly include thick, coarse, oily skin; skin tags; enlarged lips, nose and tongue; deepening of the voice due to enlarged sinuses and vocal cords; snoring due to upper airway obstruction; excessive sweating and skin odor; fatigue and weakness; headaches; impaired vision; abnormalities of the menstrual cycle and sometimes breast discharge in women; and impotence in men. There may be enlargement of body organs, including the liver, spleen, kidneys, and heart. The most serious health consequences of acromegaly are diabetes mellitus, hypertension, and increased risk of cardiovascular disease. Patients with acromegaly are also at increased risk for polyps of the colon that can develop into cancer.

When GH-producing tumors occur in childhood, the disease that results is called gigantism rather than acromegaly. Fusion of the growth plates of the long bones occurs after puberty so that development of excessive GH production in adults does not result in increased height. Prolonged exposure to excess GH before fusion of the growth plates causes increased growth of the long bones and increased height.

Acromegaly is caused by prolonged overproduction of GH by the pituitary gland. In over 90 percent of acromegaly patients, the overproduction of GH is caused by a benign tumor of the pituitary gland, called an adenoma. These tumors produce excess GH and, as they expand, compress surrounding brain tissues, such as the optic nerves. This expansion causes the headaches and visual disturbances that are often symptoms of acromegaly. In addition, compression of the surrounding normal pituitary tissue can alter production of other hormones. Most pituitary tumors arise spontaneously and are not genetically inherited. They arise from a genetic alteration in a single pituitary cell, which leads to increased cell division and tumor formation. This genetic change, or mutation, is not present at birth, but is acquired during life. Occasionally, acromegaly is caused by tumors of the pancreas, lungs, and adrenal glands. These tumors also lead to an excess of GH, either because they produce GH themselves or, more frequently, because they produce growth hormone releasing hormone (GHRH), which stimulates the pituitary to make GH.

To make an accurate diagnosis of acromegaly, multiple tests must be conducted. A single measurement of an elevated blood GH level is not enough to support a diagnosis of acromegaly because GH is secreted by the pituitary in spurts and its concentration in the blood can vary widely from minute to minute. The most accurate diagnosis is made when GH is measured under conditions in which its secretion is normally suppressed. The OGTT is used because in healthy people, ingestion of 75 grams of

This man has a large goiter caused by Graves' disease, in which the thyroid gland enlarges and produces an excess of thyroid hormones. Grave's disease is not fully understood, but it is believed to be an autoimmune disease.

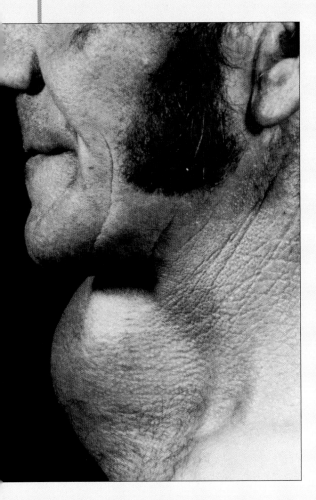

the sugar glucose lowers blood GH levels less than 2 nanograms per milliliter (ng/ml). In patients with GH overproduction, this reduction does not occur. The glucose tolerance test is the most reliable method of confirming a diagnosis of acromegaly. A test for insulin growth factor-1 (IGF-1) can also be used because elevated GH levels also increase IGF-1 blood levels. Additionally, because IGF-1 levels are much more stable over the course of the day, they are often a more practical and reliable measure than GH levels. Because of the possibility of tumors, another method of diagnosis involves imaging techniques, such as computed tomography (CT) scans or magnetic resonance imaging (MRI). Scans of the pituitary are used to locate tumors that cause the GH overproduction. Both techniques are excellent tools to visualize a tumor without surgery.

The goals of treatment are to reduce GH production to normal levels, to relieve the pressure that the growing pituitary tumor exerts on the surrounding brain areas, to improve symptoms of acromegaly, and to preserve normal pituitary function. Acromegaly may be treated by drug therapy, surgical removal, X-ray irradiation, or cryosurgery of the pituitary tumor. Two medications currently are used to treat acromegaly. These drugs reduce both GH secretion and tumor size. Medical therapy is sometimes used to shrink large tumors before surgery. Decreases in acromegalic symptoms and improvement of diabetes mellitus typically follow these therapies.

Thyroid hormone disorders

The thyroid is a small gland inside the neck, located in front of the trachea and below the Adam's apple. The thyroid gland helps set the rate of metabolism, which is the rate at which the body uses energy. The thyroid produces two hormones, tri-iodothyronine (T3) and thyroxine (T4). Both of these hormones can be either over- or underproduced.

Hyperthyroidism caused by Graves' disease affects less than 1 percent of the U.S. population, while hypothyroidism, the most common form of thyroid disorder, affects 7 million adults in the United States, mainly women over 40 years old.

When the human body is exposed to excessive amounts of thyroid hormones, the result is hyper-thyroidism. The major symptoms of hyperthyroidism include insomnia, fatigue, unexplained weight loss, weakness, heat sensitivity, increased perspiration, nervousness, itchy skin, fine, thin, or brittle hair, changes in the eyes, and enlarged thyroid (goiter). Graves' disease, the most common cause of hyperthyroidism, is an autoimmune disorder in which the body's immune system produces antibodies against its own thyroid gland, stimulating it into overproduction of thyroid hormone. This over-activity is also sometimes called toxic diffuse goiter.

When the human body does not have enough thyroid hormones, the result is hypothyroidism; the major symptoms of this condition include weakness, fatigue, cold intolerance, constipation, unintentional weight gain, depression, joint or muscle pain, thin or brittle hair and fingernails, and in children, poor growth. The most common cause of hypothyroidism is the autoimmune disorder Hashimoto's thyroiditis, in which antibodies are produced that inhibit the production of thyroid hormones.

Risk factors for developing thyroid hormone imbalances include family history, medical conditions, age, gender, ethnic background, and genetic factors. Medical conditions such as viral infections can cause the thyroid to become imbalanced. Around 5–8 percent of women are affected by postpartum thyroiditis, which is caused by pregnancy. The greatest risk is thus for women who are between the ages of 20 and 50 years of age. In addition, a person's ethnic background may increase one's risk. People of Japanese ancestry appear to be at greater risk of hyperthyroidism.

Imbalances in the thyroid gland are diagnosed by blood tests in which the hormones T3, T4, and thyroid stimulating hormone (TSH) are measured. Additionally, antibodies against the thyroid gland can also be tested. Ultrasound imaging can also help to identify disorders of the thyroid.

Once diagnosed, the level of thyroid hormones will determine the kind of treatment that is required. Typically, in hyperthyroidism, the goal of treatment is to prevent the thyroid from making too much hormone. In hypothyroidism, the goal of treatment is to supplement or replace thyroid hormones in the system.

For hyperthyroidism, anti-thyroid drugs, radioactive iodine, or surgical removal of all or parts of the thyroid gland are effective treatments. Anti-thyroid medications such as methimazole and propylthiouracil interfere with T3, T4, and TSH production, making the thyroid less efficient. Exploiting the natural properties of the thyroid gland and iodine, radioactive iodine is the most widely recommended permanent treatment of hyperthyroidism. This treatment takes advantage of the fact that thyroid cells are the only cells in the body that have the ability to absorb iodine. Thyroid cells that absorb radioactive iodine are exposed to radiation that damages or kills them. Because iodine is not concentrated by any other cells in the body, there is very little radiation exposure or side effects for the rest of the body. The majority of patients are cured with a single dose of radioactive iodine. Although not as common, surgical removal of the thyroid or parts of the gland can offer long-term cures for hyperthyroidism.

Hypothyroidism is usually quite easy to treat. The easiest and most effective treatment is simply taking a thyroid hormone pill such as Levothyroxine once a day. This medication is a pure synthetic form of T4, which is made in a laboratory to be an exact replacement for the T4 that the human thyroid gland normally secretes.

Cushing's syndrome

Cushing's syndrome, sometimes called hypercortisolism, is a hormonal disorder caused by prolonged exposure of the body's tissues to high levels of the hormone cortisol.

Cortisol is a normal hormone produced in the outer portion, or cortex, of the two adrenal glands, which are located above each kidney. The purposes of the adrenal glands are to maintain salt levels in the blood and maintain blood pressure. Each adrenal gland is actually two endocrine organs. The outer portion is called the adrenal cortex and the inner portion is called the adrenal medulla. The normal function of cortisol is to help the body respond to stress and change. It mobilizes nutrients, modifies the body's response to inflammation, stimulates the liver to raise the blood sugar, and it helps control the amount of water in the body. Cortisol production is regulated by adrenocorticotrophic hormone (ACTH), made in the pituitary gland.

Cushing's syndrome is relatively rare, and an estimated 10 to 15 of every million people are affected each year. It is four times as common in women as in men and may appear during or just following pregnancy. Although it can occur at any age, it mainly affects adults aged 20 to 50 years.

The incidence of Cushing's syndrome is 5 to 6 new cases per million per year.

General physical features of Cushing's syndrome include: a tendency to gain weight, especially on the face, which develops a typical moonlike appearance, and on the abdomen, neck, and upper back, which develops a buffalo hump; thinning and weakness of the muscles of the upper arms and upper legs; thinning of the skin, with easy bruising and pink or purple stretch marks (striae) on the abdomen, thighs, breasts, and shoulders; increased acne, facial hair growth, and scalp hair loss in women; sometimes a ruddy complexion on the face and neck; and often a skin darkening (acanthosis) on the neck.

Children show obesity and poor growth in height. Symptoms usually include fatigue, weakness, depression, mood swings, increased thirst and urination, and lack of menstrual periods in women.

In general, anything that increases the adrenal gland's secretion of cortisol will cause Cushing's syndrome, including adrenal tumors, enlargement of the outer layers of the adrenal gland, or overproduction of ACTH. Artificial induction of Cushing's syndrome includes treatment with glucocorticoid hormones such as hydrocortisone, prednisone, methylprednisolone, or dexamethasone. This iatrogenic (caused by the treatment) form is a necessary side effect when high doses of these steroid hormones must be used to treat certain life-threatening illnesses, such as asthma, rheumatoid arthritis, systemic lupus, inflammatory bowel disease, some allergies, and other conditions.

Most people who appear to have some of the classic physical features of Cushing's syndrome (cushingoid appearance) do not actually have the disease. After iatrogenic (caused by physicians as a side effect of other treatments) Cushing's is excluded, other causes of this appearance can be polycystic ovary syndrome, which is caused by androgen excess from the ovaries; ovarian tumors; congenital adrenal hyperplasia; ordinary obesity; excessive alcohol consumption; or just a family tendency to have a round face and abdomen with high blood pressure and high blood sugar.

Risk factors for developing Cushing's syndrome are an adrenal tumor or a pituitary tumor, chronic therapy with corticosteroids, and being female.

Diagnosis of Cushing's syndrome typically involves an extensive physical exam and routine blood and urine tests in which cortisol is measured by using dexamethasone suppression tests. If the pituitary is the source of the problem because it is secreting too much ACTH, then dexamethasone, the hormone that stimulated the adrenal to make cortisol, will usually lower cortisol. If there is an ectopic (that is, occurring elsewhere) ACTH-secreting tumor (such as in the lungs) or an adrenal tumor, dexamethasone will have no effect. Often a pituitary tumor is tiny and hard to find, so a special test of the release of ACTH from both sides of the pituitary (petrosal sinus sampling) might be needed. Imaging techniques such as CT or MRI are then used to localize the tumor. Small tumors producing ectopic ACTH are also sometimes difficult to localize and require repeated scans and X-rays.

Treating Cushing's disease depends upon whether the problem is in the adrenal glands, the pituitary gland, or elsewhere. Surgery or radiation therapy may be needed to remove or destroy a pituitary tumor. Tumors of the adrenal gland can often be removed surgically. Both adrenal glands may have to be removed if these treatments are not effective or if no tumor is present. If all or part of the adrenal glands is removed, corticosteroid replacement therapy is required indefinitely. Tumors outside the pituitary and adrenal glands that secrete excess hormones are usually surgically removed. Certain drugs such as aminoglutethimide, metyrapone, trilostane, and ketoconazole can lower cortisol levels and can be used while awaiting more definitive treatment such as surgery.

Conclusion

The description of a wide range of diseases like diabetes, acromegaly, thyroid disorders, and Cushing's syndrome demonstrates that although these are all classified as hormonal disorders, they are indeed their own distinct disorders. Although only a few major disorders are discussed here, it is important to know that there are several endocrine disorders that may occur. Furthermore, one endocrine disorder may have an effect on the function of another endocrine system, such as the relationship of acromegaly to the development of diabetes.

Rashmi Nemade

HPV infection

Human papillomaviruses (HPVs) are widespread in the general population. They produce epithelial lesions of the skin and mucous membranes known as warts, or condylomas, and have been closely associated with cancers of the genital tract.

HPV infects the basal epithelial cells of the epidermis in the skin and of the mucous membranes in the genital tract and leads to the development of lesions known as warts, or condylomas. Infected cells can undergo malignant transformation, replace all the layers of normal cells above, and eventually invade the tissues underneath the epithelium and complete the transition to invasive cancer. Different HPV types cause different disease: cutaneous infections (HPV 1 and 2), genital infections (HPV 6 and 11), and progression of the infected cells to cancer cells, particularly in the cervix (HPV 16 and 18). Cutaneous HPV infections are transmitted through close personal contact, whereas genital HPV infections are transmitted through sexual contact. The three main cutaneous lesions are common warts (about 70 percent of all cutaneous warts), plantar warts (about 30 percent), and flat warts (less than 5 percent) and do not usually progress to cancer. Genital HPV infections can involve both male and female external genitalia (penis, scrotum, vulva) and perianal region and internal genitalia (urethra, vagina, cervix) and anus. Genital lesions range from being small and flat (flat condyloma) to being large and spiked (acuminate condyloma) and are associated with progression to cancer. In women with external genital lesions, cervical lesions are often present as well. Patients with HIV infection are at particular risk of progression to cancer because of their poorly functioning immune system.

Symptoms and diagnosis

Both cutaneous and genital lesions are usually asymptomatic, but they may bleed and be itchy or painful if located over weight-bearing surfaces or areas of friction. About 50 percent of cutaneous lesions clear up on their own, as do 10 to 20 percent of genital lesions. The diagnosis of HPV infection is usually made clinically by physical exam. Women with external genital lesions should all undergo a Papanicolau test (Pap test). Direct visualization of the anal surface with a small camera (anoscopy) should be considered in patients with peri-

anal warts, anal symptoms, or a history of receptive anal intercourse. For lesions that are large or that bleed, a biopsy is done to rule out progression to cancer.

Treatments and prevention

Cutaneous lesions are treated locally with preparations containing salicylic acid. Treatment methods for genital lesions are many but unsatisfactory because of their high recurrence rates. Local application of trichloracetic acid, podophyllin, and imiquimod are all valid options. Cryotherapy or laser therapy are indicated during pregnancy and for treatment of cervical lesions. Avoiding contact with infectious lesions is the only method of prevention. Wearing protective footwear in swimming pools protects against foot warts; using condoms confers protection against genital HPV infections. The Pap test is essential for the screening and prevention of HPV-induced intra-epithelial neoplasia and invasive cervical cancer. Vaccines against HPV may be available in the near future.

Corrado Cancedda

KEY FACTS

Description
Viral infection that causes skin and genital warts.

Causes
Human papillomaviruses.

Risk factors
Close contact for cutaneous infections and sexual contact for genital infections.

Symptoms
Lesions usually asymptomatic.

Diagnosis
Physical examination and Pap test.

Treatment
Local applications, cryotherapy, and laser therapy.

Pathogenesis
HPV can lead to the development of invasive cancer.

Prevention
Avoiding contact with infectious lesions.

Epidemiology
5.5 million new cases per year in the United States.

See also
• AIDS • Cancer, cervical • Sexually transmitted diseases • Wart and verruca

Huntington's disease

An inherited genetic disorder, Huntington's disease destroys areas of the brain that affect movement, intellect, and emotional stability. Huntington's disease progresses gradually and can eventually cause the decline of all vital body functions.

Huntington's disease (HD) is a fatal hereditary disease that destroys nerve cells (neurons) in areas of the brain involved in the emotions, intellect, and movement. The course of Huntington's disease is characterized by uncontrollable jerking movements of the limbs, trunk, and face (also called chorea, from the Greek *choreia*, meaning "dance"); progressive loss of intellectual abilities; and the development of psychiatric problems.

Causes and symptoms

Huntington's disease is caused by a mutation in a gene called huntingtin. Normally this gene has up to 26 copies of the DNA sequence CAG; people with HD may have from 40 to more than 100 copies of CAG. It is not known why HD arises from this repeated sequence. The disease is inherited in an autosomal dominant manner; a person with the abnormal gene has a 50 percent chance of passing it on to each of his or her children.

Early signs of the disease vary from person to person. The earlier that symptoms appear, the faster the disease progresses. Usually, symptoms become apparent at midlife. The person experiences mood swings or becomes uncharacteristically irritable, apathetic, passive, depressed, or angry. HD may affect judgment, memory, and other cognitive functions. Early signs might include problems with driving, learning new things, answering questions, or making decisions. Some people may display changes in handwriting. As HD progresses, concentration becomes increasingly difficult. The disease also sometimes begins with uncontrolled movements in the fingers, feet, face, or trunk. Mild clumsiness or problems with balance may occur. Speech may become slurred; swallowing, eating, speaking, and especially walking continue to decline.

Treatments and epidemiology

There is currently no cure for HD, but specific symptoms may be relieved with drugs. Antipsychotic drugs, such as haloperidol, may help alleviate abnormal movements and help control hallucinations, delusions, and violent outbursts. These medications may have severe side effects, such as sedation.

Many community resources are available to help families, including home care services, recreation and work centers, group housing, and legal and social aid. Research is focused on determining how mutation in the huntingtin gene leads to HD. HD affects males and females equally and crosses all ethnic and racial boundaries. One out of every 10,000 Americans has HD. Around 200,000 Americans have one parent with HD, which means that they have a 50 percent chance of developing the disease themselves.

Diana Gitig

KEY FACTS

Description
A genetic disorder resulting in gradual physical, mental, and emotional decline.

Causes
Mutation in a gene.

Risk factors
Having a parent who has either the disease or the genetic mutation that causes it.

Symptoms
Uncontrolled movements, loss of intellectual faculties, and emotional disturbance.

Diagnosis
Typical cases are recognized by the combination of dementia and abnormal movements. Genetic testing confirms the diagnosis.

Treatments
Early symptoms can be managed with antipsychotic drugs and therapy.

Pathogenesis
HD slowly diminishes the ability to walk, think, talk, and reason. Eventually, the person becomes totally dependent upon others for his or her care.

Prevention
None.

Epidemiology
In the United States about 30,000 people have HD; estimates of the disease's prevalence are about 1 in every 10,000 people.

See also
• Genetic disorders • Nervous system disorders

Hyperthermia

Hyperthermia is the abnormal elevation of body temperature, unrelated to fever, as a result of an imbalance between the body's heat production and heat loss. Hyperthermia may be caused by heat-related illness such as heat exhaustion or heat stroke. Heat stroke is a medical emergency; it may lead to organ failure and death.

Hyperthermia can be caused by medications including beta-blockers, diuretics, and antihypertensives. The drugs may reduce sweating, and thus cause a reduced ability to dissipate body heat. Dehydration predisposes to heat illness. Athletes who train vigorously during heat waves are at risk, as are elderly patients or infants who do not have access to fluids. Alcoholics, the morbidly obese, and patients with multiple medical problems are also at risk.

Symptoms and diagnosis

Heat exhaustion and heat stroke occur above 104°F (40°C). Nonspecific symptoms such as headache, nausea, sweating, vomiting, dizziness, or fainting are typical of heat exhaustion. It is differentiated from heat stroke by the absence of central nervous system (CNS) symptoms. Heat stroke has associated CNS dysfunction. Physical findings with heat stroke may include excessively rapid breathing, dry skin, seizures, altered mental status, delirium, coma, and pulmonary edema. Laboratory studies may reveal multi-organ dysfunction. Heat stroke is divided into classic (nonexertional) heat stroke and exertional heat stroke. Elderly individuals with chronic medical problems are predisposed to classic heat stroke. Exertional heat stroke affects young, healthy people who exercise strenuously during extreme heat and humidity. Distinct forms of hyperthermia, not associated with environmental heat stress, include malignant hyperthermia and neuroleptic malignant syndrome. Malignant hyperthermia is a genetically predisposed condition in which patients undergoing general anesthesia experience hyperthermia and muscle rigidity. Neuroleptic malignant syndrome may occur with the use of antipsychotic medications and is associated with hypertension, muscle rigidity, and dysfunction of the autonomic nervous system.

The key treatment for hyperthermia is cooling. Fluid replenishment and rest in a cool environment is usually adequate treatment for heat exhaustion. If heat exhaustion is not treated, it may progress to heat stroke. Treatment of heat stroke involves aggressive cooling and cautious IV fluid replacement. Cooling techniques should be used until the temperature drops to 103°F (39.5°C). Clothes should be removed, fans applied, and water should be sprayed onto the patient. Ice packs to the armpits and groin are also helpful. Cold peritoneal and bladder washing and use of a heart and lung machine are invasive but effective techniques for rapid cooling. Shivering should be abated with the drugs lorazepam or diazepam. Antifever drugs are not helpful. Malignant hyperthermia is treated with dantrolene and the above methods. Treatment of neuroleptic malignant syndrome includes supportive measures and cooling.

Joanne Oakes and Jamie Flournoy

KEY FACTS

Description

Clinical condition due to elevated body temperature.

Causes

Environmental conditions, underlying medical problems, or genetic predisposition.

Risk factors

Advanced age, infancy, chronic illness, physical exertion, medications, alcoholism, obesity, dehydration.

Symptoms

Nonspecific, such as headache, nausea, sweating, vomiting, dizziness, or fainting. Same symptoms for heat stroke but with neurological dysfunction.

Diagnosis

History and physical exam.

Treatments

Cooling.

Pathogenesis

Death from environmental conditions occurs most commonly due to heat-related illness.

Prevention

Adequate amounts of fluids; keep elderly and ill cool; avoid medications that interfere with heat loss.

Epidemiology

Varies: from 1 in 4,500 to 1 in 60,000 cases of malignant hyperthermia have been reported.

See also
- Aging, disorders of • Alcohol-related disorders • Obesity

Immune system disorders

The immune system is a coordinated system of cells that protects the host from harmful, foreign organisms, called pathogens. Infectious pathogens include viruses, bacteria, fungi, and parasites. In order to protect the host, the immune system must be able to distinguish "self" from "non-self" and to respond appropriately to pathogens. Cells of the immune system can be broadly categorized as cells that provide an innate immune response or an adaptive immune response, although there is some overlap. These parts of the immune system work together to provide an immediate (innate) and highly specific (adaptive) response against pathogens.

Defects in the function of the immune system can result in immunodeficiency disorders that predispose the host to infection; allergic diseases, in which the host inappropriately responds to nonharmful substances; and autoimmune diseases, in which the host reacts against itself.

Innate immunity refers to the early immune response to a pathogen that does not require prior exposure to the organism to be effective. Innate immune responses are encoded directly into the host DNA and are therefore less specific and have limited diversity compared to adaptive immune responses. However, innate immunity has the advantage of acting quickly.

The simplest level of defense is the physical barrier provided by skin and mucous membranes, like the gastrointestinal tract. Naturally occurring antibiotics, called defensins, provide another level of defense against bacteria, fungi, and viruses. In the lungs, a layer of secreted mucus traps foreign particles, which are cleared by movement of hairlike cilia. The stomach produces digestive enzymes and acid, which can kill infectious organisms.

Cells of the innate immune system can also act specifically against pathogens through recognition of repetitive structures associated with the microbes. These pathogen-associated molecular patterns include a variant of genetic material called double-stranded RNA, found in viruses, and a component of bacterial cell membranes called lipopolysaccharide. The presence of these unique structures, which are not found in host cells, activates the innate immune response against the pathogen.

The main cells of the innate immune system are macrophages and neutrophils, which act as phagocytes, to engulf and destroy pathogens. Phagocytes are an important part of the inflammatory response, which limits tissue injury and infection to a localized area in the body. Monocytes, which develop into macrophages in tissues, as well as neutrophils, routinely circulate in the bloodstream. At sites of infection or injury, chemical signals are produced that cause phagocytes to stop their routine circulation and to migrate to the tissues where they are needed. The pathogen also becomes coated with antibody and complement (parts of the immune system that will be discussed later), which promote phagocytosis. In phagocytosis, the pathogen

ACQUIRED OR ADAPTIVE IMMUNITY

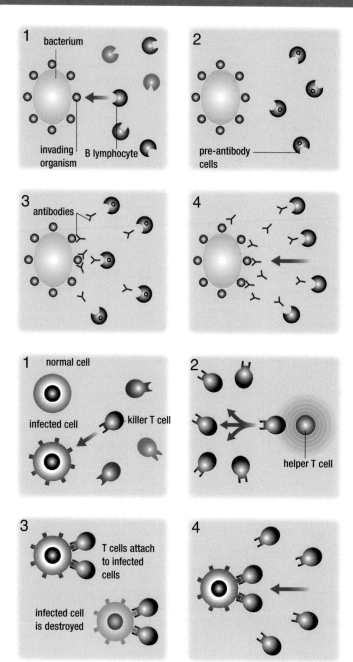

HUMORAL IMMUNITY

1. A humoral response is activated when a B lymphocyte recognizes an invader or antigen on the surface of a bacterium.

2. The B lymphocytes multiply and make cells that will become antibodies that will attack the invading bacteria.

3. The antibodies are released from the cells and home in on the antigen. More antibodies are formed and eventually the bacteria are killed.

4. If the body is reinfected by the bacteria, some B lymphocytes act as memory cells and mount an attack on the invading bacteria with large amounts of antibodies.

CELLULAR IMMUNITY

1. A cell infected by a virus is recognized by a killer T cell, prompting the T-cell activation.

2. The T cells multiply with the aid of helper T cells, which are another variety of T lymphocytes.

3. The T cells attack the infected cells by attaching to them, which destroys them. The T cells can detach themselves and kill more infected cells.

4. If any abnormal cells reappear, for example if the body is reinfected by the virus, some T cells, which are retained as memory cells, will attack and destroy the infected cells.

Acquired or adaptive immunity refers to the response that occurs when the body comes into contact with organisms that threaten its defenses. Two specific types of response can occur: humoral immunity and cellular (cell-mediated) immunity.

Humoral immunity uses B lymphocytes, which multiply once they have identified the invader, then produce antibodies to attack the invader. Cellular immunity occurs when T lymphocytes activate and attack cells that have been infected by viruses.

is destroyed inside vesicles of the phagocyte by the use of compounds produced by a complex enzyme system called the NADPH oxidase.

Other cell types of the innate immune system are mast cells, eosinophils, and natural killer cells. Mast cells and eosinophils are well known for their role in allergic diseases, but they are also critical for the immune response against parasitic worms. Mast cells and eosinophils are commonly found in tissues with potential exposure to these organisms, such as the gut, respiratory tract, and skin. Antibodies, a part of the adaptive immune response, bind to the parasites. This signal activates mast cells and eosinophils to release their internal granule contents, which include proteases and toxins that help kill the pathogen. The mast cells and eosinophils also produce signals, called cytokines, which recruit other immune cells to the area.

Natural killer cells are named for their ability to kill cells without previous activation. They specifically target cells that lack the expression of major histocompatibility type I (MHC I) receptors, which are molecules expressed on the surface of all normal host cells. Virus-infected cells and cancer cells often reduce their expression of MHC I receptors in an attempt to escape detection by the immune system. Natural killer cells also produce the cytokine called interferon-gamma, which enhances killing of virus-infected cells and inhibits virus production. Natural killer cells can also destroy infected cells by forming pores in the cell membrane and secreting proteins that degrade DNA.

In addition to the cell types described above, there is a system of proteins in the bloodstream, called the complement system, that destroys pathogens in the circulation. The complement system enhances activity of both the innate and adaptive immune responses. Complement can be activated either directly by pathogens or by the antibody complexes formed against the pathogens. The complement pathways ultimately result in the formation of a membrane attack complex, which is a group of proteins that insert into the cell membrane to destroy the microbe.

Adaptive immunity

The adaptive immune response refers to the highly diverse and very specific immune response produced by T lymphocytes (also called cell-mediated immunity) and antibodies (also called humoral immunity).

Adaptive immune responses occur more slowly than innate responses, because they require the activation and expansion of these cells. In contrast to innate immune responses, adaptive immunity also exhibits immunological memory, in which previous exposure to a specific pathogen leads to an enhanced immune response to that pathogen in the future. This memory results from persistence of long-lived lymphocytes in the host, called memory B and T cells, which respond quickly when the pathogen is encountered again.

B and T lymphocytes arise from a common ancestor cell located in the bone marrow. T cells complete their development in the thymus, an immunological organ in the chest, whereas B cells mature in the bone marrow. During development, B and T cells undergo a complex system of genetic recombination, which is a process of cutting and rejoining of DNA segments, to produce genes that code for a tremendous diversity of cell surface receptors. These receptors bind to antigens, which are substances that stimulate an immune response, and they enable the lymphocytes to recognize many different pathogens.

B cells produce an antibody, also called immuno-globulin, which can either be bound to the surface of the B cells to function as their antigen-binding receptor, or secreted outside the cells. In general, antibodies are specialized to target bacteria and their toxins, which circulate outside the host cells.

An antibody's structure can be divided into two parts: the variable region is the portion that binds to an antigen; the constant region of the antibody determines its class, also called isotype, and the response it will have to the antigen. The immunoglobulin isotype IgG is the most abundant in the body. It can neutralize toxins and pathogens to make them ineffective, and it promotes phagocytosis. IgM and IgG can activate the complement pathway. IgA is found in secretions, such as tears and saliva, as well as the intestinal tract, where it neutralizes toxins and prevents binding of pathogens to the host cells. IgE plays an important role in the immune response against parasitic worms and in allergic reactions.

T cells recognize antigens using T cell receptors located on their cell surface. Expression of a functional T cell receptor is required for T cell development. The major subtypes of T cells are helper CD4+ and cytotoxic CD8+ cells. More recently, regulatory T cells

IMMUNIZATION

Active immunization refers to the specific and protective immune response against a pathogen that is stimulated by administration of a vaccine into the host. A vaccine is a preparation of weakened or killed microorganisms, such as bacteria, viruses, or antigenic proteins derived from microorganisms, which are given to prevent, improve, or treat an infectious disease. In contrast, passive immunization refers to administration of protective antibodies against a specific pathogen in order to provide temporary immunity, such as administration of rabies immune globulin that is given after exposure to the rabies virus.

Active immunization induces long-term antibody and cell-mediated immunity through induction of memory B and T cells. Live attenuated vaccines contain a modified virus strain that is not pathogenic but stimulates a robust immune response by mimicking an infection. In rare instances, viral mutations can lead to viral strains that cause disease, as in the case of oral polio virus. The oral live polio virus has been replaced by inactivated polio virus in the United States.

Live vaccines should generally be avoided in hosts who are immunocompromised, that is, people with a weakened immune system, and they also should be avoided in pregnant women.

Components of microorganisms or their toxins can be used as vaccines without risk of causing active infection. However, these subunit vaccines often induce a limited immune response. Subsequent immunizations, often called "booster immunizations," can be given to further enhance someone's immunity. The response against polysaccharide antigens can also be improved in young children by conjugating, or joining, these polysaccharides to proteins, such as in the vaccine for *Hemophilus influenzae*. Substances called adjuvants, such as aluminum, are included in the tetanus toxoid vaccine to enhance the immune response.

Although most immunizations do not produce severe side effects, risks are associated with some vaccines. The person may develop redness and soreness at the site of the injection and flulike symptoms and fever. In some people, a mild form of the disease follows vaccination; rarely, the person is allergic to the vaccine and has a severe reaction. Those people should not receive subsequent immunizations.

In addition to providing individual protection, an effective immunization program can result in herd immunity, which refers to the reduced chance of an infection being spread in a population that has a high level of immunity. As well as routine childhood immunization programs, extra immunizations may be necessary before people travel in foreign countries.

An effective vaccine against the human immunodeficiency virus (HIV) remains elusive because of the virus's frequent mutations, destruction of CD4+ T lymphocytes, and the ability to remain latent to evade detection by cells and chemicals of the immune system.

have been identified that suppress, rather than enhance, immune responses against specific antigens. CD4+ T cells provide "help" or costimulatory signals to other cells of the immune system and can be further characterized as T helper type 1 or type 2. Helper type 1 cells produce signals that enhance phagocyte responses, whereas helper type 2 cells promote antibody production by B cells. Cytotoxic CD8+ T cells are named for their ability to kill cells through a process similar to that of natural killer cells. They release toxic granules that destroy the cell membrane, or activate pathways leading to DNA degradation. As part of their maturation process in the thymus, T cells undergo a selection process, which eliminates cells that react too strongly against the host's own proteins.

Vaccination and immunization

Vaccination refers to the administration of a vaccine, which is a preparation containing a modified pathogen or its components intended to induce an immune response against that pathogen. Vaccinations are most commonly given as injections. Immunization refers to the process through which the immune response against a pathogen is achieved; immunization is subdivided into active and passive forms.

In active immunization, a protective long-term immune response against a microbe is stimulated by vaccinating the host. The initial immune response is composed of IgM antibodies that can be detected within days of immunization, but it is short-lived. In contrast, the IgG antibody response occurs within weeks of vaccination and can persist for years. This long-term immunity is achieved through induction of memory B and memory T cells that recognize the microbial antigens. Live attenuated vaccines contain a modified virus strain that does not cause disease but stimulates a strong immune response by mimicking an infection with that pathogen. In rare instances, viral mutations can lead to virus strains that cause disease, as in the case of oral polio virus. The oral live polio virus has been replaced by inactivated polio virus in the United States. Live vaccines are generally avoided for immunocompromised people and for pregnant women because of the risk of serious complications. Components of the microbes or their toxins can be used as vaccines without risk of causing an active infection. However, these subunit vaccines often induce a limited immune response. Subsequent booster shots can be given to enhance and prolong immunity. Another approach is to add an adjuvant to the vaccine, such as aluminum salts, to enhance the immune response to the antigens. The immune response against polysaccharide antigens can also be improved by modifying them with a protein carrier, to produce a conjugated vaccine.

In contrast to active immunization, passive immunization refers to the administration of protective antibodies against a specific antigen to provide temporary immunity. For instance, administration of antibodies specific to rabies virus can be given immediately after an exposure to the virus to provide temporary protection. A major advantage of passive immunization is that it is effective immediately, and does not require the host to develop its own adaptive immune response. Passive immunity also provides infants with protection from many types of infections in early life through the acquisition of IgG antibodies from their mothers during pregnancy.

Effective immunization programs induce protective immunity in the individuals receiving the vaccines. From a public health standpoint, an additional benefit to the public is herd immunity. Herd immunity refers to the reduced likelihood of an infection being spread from person to person in a population that includes many people who are immune. Therefore, even people who have not been immunized attain some benefit. Routine immunization in childhood has significantly reduced the incidence of previously common infections, such as mumps, measles, and most recently varicella, usually called chicken pox. Smallpox infection was eliminated throughout the world as a result of a widespread immunization program, with the last natural case occurring in 1977. However, difficulties still exist with vaccine development today. A new influenza vaccine must be developed every year because significant genetic differences in the strains that are prevalent in any given year result from genetic mutations in the virus, called antigenic drift. An effective HIV vaccine has not yet been developed, partly because of the virus's frequent genetic mutations.

Allergic diseases
Allergy, or hypersensitivity, refers to an inappropriate immune response to a nonharmful antigen, called an allergen, leading to adverse effects in the host. Common allergens are found in pollens, animal danders, foods, and medications. Allergy leads to typical symptoms that range from mild to potentially life-threatening reactions. Allergic diseases affect more than 50 million Americans in the form of allergic rhinitis, asthma, food allergies, dermatitis rashes, and other conditions, and the prevalence rate is rising.

Type I hypersensitivity reactions refer to the classical, immediate-type allergic responses involving IgE antibodies. IgE molecules bind both to the allergen and also to the surface of mast cells. This signal activates mast cells to release chemicals, such as histamine, which can cause mild allergic symptoms like wateriness and itching of the nose and eyes to life-threatening symptoms of airway constriction and vascular shock that occur in anaphylaxis. Acute allergic symptoms can start within minutes of exposure to an allergen and may be followed by late-phase reactions occurring hours later, owing to the action of T lymphocytes. Type II hypersensitivity reactions occur when antibodies bind to cell surface antigens, which leads to complement activation and destruction of the cells, such as in some types of anemia. Type III hypersensitivity reactions occur when antibodies bind to circulating antigens, causing formation of antibody-antigen complexes in the circulation. These immune complexes can lodge in small blood vessels and cause damage to organs such as the kidney. Type IV reactions, also called delayed-type hypersensitivity reactions, are produced by T cells. Upon exposure to an allergen, for example, poison ivy, T cells release cytokines that stimulate and recruit T cells and macrophages to the area, producing a characteristic rash, which is called allergic contact dermatitis.

The most effective treatment for an allergy is to strictly avoid the offending allergen. When this cannot be done, medications can be used, including antihistamines, which block the effect of histamine released by mast cells, and corticosteroids, which control late-phase allergic responses. In the case of allergy to environmental components such as pollens and insect venoms, specific allergen immunotherapy can also be performed. Allergen immunotherapy, commonly called allergy shots, involves injections of gradually increasing doses of an allergen in order to modify the immune response to that allergen. Successful immunotherapy leads to a shift from a predominantly IgE to an IgG response and to generation of regulatory T cells that enhance tolerance to the allergen. When use of an alternative medication is not possible, a desensitization procedure can be performed in some cases to induce a temporary tolerance to the medication. Both desensitization procedures and allergy shots carry a risk of causing a severe allergic reaction such as life-threatening anaphylaxis. Anti-IgE is an injectable medication that blocks the binding of IgE molecules to the surface of mast cells. It is a new treatment approach for severe asthma and is also being investigated for treatment of other IgE-mediated allergic diseases.

Immunodeficiency disorders

Defects in the immune system can result in an increased susceptibility to infection, called immunodeficiency. In some cases, the abnormal functioning of the immune system also predisposes the patients to autoimmune disease and cancer. Immunodeficiency disorders are classified according to the type of immune response that is affected: innate, humoral, cell-mediated, or combined disorders. Primary immunodeficiency disorders are genetically determined and often present in childhood. There are nearly 100 recognized disorders, which affect from 1 in 700 people in the case of the most common defect, up to 1 in a million people for the rarest conditions. In contrast, secondary immunodeficiency disorders result from external factors such as infection by the human immunodeficiency virus (HIV) or toxicity to the immune system from chemotherapy or radiation.

Defects in innate immunity

Chronic granulomatous disease is the most common immune deficiency to affect phagocytes. The underlying defect occurs in the NADPH oxidase complex, which generates the molecules used for killing by phagocytes. These patients are unable to eliminate infections caused by some bacteria and fungi. The diagnosis is made by demonstrating inability of the phagocytes to produce products of the NADPH oxidase system. Antibiotics are used to prevent and treat these infections. More recently, the cytokine interferon-gamma has also shown benefit.

Leukocyte adhesion deficiency results from abnormal cell trafficking, in which leukocytes cannot leave the blood circulation to enter the tissues at sites of infection. The white blood cell count in the bloodstream is very high—up to 10 times the normal level. Affected children have recurrent infections and poor wound healing. Severe cases need a bone marrow transplant.

Deficiency of complement can lead to very different symptoms, depending on the specific proteins affected.

Scleroderma, or systemic sclerosis, is an autoimmune condition in which the body's immune system attacks its own tissues. The condition can affect any part of the body but is seen here on the hand, where it has produced red, shiny, and tight skin. Scleroderma may spread and prove fatal, and as yet there is no effective treatment.

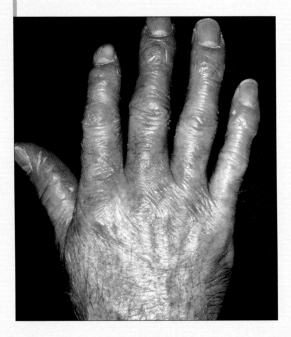

Deficiency of the late complement components, which form the membrane attack complex, predisposes to recurrent bacterial infections. Deficiency of some of the early components predisposes to development of autoimmune disease rather than to infections.

Humoral deficiency

Agammaglobulinemia refers to antibody deficiency occurring due to the absence of B cells. Infants are protected from infections until about the age of 6 months by maternal antibodies that are passed through the placenta. After this time, infants with agammaglobulinemia develop recurrent bacterial infections of the lungs, sinuses, and ears. Typical organisms are bacteria, such as *Streptococcus pneumoniae* and *Hemophilus influenzae*, which require an antibody response against their outer polysaccharide coat to be effectively cleared. Severe viral infections can also occur. Most cases of agammaglobulinemia occur in males because the genetic defect occurs in Bruton's tyrosine kinase, which is a gene located on the X chromosome that is required for B cell maturation. Unlike females, males have only one X chromosome. The affected males do not have a normal copy of the gene that could prevent the disease.

Hypogammaglobulinemia refers to antibody deficiency occurring in the presence of normal B cell numbers. Common variable immunodeficiency (CVID) is a type of hypogammaglobulinemia that can present in childhood or adulthood. CVID refers to a group of disorders defined by low IgG levels and decreased antibody production against specific pathogens. There is also some impairment of T cell immunity. CVID can present at any age with recurrent bacterial infections similar to those seen in agammaglobulinemia. There is also an increased risk of some viral infections, autoimmune disease, and cancers.

IgA deficiency is the most common immune defect, affecting up to 1 in 700 Caucasians. However, most patients are asymptomatic. Some patients develop recurrent bacterial infections, especially if they have other problems with their immune system, such as CVID. When there is complete deficiency of IgA, patients may produce IgE antibodies against IgA. If these patients receive blood products containing IgA, they can potentially have a severe allergic reaction.

To evaluate for antibody disorders, blood tests are performed to quantify immunoglobulin levels and B cell numbers. To assess the function of the immune system, antibody titers are checked before and after administration of vaccines such as the pneumococcal and tetanus vaccines, to measure the immune response against polysaccharide and protein antigens.

Treatment of antibody disorders is aimed at the control and prevention of infections. This can be done in part through the use of antibiotics. For CVID and agammaglobulinemia, patients also require replacement of IgG antibodies through intravenous infusions of immunoglobulins obtained from blood donors. These patients are also monitored for evidence of chronic lung disease that can result from recurrent respiratory infections and for development of other potentially associated conditions.

T cell disorders and combined disorders

T cell disorders predispose patients to many infections, because T cells have a critical role in the immune system. T cells mount an immune response to intracellular organisms, such as viruses. They also provide signals to B cells to facilitate antibody responses to proteins and to switch from one antibody class to another. Disorders predominantly affecting T cell function are separated from "combined disorders" that significantly diminish both B and T cell responses.

To evaluate for T cell or combined disorders, total lymphocyte counts and specific T cell subsets can be measured in the blood. T cell function can be assessed in a patient by introducing mumps or candida antigens into the skin to produce a delayed type hypersensitivity reaction, which is a T cell–dependent process. Another method to assess T cell function is a mitogen assay, in which T cells obtained from the patient are incubated with a known stimulus in a test tube to measure their proliferation response.

DiGeorge syndrome is a disorder of T cell development as a result of a genetic defect in the formation of the thymus gland, which is the site of T cell maturation. Other features of the syndrome include cardiac defects and low calcium levels because of malformation of other structures located adjacent to the thymus. In patients with complete DiGeorge syndrome, thymus transplantation has been performed to restore T cell function.

Wiskott-Aldrich syndrome is an X-linked combined deficiency that causes a characteristic skin rash, bleeding due to low platelets, and recurrent bacterial and viral infections. There is also an increased risk of cancer and autoimmune disease. The disorder results from a defect in a protein that regulates the cell structure and results in defective platelets, B cells, and T cells. Blood tests show small, abnormal platelets. Treatment includes management of the bleeding and infections and maintenance of adequate platelet counts. Bone marrow transplantation offers a potential cure.

HIV/AIDS

The human immunodeficiency virus (HIV) is the retrovirus that causes the acquired immune deficiency syndrome (AIDS). HIV can be transmitted through contaminated blood, sexual contact, and breast milk and is a worldwide health problem, particularly in developing countries. According to the World Health Organization, more than 1 million people in the United States are HIV positive; globally, an estimated 40 million people are infected. Another 25 million people have already died from AIDS worldwide.

HIV causes profound immunodeficiency through infection and destruction of CD4+ T cells. In the host cell, viral RNA is reverse-transcribed into DNA, which inserts into the host genome. These genetic instructions lead to production of viral proteins that are cleaved by a viral protease and packaged along with viral RNA to produce new virus particles.

HIV infection is identified by blood tests that demonstrate the presence of antibodies to HIV. The progression of disease is monitored by measurement of CD4+ T cell counts and viral copies.

HIV infection may not cause any noticeable symptoms for years. AIDS occurs when HIV infection progresses to reduce CD4+ T cells counts to less than 200 per cubic millimeter (mm^3) in association with the development of characteristic infections or cancers. Opportunistic infections occur from pathogens, such as *Pneumocystis carinii* and *Mycobacterium avium*, which are normally controlled by a functional immune system. Typical cancers occurring in AIDS are Kaposi's sarcoma and non-Hodgkin's lymphoma.

HIV treatment is directed at prevention of opportunistic infections using prophylactic antibiotics and antiviral medications that inhibit the viral reverse transcriptase and protease enzymes. Although the life expectancy and quality of life of HIV/AIDS patients have significantly improved in recent years, an HIV cure has not yet been achieved. Significant limitations to HIV eradication include the poor immune response to the virus, as well as the ability of the virus to remain dormant within host cells to evade detection. Furthermore, frequent viral mutations can lead to resistance to antiviral medications, and these medications are also associated with high cost and side effects. Prevention of HIV infection is emphasized through education about its transmission and avoidance of high-risk behaviors. Prophylactic antiviral therapy can also be given during childbirth to reduce viral transmission from mother to child. An effective HIV vaccine has not yet been developed, but it is a very active area of research.

SCID

Severe combined immunodeficiency (SCID) refers to a group of rare inherited disorders with severe deficiency of both antibody and cell-mediated immunity. SCID presents early in infancy with failure to thrive, chronic diarrhea, skin rashes, and recurrent, life-threatening infections. The infections can occur as a result of bacteria, fungi, or viruses, and involve opportunistic organisms. The most common form of SCID, affecting about half of SCID patients, occurs because of a genetic defect in the common gamma chain receptor. This receptor participates in several important cytokine signaling pathways that are necessary for T cell–mediated immune responses. This type of SCID affects males because the gene is located on the X chromosome. A genetic defect in Jak3, which is a member of the same cytokine signaling pathway as the gamma chain receptor, also leads to SCID. However, Jak3 deficiency affects males and females equally because the genetic mutation occurs on a different chromosome. In both gamma chain and Jak3-deficient SCID, there are normal numbers of B cells, but absent antibody production, T cells, and natural killer cells. Deficiency of adenosine deaminase, which is an enzyme needed for DNA metabolism, leads to accumulation of toxic products in lymphocytes and natural killer cells. Deficiency of the recombination-activating enzymes, which are critical for the formation of B cell and T cell antigen receptors, results in SCID

AIDS IN AFRICA AND ASIA

Since the HIV/AIDS pandemic began in the early 1980s, approximately 65 million people worldwide have become infected with HIV; more than 25 million have died. The region that has been most affected by HIV/AIDS is sub-Saharan Africa. In 2006, around two-thirds of all people (almost 25 million) living with HIV were in that region. In the same year, there were 2.8 million new infections and 2.1 million deaths from AIDS. Around 6 percent of adults are infected with the virus. Low condom use exacerbates the problem. Programs are available to provide anti-retroviral drugs (ARV), which can protect people from HIV infection and prevent the virus being passed to unborn babies. However, there is resistance in some African countries to sustaining such programs. In South Africa, where around 1,500 people are infected daily with HIV, there has been a debate over whether HIV ac-tually causes AIDS. The South African government is reluctant to provide ARV drugs in the public health service, consequently, there is no sign that the rate of infection is slowing down.

In Asia and the Pacific, around 8 million are living with HIV/AIDS. Although the prevalence is low, because of the large population (about 60 percent of the total world population), very large numbers of people are affected. Sex workers and drug users are most seriously affected, leading to infection of partners, then newborns. Because men are more likely to indulge in extramarital sex, the rate of infection rises for women on marriage. Poor education or access to information can result in women not being tested, and hence not being treated. As the number of people infected increases, so will the demand for treatment, which will be a challenge for health care budgets in Asia.

with absence of T and B cells. Several other less common genetic defects have been identified as causes of SCID.

SCID is diagnosed by measuring lymphocytes in the blood. All SCID subtypes share in common a deficiency of T cells and antibodies, but they vary in the numbers of B cells and NK cells present. On X-ray, the thymus cannot be seen. The specific genetic defects can also be assessed in the patient's cells. SCID is fatal in childhood unless it is appropriately treated. Prior to the onset of successful bone marrow transplantation, life-threatening infections still occurred despite treatment of frequent use of antibiotics, immunoglobulin infusions, and strict avoidance of microbes, as demonstrated by "the boy in the bubble," who lived from birth in a microbe-free plastic tent and died at 12 after surgery, when he left the bubble for the first time. The current treatment of choice is bone marrow transplantation. In this procedure, bone marrow stem cells are obtained from a compatible donor and transfused into the patient to reconstitute a functional immune system. The best outcomes occur when the transplant is done early in life using cells from well-matched donors. However, transplantation still carries a risk of life-threatening complications, even when a matched donor is found. Gene therapy is an experimental procedure for SCID, in which the genetic

defect is corrected by inserting a good copy of the gene into the patient's cells. However, severe complications like leukemia have occurred, albeit rarely, when the procedure unintentionally disrupted other genes. In the case of adenosine deaminase deficiency, the missing enzyme can be infused to improve immune function.

Tolerance and autoimmunity

Autoimmunity refers to an immune response directed at self-antigens. As a result of the random generation of antibodies and T cell receptors, some antigen receptors are produced that can bind to self-proteins. Under normal circumstances, lymphocytes bearing self-reactive receptors are eliminated or made non-responsive to achieve a state of self-tolerance. When this tolerance fails, autoimmune disease can occur. Central tolerance is predominantly achieved by deletion of self-reactive lymphocytes in the thymus or bone marrow. Self-reactive B cells can also undergo modification of their antigen receptors to change their antigen specificity. Peripheral tolerance is achieved when lymphocytes are inactivated after binding to antigen in the absence of necessary costimulatory signals. Regulatory T cells recognize self-antigens and inhibit immune responses against these antigens.

Type I insulin-dependent diabetes mellitus occurs as a

result of antibody-mediated destruction of the beta islet cells of the pancreas, which produce insulin. Insulin is a hormone that regulates blood sugar levels. In this condition, the blood sugar levels rise, owing to inadequate insulin production. The development of antibodies against the beta islet cells is thought to be triggered by a similarity in their proteins to viral proteins, in a process called molecular mimicry. Acute symptoms of type I diabetes mellitus include frequent urination, dehydration, nausea, and abdominal pain. If insulin is not replaced, the patient may experience diabetic ketoacidosis, a medical emergency in which toxic substances called ketones build up in the body. Over the long term, poor control of blood sugar levels can lead to blood vessel damage, causing disease in the cardiovascular system, kidney, retina, and nerves. The treatment for type I diabetes is insulin replacement, diet, and exercise. Transplantation of the beta islet cells is an experimental treatment that has the potential to cure the disease, but it requires lifelong use of immuno-suppressive medications to prevent transplant rejection.

Systemic lupus erythematosis, or lupus, is an autoimmune disease that can affect the skin, lungs, joints, kidney, heart, blood, and brain. Classic symptoms include a butterfly-shaped rash on the face, arthritis, inflammation of the lining of the lungs and heart, and kidney disease, but many other symptoms have been described. The disease course can involve symptom flares or periods of remission. Lupus is much more common in women than men. In most cases, lupus is associated with the presence of antibodies (called antinuclear antibodies) directed at the nuclear material inside cells; the presence of antinuclear antibodies is nonspecific, although high levels of the antibodies are more predictive. Other markers, such as antibodies against double-stranded DNA, are more specific for the disease. Treatment of lupus aims to suppress the immune response with corticosteroids and other agents. Treatment is based on the severity of organ involvement and potential side effects of treatment.

Wegener's granulomatosis is a rare disease of inflammation of the blood vessels, called vasculitis. It affects adult men and women equally. Symptoms can affect many organ systems, but most commonly, there is nasal and sinus inflammation, sometimes causing a classical "saddle nose" deformity. Vasculitis involving the kidneys or lungs can result in severe organ damage if it is not appropriately treated. Wegener's granulomatosis is frequently associated with the presence of specific antibodies, called antineutrophilic cytoplasmic proteins, but this is not sufficient for diagnosis. Diagnosis is confirmed by tissue biopsy demonstrating characteristic inflammation of the blood vessels. Treatment involves corticosteroids and other immunosuppressive drugs.

Sjogren's syndrome is an autoimmune disease with infiltration and destruction of glands in the body. Like lupus, the disease is much more common in women than men. Typically, the parotid, lacrimal, and salivary glands are affected, causing gland enlargement and the classic symptoms of dry mouth and eyes, also called sicca syndrome. The disease can also affect the joints, respiratory tract, gastrointestinal tract, or nerves, and there is an elevated risk of lymphoma. Biopsy may show lymphocytes, while blood tests frequently show antibodies against specific proteins, called Ro/SSA and La/SSB. Sjogren's syndrome can also occur in association with other autoimmune diseases, such as lupus or rheumatoid arthritis. Treatment is generally directed at controlling sicca symptoms, such as by moisturization of the eyes. When more severe symptoms occur, immunosuppressive medications are given.

Myasthenia gravis is a disorder in which antibodies are produced against the acetylcholine receptor. This receptor is a critical component of the signaling pathway that is required to produce muscle contractions. The classic symptom of myasthenia gravis is muscle fatigue that worsens with use and improves with rest. When the eye muscles are affected, this results in droopy eyelids or double vision. Involvement of other muscle groups can cause difficulty speaking, swallowing, or breathing. The diagnosis is confirmed by detection of antibodies against the acetylcholine receptor, specific findings on nerve studies, and improvement of symptoms when acetylcholine levels are increased. Most patients with myasthenia gravis have abnormalities of the thymus gland, such as tumors of the thymus, but the precise role of the thymus in the disease is unclear. Treatment includes use of medications that increase acetylcholine levels and surgical removal of the thymus.

Debby Lin

Impetigo

Impetigo is a common bacterial infection of the superficial layers of the skin. It is characterized by draining inflammatory skin lesions that most commonly occur on the face (especially around the nose and mouth). This condition can become quite severe without appropriate treatment.

Impetigo is always caused by bacteria. *Streptococcus pyogenes* and *Staphylococcus aureus* are the most common causative agents. Other less common types of streptococci can cause impetigo as well.

Impetigo usually occurs in young children. The infection often arises from sites of minor skin trauma such as cuts or abrasions. It is frequently spread from person to person in settings where there is close contact, such as within families and schools. Poor personal hygiene may also promote the spread of infection.

Symptoms and signs

In its classic presentation, the infection begins as localized inflamed lesions over the skin which may enlarge, become fluid-filled, and rupture. Pus may drain from the ruptured lesions. The purulent drainage dries to form a characteristic yellow crust over the skin, described as yellow-amber in appearance. Patients typically have little pain, and fever is usually absent.

Diagnosis and treatments

The diagnosis is typically made based on the characteristic appearance of the skin lesions. Culture of the draining fluid may also grow the bacteria.

In uncomplicated cases, topical antibiotics may be effective. In more severe cases, oral or intravenous antibiotics are recommended. Standard first-line medications include dicloxacillin, cephalexin, and erythromycin. Other antibiotics are equally effective.

The bacteria usually gains entry to the skin through skin trauma, such as a minor cut. Depending on the type of bacteria, it attaches to host cells through various proteins on its surface. It also may produce toxins that damage host tissues and lead to more severe infection.

There is no available vaccine to prevent this infection. Appropriate hygienic measures and avoidance of people who are already affected may prevent the spread of impetigo from person to person.

Epidemiology

Young children are most commonly affected, although all age groups can potentially acquire the infection.

Due to crowding and poor hygiene, the condition may also afflict the homeless population. More cases occur during warmer months of the year. Impetigo is a common complaint of patients in outpatient clinics and hospitals, and several million cases occur every year in the United States.

Joseph Fritz and Bernard Camins

KEY FACTS

Description
Bacterial infection of superficial layers of skin.

Causes
Most commonly the bacteria *Streptococcus pyogenes* or *Staphylococcus aureus*.

Risk factors
Overcrowded living conditions, poor hygiene, close contact with those already affected.

Symptoms
Red, inflamed lesions over the skin, usually on the face. The lesions enlarge, become fluid-filled, and eventually rupture and drain pus.

Diagnosis
Based on appearance of skin lesions. Bacteria may be detected by culture of draining fluid.

Treatments
Antibiotics, both topical and systemic, depending on the severity.

Pathogenesis
Entry of bacteria through minor skin trauma; bacteria adhere to skin cells and produces damaging toxins, leading to severe infections.

Prevention
Appropriate hygiene. No vaccine is available.

Epidemiology
Usually affects children of all ages and can be spread person to person through contact. Males and females are affected equally. Several million cases occur annually in the United States.

See also
• Antibiotic-resistant infections • Infections, bacterial • Skin disorders

Infections

Infection is defined as invasion by and multiplication of microorganisms within the body. The course of human history has been shaped by infectious diseases such as plague, influenza, dysentery, typhus, malaria, and most recently, emerging infections like HIV. Infections are currently the leading cause of death worldwide, causing a third of all deaths. In the United States, pneumonia is the fifth overall leading cause of death.

The agents that cause infections range from viruses to parasites. They include bacteriophages (viruses that can disrupt bacterial cells), plasmids (structures in bacterial cells that carry genes), and transposons, which are mobile clumps of genes that infect bacteria and modify their ability to cause disease. Prions are proteinaceous infectious particles that cause infections like Creutzfeldt-Jakob disease.

It is important to differentiate infection from infestation, which is the presence of animal parasites on or in the body. Carrier state is defined as a condition in which a person harbors microbes but does not become sick because of them; however, the microbes cause infection in a person to whom the organisms are transmitted. Opportunistic infections are infections that occur in patients with low immunity by organisms that do not normally cause infections in a healthy host.

Routes of spread

Infectious agents can enter the body through several routes. Many skin infections and the common cold spread through direct contact. Influenza and tuberculosis spread through air. Contaminated food and water are the usual vehicles for spread of dysentery and typhoid fever. Syphilis, gonorrhea, HIV, and hepatitis B and C spread through unprotected sex, as well as contact with blood and blood products. Transmission can occur to the fetus through the placenta. Infections that are transmitted from animals to humans are called zoonotic infections; examples include rabies through dog bite and malaria through mosquito bite. Infections transmitted in a hospital setting are called health care–associated infections.

Pathogenesis

Infection occurs in a person through a complicated interplay of factors involving the microbe, the human body, and the environment. Several natural body defenses exist in the human host that the microbes would need to overcome before causing infection. The mechanisms include physical barriers such as the skin and mucosal membranes; the presence of cells

RELATED ARTICLES

in the tissues called phagocytic and natural killer cells, which can destroy the invading microbes; and specialized immune mechanisms mediated through white blood cells called lymphocytes. The microbes also have complex mechanisms through which they invade the body and cause disease. They include the ability to attach to appropriate cells, the ability to invade cells and cause cell destruction, and strategies to avoid recognition or destruction by the immune system. The environment plays an important role in infection, both in transmission and in the ability of the host to combat the invader. Microbes multiply locally at the site of invasion or travel to other parts of the body through blood, lymph, or via the nerves. Once the organisms reach the target sites, they induce inflammation that results in tissue necrosis and perhaps formation of pus. The symptoms of infection are a result of products of inflammation circulating in the body.

Clinical features, diagnosis, and lab tests

The clinical features of infections are diverse. Fever, chills, and night sweats are the most common systemic symptoms of infection. Pain, pus discharge, redness, swelling, and tenderness may be present in the infected area. The infected persons also have symptoms that are related to the organ system involved (for example, cough and sputum in someone with pneumonia). Septicemia is said to occur when there is a sudden-onset, catastrophic illness with very high, raging fevers or very low body temperature, low blood pressure, and the offending microbes are identified in the blood. The onset of illness may be acute (occurring within days), subacute (occurring over weeks), or chronic (occurring over months).

Most diagnoses are based on clinical features, and laboratory tests may not be necessary. The white blood cell count is commonly elevated. The microorganisms are commonly identified from specimens of blood, urine, sputum, stool, cerebrospinal fluid, or joint fluid obtained from the body sites that are suspected to have infection. The specimens are stained and grown in culture media. Specimens from patients, most commonly blood, can be tested for the presence of antigens, which are molecules from the pathogens, and antibodies, which are molecules produced by the human body in response to the presence of antigens.

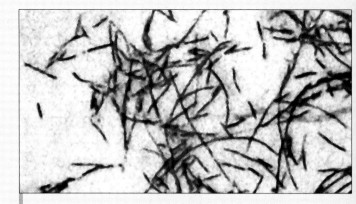

A colored micrograph shows Legionella *bacteria, which cause a lung infection called Legionnaires' disease. The major source of* Legionella *organisms is in water systems.*

Radiological tests such as X-ray, ultrasonography, CT (computed tomography) scan, and MRI (magnetic resonance imaging) help locate the site of infection and its extent. A biopsy may be necessary.

Treatments

Many infections are self-limiting. The mainstay of treatment of infections is the use of drugs called antimicrobials that can kill the pathogens. Some examples of antimicrobials are antibacterial agents such as the penicillins, antiviral agents such as acyclovir, antifungal agents like fluconazole, and anti-parasitic drugs such as albendazole. Resistance of the organisms to the drugs may be an issue if the infections do not improve with antimicrobial treatment.

Surgery may be necessary to drain pus, remove dead tissue, or eliminate large parasites. The infected persons may also need drugs to treat symptoms such as fever and pain. Drugs that suppress the immune system (steroids) may be useful, and so are drugs that interfere with the clotting system, such as activated protein C.

Prevention

Improvements in sanitation and living conditions and health education can eliminate most infections all over the world. Vaccines, if available, are important in the prevention of infections. In the setting of exposure to certain infections, antimicrobial drugs may be used to prevent disease. Scientific advances in genetic technology also offer means of infection prevention.

Pranavi Sreeramoju

Infections, animal-to-human

Infections that are transmitted from animals to humans are called zoonoses. All members of the microbial classes, such as bacteria, viruses, fungi, and parasites, can cause these infections. There are more than 200 such infections that occur worldwide, and any vertebrate animal or animal product encountered by humans may be involved.

Notable examples of zoonotic infections include: brucellosis, which presents with fevers and chills and is acquired through ingestion of unpasteurized cheese and other dairy products; anthrax, which may present as a fatal form of pneumonia, caused by inhalation of bacterial spores from infected animals; and leptospirosis, which is a disease with symptoms of fever and jaundice that is contracted by swimming in water contaminated with the urine of infected animals. Salmonellosis is an important zoonotic infection transmitted from many animals and birds in tropical countries, and it is characterized by high fevers and involvement of many organ systems.

Common animals involved in causing zoonotic infections are birds, dogs, cats, rabbits, horses, cattle, pigs, and monkeys. The animals may have the symptoms of disease, or they may simply act as reservoirs and vectors for these infectious organisms without having any symptoms. These infectious agents usually spread from one animal to the other. Humans acquire them when they are exposed in some way to the animal. The exposure may occur through direct animal contact, outdoor activities, exposure to and inhalation of infectious air particles, insect bites, contact with previously infected human blood products, and contact with and ingestion of infectious agents transmitted by animal-contaminated water and insufficiently cooked meat, eggs, fish, and shellfish, or unpasteurized dairy products.

Zoonotic infections occur in strange and often interesting ways. They can be severe, life threatening, and contagious, and may even warn of an emerging epidemic or a possible bioterrorist act.

Q fever was discovered after a group of poker players in Nova Scotia came down with pneumonia after exposure to the infected placenta of a house cat that had just delivered kittens.

More than 80 people in the midwestern United States developed monkey pox in the spring of 2003, and the exposure was traced to exposure to pet prairie dogs. These prairie dogs arrived at a pet shop along with a shipment of exotic pets from West Africa. West Nile viral encephalitis is thought to have been imported

RELATED ARTICLES

COMMON ANIMAL SOURCES OF INFECTIONS IN HUMANS

Disease	Birds	Cat	Dog	Rat	Rabbit	Horse	Goats and sheep
Anthrax		x	x			x	x
Brucellosis			x	x			x
Leptospirosis			x	x	x		x
Listeria infection	x				x		x
Lyme disease			x	x		x	
Plague		x		x	x		
Rabies	x	x	x	x	x	x	x
Toxoplasmosis		x					x
Tularemia	x	x	x	x	x	x	x
West Nile encephalitis	x		x			x	

into the United States through migratory birds or intercontinental air travel. Histoplasmosis is a fungal infection that occurs in cave explorers that are exposed to bat guano.

SARS (severe acute respiratory syndrome), which is a frequently fatal form of respiratory infection, is a recent example of a zoonotic infection. The virus originated from the masked palm civet in Southeast Asia but acquired the ability to spread from humans to humans. HIV (human immunodeficiency virus) and influenza are examples of infections that may have begun as zoonoses. When the virus becomes fully adapted to humans, it no longer requires an animal reservoir for continuing transmission. Letters that were deliberately contaminated with anthrax spores were responsible for up to a dozen infections, at least one death, and a massive public scare in the United States in 2001.

Epidemiology and risk factors
The vast variety of infections makes it difficult to count the number of zoonotic infections. It is estimated that about 15,000 such infections probably occur in the United States every year. There are about 50 million dogs in the United States, and they are associated with transmission of over 50 organisms. There are an even greater number of cats in the United States, and they are associated with transmission of over 40 organisms.

People at risk for acquiring these infections are those in certain occupations, such as veterinarians, hunters, farmers, and laboratory researchers; those who own pets, including dogs, cats, hamsters, and exotic pets such as reptiles and monkeys; people who are active outdoors, such as hikers, and those who travel to exotic places; and people with low immunity. For example, rabies occurs in travelers to Southeast Asia who are bitten by stray dogs; tularemia, plague, and anthrax occur in farmers and hunters who handle infected animals; brucellosis is common in travelers to Mexico who eat unpasteurized goat cheese.

In the modern era, there are more opportunities for increased human contact with animals. Changes in global temperature, rainfall, nature of soils, regrowth of forests, global trade, migration patterns of animals and birds, and increased travel to exotic areas all contribute to the increase. An example is the increase in populations of white-tailed deer, white-footed mice, and ticks due to reforestation, which contributed to an increase in Lyme disease in the northeastern United States.

The criteria used to define a zoonotic infection are: first, the animal reservoir should be a vertebrate other than humans; second, the agent is transmitted from the animal directly to people or from products derived from the animal or through an insect; and third, there is a recognizable pattern of clinical features in humans. Many animals that carry zoonotic pathogens can develop clinical disease. Other noninfectious diseases acquired from animals and insects, such as tick paralysis and the fish toxin illnesses, do not represent zoonoses. Malaria is not considered a zoonotic infection because the disease exclusively cycles between humans and mosquitoes, and there is no vertebrate host involved.

Diagnosis

Zoonotic infections are best diagnosed by an approach of recognition of a specific pattern of clinical features (called a syndromic approach), history of exposure to animals, and laboratory testing.

Zoonoses that present with symptoms of pneumonia such as fever, cough, and shortness of breath include psittacosis, Q fever, tularemia, plague, hantavirus, rhodococcus, histoplasmosis, and anthrax. Zoonoses presenting as rashes include ehrlichiosis, leptospirosis, Lyme disease, scabies, typhus, Rocky Mountain spotted fever, and anthrax. A characteristic ulcer occurs in anthrax and tularemia. Central nervous system involvement with altered consciousness or paralysis occurs in listeria infection, leptospirosis, and herpes B encephalitis, Lyme disease, lymphocytic choriomeningitis, rabies, cysticercosis, and Creutzfeldt-Jakob disease. Zoonotic illness may also result in arthritis, jaundice, diarrhea, sepsis and shock, kidney failure, fever of unknown origin, and infection of the lining of the heart.

An individual's at-risk activity or animal contacts can help narrow the possible causes of the infection. The potential modes of spread can be evaluated through questions regarding direct contact with animals or animal products, animal bites, and insect bites. Careful attention must be paid to the places a patient lived in or traveled to, as many zoonoses are confined to specific geographic areas. History of at-risk behaviors should be obtained from the person affected. This includes occupation (for example, veterinarian or farmer) and outside interests (for example, hunting, hiking, or exploring caves).

Laboratory studies are aimed at searching for specific parasites, as well as evaluating target organ involvement. Studies include cultures, tests for antibodies, and rapid diagnostic tests such as polymerase chain reaction (PCR), which is a method of copying DNA; and enzyme-linked immunosorbent assay (ELISA), which is used in the diagnosis of infectious diseases.

Despite the large number of infections that are transmitted from animals to humans, clinicians evaluating an individual patient usually need to consider only a limited number of historical details to arrive at a diagnosis.

Treatment and prognosis

In acute circumstances, treatment should be started based on clinical suspicion and available data, while awaiting confirmation with laboratory testing. Therapy is currently available for the majority of nonviral zoonotic infections and even for a few viral zoonoses. The mainstay of treatment is antibiotics targeted against the specific pathogen and supportive care.

Highly fatal zoonoses include Creutzfeldt-Jakob disease, rabies, anthrax, ebola fever, hantavirus, eastern equine encephalitis, plague, yellow fever, tularemia, and Rocky Mountain spotted fever. These

TULAREMIA

Tularemia is a potentially serious illness that is caused by the bacterium *Francisella tularensis* found in animals (especially rodents, rabbits, and hares). The symptoms of tularemia could include sudden fever, chills, headaches, diarrhea, muscle aches, joint pain, dry cough, and progressive weakness. People can also catch pneumonia and develop chest pain and bloody sputum. They can have trouble breathing and even sometimes stop breathing. Other symptoms of tularemia depend on the way in which a person was exposed to the tularemia bacteria. These symptoms can include ulcers on the skin or mouth, swollen and painful lymph glands, swollen and painful eyes, and a sore throat. Symptoms occur between 3 to 14 days after exposure. People can get tularemia many different ways, such as being bitten by an infected tick, deerfly, or other insect; handling infected animal carcasses; eating or drinking contaminated food or water; or breathing in the bacteria. Tularemia is not known to spread from person to person. People who have tularemia do not need to be isolated. Those who have been exposed to the tularemia bacteria should be treated as soon as possible. The disease can be fatal if it is not treated with the appropriate antibiotics.

organisms are also prime candidates for biological weapons. There is a great deal of ongoing research to develop vaccines and newer forms of treatment to combat these infections.

Prevention

There are many simple measures that can be taken to prevent zoonotic infections. Pets must be routinely immunized and neutered if necessary. Hands should be washed thoroughly with soap and warm water, especially after handling animal litter or carcasses.

Any change in the behavior of pets, especially rodents and rabbits, or livestock should be taken seriously; a veterinarian should be consulted if they develop unusual symptoms. It is important to make sure that meat, fish, and eggs are cooked well, and that drinking water is from a safe source. Unpasteurized dairy products should be avoided.

To prevent insect and tick bites, insect repellant containing DEET should be applied to the skin prior to entering a wooded area. Clothing should entirely cover the body; or, clothing can be worn that is treated with repellent containing permethrin.

In the hospital, special isolation precautions should be implemented, such as wearing gown and gloves, special types of masks, and placing the patient in a specially designed room may be necessary to

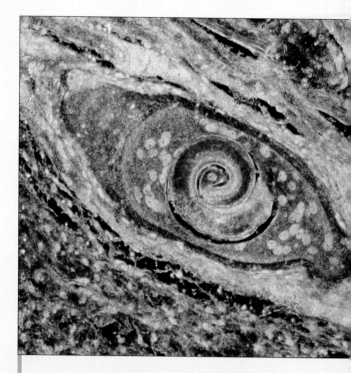

This light micrograph shows a larva of a Trichina spiralis *encysted in human muscle. The oval cyst is dark green; the single coiled larva is stained dark pink. Trichina spiralis is a species of roundworm, which is the cause of trichinosis in humans. The parasite is also found in dogs, cats, foxes, badgers, pigs, and rats.*

prevent spread of certain infections, such as viral hemorrhagic fever and plague.

Anyone planning exotic travel should get medical advice regarding precautions, travel alerts, medications to prevent diseases, and also to get appropriate vaccinations. For example, a yellow fever vaccine is recommended before traveling to certain parts of Africa. Some vaccines, like the rabies vaccine, are effective even after exposure (such as a dog bite), provided it is given soon after exposure.

Specific immunoglobulins that can be used for prevention are available for certain diseases like rabies. Certain bacterial infections like brucellosis or anthrax may be prevented with specific antibiotics if exposure has occurred. People in occupations that carry a particular risk, such as laboratory researchers and veterinarians, are advised to get additional vaccinations as a preventive measure.

Pranavi Sreeramoju

BRUCELLOSIS

Brucellosis is an infectious disease caused by various strains of bacteria of the genus *Brucella*. These bacteria are primarily passed among animals, such as sheep, goats, cattle, deer, elk, pigs, and dogs. Humans become infected by coming in contact with animals or animal products that are contaminated with these bacteria. In humans, brucellosis can cause a range of symptoms that are similar to influenza and may include fever, sweats, headaches, back pains, and physical weakness. Severe infections of the central nervous system or lining of the heart may occur. Brucellosis can also cause long-lasting or chronic symptoms that include recurrent fevers, joint pain, and fatigue. Treatment is with long-term antibiotics such as doxycycline and rifampin. About 100 to 200 cases of brucellosis occur in the United States every year.

Infections, bacterial

Bacteria are single-celled microorganisms that live in the air, in water, and in soil and can also live in the human body. Not all bacteria are harmful, but some bacteria can cause serious diseases.

Bacteria are single-cell organisms. Their small size renders them invisible to the human eye, yet the earth and its inhabitants are full of these microorganisms. Most bacteria are harmless to humans, whereas others can cause serious illness, even death. The discovery of penicillin led the way to the successful antibiotic treatment for many bacterial infections.

Most bacteria do not cause human disease and many are beneficial. Disease-causing bacteria are called pathogens. Bacteria can gain entry to the body by inhalation, and they can be ingested by eating contaminated food. Bacteria are transmitted to people both by direct and indirect contact. Direct physical contact includes shaking hands and intimate contact such as kissing and sexual activity, when infected body fluids such as saliva, mucus, or blood may be transferred to another person. Bacteria can also spread indirectly between people, for example, when they share or touch a common object such as a drinking glass or a telephone.

Prevention of bacterial infections

One simple way to prevent bacterial infections is to wash the hands often. If soap and water are not available, alcohol-based hand sanitizers can be used. Surfaces around the home should be cleaned and disinfected regularly, particularly in the bathroom and the kitchen, where sources of bacteria are more likely to be lurking. Bacteria are present on many foods: fresh fruits and vegetables, meat, and eggs. It is also important to wash the hands before eating. If someone touches a contaminated surface and then handles food, there is a chance of transferring bacteria to the food. Cleaning with soap and water removes many germs. For some bacteria, stronger disinfectants such as sodium hypochlorite (household bleach) and alcohol-based solutions are needed to kill the germs on surfaces. Ultraviolet rays from the sun are also deadly to many germs. Light, moisture, and temperature are some of the factors that determine how long bacteria can live on inanimate objects and surfaces.

Until the late 1940s, when antibiotics began to be produced on a mass scale and made routinely available, the main leading causes of death were bacterial in origin and included pneumonia, tuberculosis, and nephritis. In 1949 U.S. regulatory

RELATED ARTICLES

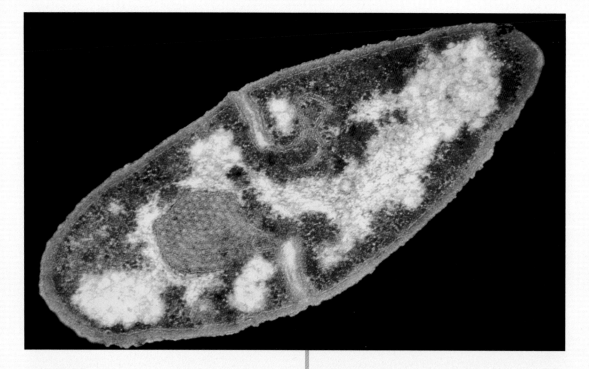

authorities licensed the first combination vaccine, which targeted three common and deadly diseases: diphtheria, tetanus, and whooping cough (pertussis). Diphtheria (*Corynebacterium diphtheriae*) can cause serious respiratory disease and skin infection. Whooping cough (*Bordetella pertussis*) can vary from a mild to a serious upper respiratory disease. Tetanus is caused by *Clostridium tetani*, which is present in the soil and typically enters the body through a break in the skin. Tetanus is also called "lockjaw," which is an early symptom of the bacterial infection. Death occurs in about 11 percent of cases, especially in older people.

More recently, three additional important childhood vaccines became available and recommended for routine use to prevent serious illness and death from these bacteria: *Hemophilus influenzae* type b, *Neisseria meningitidis*, and *Streptococcus pneumoniae*. *Hemophilus influenzae* type b bacterial infection causes a variety of serious diseases such as meningitis (an infection of the membranes covering the brain), epiglottitis (swelling in the throat that can cause life-threatening airway blockage), and pneumonia. *S. pneumoniae* is the most frequent cause of pneumonia, bacteremia, and acute otitis media (ear infection). Meningogoccal disease (caused by *N.*

This colored transmission electron micrograph shows a section through a **Corynebacterium diphtheriae,** *which is the cause of diphtheria in humans. It is a rod-shaped bacterium spread by inhalation of airborne bacteria.*

meningitidis) is also very serious, with death occurring among 10 to 15 percent of infected persons and a similar percentage of survivors having long-term effects such as brain damage, hearing loss, and amputation of limbs.

Respiratory infections
According to the Centers for Disease Control and Prevention (CDC), despite antibiotics and immunization, bacterial respiratory infections continue to threaten public health. Examples are pneumococcal infections, Legionnaires' disease, streptococcal infections, community-acquired pneumonia, and infections with *Hemophilus influenzae*. Impetigo, strep throat, necrotizing fasciitis, rheumatic fever, and toxic shock syndrome represent the range of disease caused by group A streptococcal infections.

Legionnaires' disease is caused by a type of bacteria called *Legionella* and is an example of bacterial transmission occurring simply by inhalation. *Legionella* grows best in warm water environments

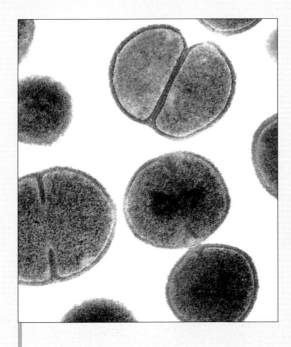

Methicillin-resistant Staphylococcus aureus (MRSA) bacteria are shown dividing on an electron micrograph. MRSA is of concern in hospitals, where outbreaks are difficult to control among vulnerable patients.

systems, or components of the air-conditioning systems of large buildings. The bacteria was first identified and named after an outbreak of pneumonia that occurred in 1976 among attendees of an American Legion convention. According to the CDC, each year at least 8,000 people are hospitalized with Legionnaires' disease in the United States, and death occurs in 5 to 30 percent of reported cases. The majority of people with *Legionella* infection recover following treatment with antibiotics.

Tuberculosis (TB) is caused by an infection with the bacterium *Mycobacterium tuberculosis*. TB is transmitted through the air, typically in close quarters in air contaminated by a person with untreated TB who is coughing. TB is no longer a leading cause of death in the United States; however, in many other countries, tuberculosis is an increasingly serious public health problem because *M. tuberculosis* is becoming resistant to multiple antibiotics.

Gastrointestinal infections

The majority of gastrointestinal infections are caused by food-borne bacteria and their toxins. According to

the CDC, the process of infection proceeds as follows. After the disease-causing bacteria are swallowed, there is a delay, called the incubation period, before the symptoms of illness begin. This delay may range from hours to days, depending on the organism, and on how many were swallowed. During the incubation period, the bacteria pass through the stomach into the intestine, attach to the cells lining the intestinal walls, and begin to multiply there. Some types of microbes stay in the intestine, some produce a toxin that is absorbed into the bloodstream, and some can directly invade the deeper body tissues.

Many bacteria and viruses cause similar symptoms, especially diarrhea, abdominal cramps, and nausea, so it is difficult to determine the cause of the infection. Typically, it is necessary to conduct laboratory tests to identify the source and cause of food-borne infections. The most commonly recognized food-borne infections are those caused by the bacteria *Campylobacter*, E. coli O157:H7, and *Salmonella*. *Salmonella* is widespread in the intestines of birds, reptiles, and mammals. E. coli O157:H7 is a bacterial pathogen that has a reservoir in cattle and other similar animals. In addition to disease caused by direct infection, some food-borne diseases are caused by the presence of a toxin in the food that was produced by bacteria in the food. *Staphylococcus aureus* is an example of a bacterium that produces a toxin in food. Another emerging food-borne bacterial infection is listeriosis. Listeriosis is caused by an infection with the bacterium *Listeria monocytogenes*, which is found in soil and water. Animals also are carriers of the bacteria. Listeria has been found in both raw foods and processed foods, such as soft cheeses and cooked meats. Listeria is killed by pasteurization and cooking. A serious consequence of listeriosis involves infections during pregnancy, which can lead to miscarriage or stillbirth, premature delivery, or infection of the newborn.

In developing countries, cholera and typhoid fever (caused by *Salmonella typhi*) are spread through fecal contamination of water, beverages, or food. These gastrointestinal bacterial infections are rare in regions where clean water and sanitation systems are in place. Also, cholera bacteria reside naturally in warm coastal seawater and can contaminate resident fish and shellfish. Typhoid fever is a life-threatening illness.

In the United States about 400 cases occur each year, and 75 percent of these occur while traveling. Typhoid fever is still common in the developing world, where it affects about 21.5 million people each year. Improved vaccines are in development for both diseases.

Rickettsial diseases

Lyme disease is caused by the bacterium *Borrelia burgdorferi* and is transmitted to humans by the bite of infected ticks. Symptoms include fever, headache, and a characteristic skin rash called erythema

VACCINES

Vaccines provide immunity to specific infectious diseases. They are typically made up of the disease-causing microorganisms that have been modified or killed. Certain bacteria and viruses produce toxins or antigens that alone can be given in doses that provide protection against disease. Health providers follow the recommendations of the Centers for Disease Control and Prevention in administering vaccines to children and adults. Most vaccines are given by injection, but some are given by mouth or through a nasal spray. There are several types of vaccines.

The table below shows vaccines that are in common use in the United States and in many other developed countries.

Type of vaccine	Description	Example of vaccine product
Live-attenuated	Prepared from live microorganisms or viruses that have been modified to prevent illness but that stimulate an immune response	Measles, mumps, and rubella (MMR)
Inactivated	Prepared with a microorganism or virus that has been killed, usually with a chemical agent such as formaldehyde	Poliovirus
Toxoid	Prepared from the inactivated bacterial exotoxin that has lost its toxicity but retains its antitoxin-producing properties	Diphtheria toxoid
Protein conjugate	Made from the coupling of antigens that make up the capsular portion of encapsulated bacteria with a carrier protein that provokes a stronger immune response for the antigen	*Hemophilus influenzae* type b (Hib) conjugate
Recombinant subunit	The proteins are produced by recombinant DNA technology using genetically engineered cell cultures that produce specific protein subunits of the virus	Hepatitis B

migrans. The majority of people diagnosed with Lyme disease recover from the disease following treatment with antibiotics. Untreated Lyme disease can spread to the joints, heart, and nervous system. Other tick-borne diseases include babesiosis, Crimean-Congo hemorrhagic fever, ehrlichiosis, Rocky Mountain spotted fever, southern tick-associated rash illness, tick-borne relapsing fever, and tularemia.

Sexually transmitted diseases

Sexually transmitted bacteria and the diseases they cause include: *Neisseria gonorrheae* (gonorrhea), *Chlamydia trachomatis* (chlamydial infections), *Treponema pallidum* (syphilis), *Hemophilus ducreyi* (chancroid), and *Klebsiella granulomatis*. The sexually transmitted bacterial infections are curable with antibiotic treatment. Worldwide, 62 million of cases of gonorrhea and 92 million cases of chlamydial infections occur yearly. Possible complications in women include infertility and chronic pelvic pain. Transmission of gonorrheal infections in newborns can lead to blindness if not treated promptly.

Other bacterial infections

Leprosy or Hansen's disease is a chronic infection of the skin, mucous membranes, and peripheral nerves. The bacterium *Mycobacterium leprae* causes leprosy and is usually spread from person to person in respiratory droplets. Globally, leprosy permanently disables 1 to 2 million people. Multidrug antibiotic treatment is necessary to prevent relapse of the disease, which is not readily available in endemic areas, such as Brazil, Mozambique, and Nepal.

Another mycobacterial infection, Buruli ulcer, is caused by *Mycobacterium ulcerans*. This presents as a cotton wool-like appearance and causes thickening and darkening of the skin surrounding the ulcer. The healing process of Buruli ulcers often results in severe deformity and scarring of the skin. Cases of Buruli ulcer have been reported worldwide. The reservoir of the bacterium has not been identified, which impedes prevention of the infection.

Trachoma is a chronic disorder that leads to scarring of the conjunctiva and cornea in the eye, resulting in decreased vision and blindness. Infections occur frequently in children. Trachoma is caused by infection with *Chlamydia trachomatis*, serovars (subdivisions of bacteria) A, B, Ba, and C. The disease was first described in the sixteenth century BCE.

The World Health Organization estimates that approximately 6 million cases of blindness occur as a result of trachoma each year. The disease is spread by secretions from the eye and respiratory tract, which can be spread through insects like house flies. Emerging resistance to antibiotics challenges global public health efforts to eradicate trachoma.

Spread and transmission of bacterial infections

Bacteria are spread and transmitted in many ways. They enter the body via the lungs, where they are inhaled in infective droplets. They can also be transmitted through the skin, in burns, cuts, or deep wounds.

Direct physical contact is another method of transmission; for example, bacteria can be transmitted during person-to-person contact such as shaking hands. Infected body fluids such as saliva, mucus, or blood may be transferred to another person during intimate contact, such as kissing and sexual activity.

Bacteria can be transmitted by respiratory droplet spread; bacteria are often present in saliva, in the mucus from the nose and lungs, which can be sent airborne through talking, sneezing, or coughing. Some bacteria such as *M. tuberculosis* produce spores that can remain suspended in the air. The amount of air movement influences how easily the spores can spread from person to person.

The fecal-to-oral route of transmission occurs when an infected person fails to adequately wash his or her hands after going to the bathroom and then contaminates a shared common object or prepares food that contains bacteria that is eaten by another person. Restaurant workers and food handlers can transfer the bacteria from their unwashed hands to food products.

Bacteria can also spread indirectly between people, for example, when they share or touch a common object such as a drinking glass or a telephone. This method is called common-vehicle spread. Contaminated water or food can transmit bacteria and toxins to large numbers of people.

Vector-borne spread occurs when insects and other animals transmit bacterial infections from direct contact or a bite. For example, Lyme disease is transmitted from an infected tick that carries the bacterial spirochete *B. burgdorferi*.

Bacteria versus viruses

Viruses and bacteria are distinct. Bacteria are single-celled and are one of the smallest life forms, yet they are 1 million times the size of a typical virus. Bacteria resemble houseguests in the body, while viruses can be likened to alien invaders.

Bacteria are found throughout the Earth, in air, water, soil, ice, even in the most inhospitable areas such as geothermal springs and the intestinal tracts of animals. Bacteria live inside and outside the human body. Many bacteria are beneficial to humans, whereas others cause disease and are pathogenic.

Under optimal conditions, bacteria can divide and multiply rapidly in the human body. Antibiotics treat bacterial infections by interfering with the growth of new bacterial cells and halting further infection.

Viruses are mostly genetic material, that is, DNA or RNA, and often have a protective coat surrounding their genes. Outside the body's cells, a virus cannot survive for long. Viruses cannot reproduce without the help of a host such as a human or animal cell. Viruses invade cells. They use the machinery of body cells to make new viruses. Typically, the progeny viruses destroy the cell as they leave to infect new cells. Freeloading viruses rather than bacteria are the more frequent culprits of respiratory illnesses like colds, sore throats, and coughs, according to the CDC.

Bacterial toxins

In addition to disease caused by direct infection with bacteria, some bacteria produce toxins. Toxins can make people very sick; for example, *Clostridium botulinum* produces a deadly neurotoxin in contaminated food. This form of food poisoning is called botulism. *Clostridium* bacteria are commonly present in the soil where food crops are grown; however, the bacteria are killed at high temperatures. With the advent of commercial food canning and preparation, botulism is a rare occurrence today.

Escherichia coli and *Staphylococcus aureus* are also toxin-producing bacteria that commonly contaminate food. E. coli O157:H7 resides in the intestinal tract of cattle. This bacterium travels with cow feces and can contaminate food products from cattle and water that comes in contact with these animals. Staphylococcal bacteria reside in our nasal passages. By touching the nose during food preparation, people may inadvertently transfer these bugs into an ideal environment where they will grow rapidly and produce toxin. Both E. coli and staphylococci are killed at cooking temperatures, but their toxins are often more heat resistant and survive in the food. When ingested, the toxins cause vomiting, diarrheal disease, and occasionally more serious illness. The toxins from staphylococci can make someone ill very quickly, sometimes within 30 minutes.

Flesh-eating bacteria

Flesh-eating bacteria may sound like a product of medical fiction, but they are a real yet rare complication of an infection with group A beta-hemolytic streptococcus. The same bacteria that is responsible for strep throat and the common skin infection impetigo leads to necrotizing fasciitis, which is the correct term for the flesh-eating bacterial infection.

In the United States, less than 1,000 cases of necrotizing fasciitis are reported annually, compared with several million cases of strep throat and impetigo each year. Invasive group A streptococcal infections occur when the bacteria breach the defenses of the person who is infected. This may occur when a person has sores or other breaks in the skin that allow the bacteria to get into the tissue, or when the person's ability to fight off infection is decreased because of chronic illness or immune system suppression.

The bacteria infect the skin and underlying soft tissue called fascia. Early symptoms of necrotizing fasciitis include fever, as well as severe pain, swelling, and redness at the wound site.

Necrotizing fasciitis destroys muscles, fat, and skin tissue. Prompt diagnosis and treatment are essential to control the rapidly spreading infection and death of soft tissue. Treatment includes surgical removal of the dead (necrotic) tissue and antibiotic therapy.

According to experts, early diagnosis and treatment of necrotizing fasciitis may reduce the risk of death from invasive group A streptococcal disease. However, even the best medical care does not prevent death in every case. Despite medical interventions, about 20 percent of patients with necrotizing fasciitis do not survive the infection.

Mary Quirk

Infections, fungal

Fungi are a vast group of organisms. Fungi can cause infection in humans, other animals, and plants. Human infections usually occur in people whose immune system is compromised. To prevent sickness and death, an early diagnosis is important. Although there are about 1.3 million species of fungi, most do not cause disease in people.

Human pathogenic fungi belong in two groups: molds and yeasts. They are either endogenous fungi associated with humans, or exogenous (from outside the body). Molds are fungi that grow vegetatively as hyphae, which are long filaments divided into cells by cross walls called septa. The size, shape, color, and presence of septa help identify the various types of hyphae in specimens such as skin scrapings, sputum, and sections of tissue. In contrast to molds, some fungi grow vegetatively as solitary cells that reproduce by budding. These fungi are yeasts, some of which may be normal flora on the skin and in the gastrointestinal tract. Size, shape, budding pattern, presence of capsules, color, and pseudohyphae can be used to classify yeasts.

One group of fungi are dimorphic, that is, the fungus can grow in two different morphological forms depending upon temperature. Most dimorphic fungi grow as a mold at 77°F (25°C), and as a yeast in tissue when they are causing an infection. *Coccidioides immitis* is an exception because it grows as spherules that form endospores in tissue or at 98.6°F (37°C) in the lab, and as a mold at 77°F (25°C).

Infections are caused by fungi such as molds, yeasts, or dimorphic pathogens. Infections occur when a yeast or mold grows on the surface of hair, nail, or skin. There may be some inflammation, but the fungus does not invade deeper. The fungus black piedra (*Piedraia hortae*), which forms nodules around the hair shaft, is a classic example of this type of infection.

Cutaneous infections can be caused by molds or yeast. The fungus typically grows in the surface layer of the skin, in nail tissue, or in hair. Dermatophyte infections called dermatophytosis, tinea, ringworm, or jock itch are often seen in children and adults. The fungi that cause these infections are anthropophilic (from people), zoophilic (from animals such as cats and dogs), or geophilic (originating from soil). In contrast, there is a group of lipophilic yeasts called malassezia that are associated with the skin, which cause pityriasis versicolor. This infection is easily seen on the skin during summer because the yeast acts as a sunscreen, with the result that infected areas have a different color from the surrounding skin.

Subcutaneous infections usually occur because the fungus is introduced into the subcutaneous tissue on a splinter or other wound. These types of infections typically remain localized and do not spread to other organs. In all of the infections discussed so far, dissemination does not occur for various reasons. Essentially they occur in people who have active immunological defense mechanisms in place.

Disseminated systemic infections are more serious because the patient is usually immunocompromised owing to a disease such as cancer or immuno-suppressive therapy. The fungus is inhaled into the lungs, or enters the circulatory system. With systemic infections, the fungus may cause skin disease, subcutaneous infections, and involve multiple organs.

Factors affecting fungal infection development
Factors that influence the development of fungal infections include the virulence of the fungus and host defense mechanisms. Virulence factors allow the fungus to grow, reproduce, and evade normal host defense mechanisms. In tissue, the yeast form of

Histoplasma capsulatum grows and reproduces within macrophages. The polysaccharide capsule of *Cryptococcus neoformans*, as well as the presence of melanin, aids its ability to grow in human tissue. The capsule protects the yeast cells against phagocytosis. Before *Candida albicans* invades tissue, it must adhere to the endothelium of blood vessels. Host defense mechanisms help prevent infections as does intact skin. Hydration of the skin and abrasion allow yeast infections called diaper rash to develop. For pulmonary pathogens such as *Aspergillus fumigatus*, secretions from the nasal passage and cilia can capture fungal conidia and remove them before they reach the lungs. The normal skin, mucosal surfaces, and gut flora can inhibit fungal growth.

The bacteria of the vagina are important in the development of yeast vaginitis caused by *C. albicans*.

Common fungal infections

Patients with certain conditions are at risk for fungal infections. These include HIV and AIDS, solid organ and bone marrow transplantation, cancer, diabetes mellitus, burns, chronic lung disease, chemotherapy, radiotherapy, and steroid use.

Yeasts. The most common yeast infection is candidiasis; the second is *Cryptococcus neoformans*, which was a serious cause of cryptococcal meningitis. The yeast is protected from the host by a capsule. The yeast originates from soil enriched by bird droppings. It is transmitted in the air, where it is inhaled. It affects the lungs, then may disseminate in the body. AIDS patients are more prone to this infection once the CD4 cell count is below 100. (CD4 receptor molecules are on the surface of helper cells or T cells; HIV molecules attach to the CD4 molecule, allowing the virus to enter the cells.) The diagnosis is usually by serology, and the measurement of antibody has prognostic value. The presence of a capsule around a round yeast cell suggests *Cryptococcus*. In AIDS patients it is important to control the disease. Patients with limited pulmonary disease and normal immunity will usually recover.

Molds. Mold infections include dermatophyte infections and aspergillosis in the immunocompromised patient. A dermatophyte is a fungus that invades hair, nail, or skin on the living host. The diagnosis of ringworm is based upon the presence of hyphae in keratinized tissue, or arthroconidia in hair, or by culturing the fungus on laboratory media. The identification of the dermatophyte helps determine its origin. For example, the isolation of *M. canis* would suggest that the fungus came from a pet cat or dog.

Aspergillus species are molds that can cause severe disease in healthy and immunocompromised hosts. The most common species of Aspergillus causing disease in humans are *A. fumigatus*, *A. flavus*, *A. niger*, and *A. terreus*. Aspergillus is found worldwide; it is a decomposer of plant material. Conidia of the mold are inhaled by the host. In patients with cystic fibrosis, the incidence of colonization is high. Diagnosis is often difficult. Computed tomography (CT) and magnetic resonance imaging (MRI) are useful tools, as well as the presence of fever. The infection can be treated with drugs, and surgical intervention may be helpful.

Dimorphic. Four important dimorphic fungal infections include blastomycosis, coccidioidomycosis, histoplasmosis, and sporotrichosis. The first three are most common in the United States. Blastomycosis is caused by *Blastomyces dermatitidis*. The fungus has been isolated from decaying wood, and there is a high incidence in hunting dogs because they constantly sniff the environment. The incidence in men is more than that in women and there is strong occupational exposure. Infections in immunocompromised patients are more severe and often involve the central nervous system.

Coccidioidomycosis is a unique dimorphic infection because the causative agent, *Coccidioides immitis*, grows in tissue.This dangerous fungus is the only fungus listed as a Biological Safety Level (BSL) 3 pathogen. Special safety precautions are used when working with this fungus. *Histoplasma capsulatum* is a dimorphic fungus in which the yeast form grows and replicates within macrophages and giant cells. The infection is caught from soil enriched with avian feces or bat guano. Finally, *Sporothrix schenckii is a* dimorphic fungus that gains entry to subcutaneous tissue after the implantation of the fungus on thorns or plant debris.

Antifungal agents

Many antifungal agents are effective in managing fungal infections. There has also been success in treating infections by modulating the immune system. Antifungal agents target any fungal biosynthetic pathways and cellular components not present in humans.

Bilal Sarvat and Michael McGinnis

Infections, parasitic

Parasitic infections are caused by organisms called parasites that live on or inside another organism called the host. Parasites enter the body through the skin or mouth and generally cause harm to the host. Parasites are common in rural parts of Africa, Asia, Latin America, and the United States. People traveling abroad may acquire these parasites, which a doctor may not diagnose once they return home. Some parasites are carried in contaminated food, drink, and water in regions with poor sanitation. When eating in developing areas, travelers are advised to drink only bottled water and to check that food has been thoroughly cooked. Because parasites may survive freezing, even ice cubes may be contaminated. Parasites that penetrate the skin often enter through the soles of the feet, when a person swims or wades in water.

Many kinds of parasites infect animals and humans. The general types include one-celled organisms such as amoebas or other protozoa; roundworms, such as hookworms and threadworms; flatworms, such as tapeworms and flukes; and insects such as lice.

If a doctor suspects a parasite, he or she may take samples of blood, stool, or urine for laboratory analysis and may also take a sample of the infected tissue. Antibiotics, laxatives, and antacids can reduce the number of parasites and make detection more difficult. Most parasites respond to treatment with medication; however, if the condition has damaged major organs and tissues, effects may be permanent.

Parasites that infect humans are much more prevalent and widespread than most people realize, despite the availability of accessible information. On their Web sites, the National Institute of Allergy and Infectious Diseases and the Centers for Disease Control and Prevention (CDC) provide information about parasitic infections. Most health departments have specialists who advise travelers about conditions in certain areas and how to avoid them, and they may prescribe preventive medicines. Travelers need to be aware that they may unknowingly become infected with parasites.

Diseases caused by protozoa

Protozoa (one-celled organisms) cause many diseases. The most commonly encountered diseases caused by protozoa are amebiasis, babesiosis, cryptosporidiosis, cyclosporiasis, giardiasis, malaria, toxoplasmosis, sleeping sickness, and Chagas' disease.

Amebiasis is an infection of the large intestine and is caused by *Entamoeba histolytica*. Common in areas where sanitation is poor and human feces are used as fertilizer, amebiasis is acquired through food, water, and sexual practices. *Entamoeba histolytica* has two forms: an active state, called a trophozoite, and a dormant cyst. When cysts are swallowed, the warmth of the intestine causes the membrane of the cyst to break open, creating an active medium in which protozoa multiply and penetrate the lining of the intestine. These protozoa cause diarrhea or amebic dysentery. The amoebas may infect the abdominal cavity, liver, genitals, lungs, and brain. Diagnosis involves finding the trophozoites or cysts in the stool of the person. The antiamebic drug metronidazole is used for treatment.

Babesiosis is an infection of red blood cells and is caused by the *Babesia* genus of protozoa. The same deer tick that transmits Lyme disease carries these parasites. They live inside human red blood cells and eventually destroy them, producing fever, headache, muscle aches, and anemia. Diagnosis is made by examination of a blood sample under the microscope. The drugs quinine and clindamycin are used to treat this infection.

Cryptosporidiosis is a diarrhea-producing infection caused by *Cryptosporidium parvum*. This infection is acquired by ingesting contaminated water or food. The cysts are very hardy and frequently are found in surface water in the United States, especially in areas where there are farm animals. Usual levels of chlorine in drinking water or swimming pools do not kill the organism, so it is important to take preventive care. No drugs have been found that kill the organism in people, so the affected individual is usually permanently infected.

Cyclospora cayetanensis is a small protozoan that causes cyclosporiasis. It is spread through ingestion of food or water contaminated by infected feces. The first cases were reported in 1979 and then more frequently in successive years. One famous outbreak occurred when contaminated raspberries from Chile caused outbreaks among people who ate the raspberries. *Cyclospora* affects the small intestine and causes watery diarrhea with explosive bowel movements. Recommended treatments for cyclosporiasis include sulfa drugs and antibiotics.

The protozoan *Giardia lamblia* causes giardiasis, the most common parasitic infection in the United States. Most people get this infection from drinking contaminated water from lakes and streams that appear clean. Backpackers and hikers who drink untreated water are at risk. It is a major cause of traveler's diarrhea. Symptoms are gas, cramps, and foul-smelling diarrhea. Microscopic examination of stools may reveal the parasite. The drug metronidazole, taken orally, is effective against this parasite.

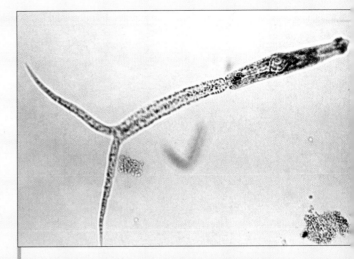

This photomicrograph shows the larval stage of the parasite Schistosoma cercaria, *which can live in lakes and rivers. The larvae can penetrate human skin and then develop in the body into flukes (adult forms), which cause severe illness.*

Protozoa of the genus *Plasmodia* cause malaria, an infection of red blood cells, which leads to fever, an enlarged spleen, and anemia. The complex cycle of infection begins when an infected female mosquito bites a person with malaria and ingests blood that contains parasites. Inside the mosquito, the parasite multiplies and migrates to the salivary glands; when the mosquito bites another person, that person becomes infected with the parasites. Parasites then move to the host's liver and begin to multiply again and invade the red blood cells. As the infected blood cells rupture and release parasites, the person develops shaking chills, followed by a very high fever. Headaches, body aches, and heavy sweating are common. It is important to prevent mosquito bites, especially when traveling to areas where the infections are common. Chills and fevers, especially for those who have traveled to areas where malaria is endemic, usually indicate malaria. Drugs to prevent malaria are recommended for those planning to travel to infected areas. Chloroquine is the preferred drug for treating malaria.

Insects are also the carriers of several serious conditions. The infamous tsetse fly carries *Trypanosoma brucei*, a protozoan that causes African sleeping sickness. The assassin bug, or kissing bug, carries *Trypanosoma cruzi*, which causes Chagas' disease, an infection that affects people who live in South and

MALARIA

Malaria is one of the greatest plagues of mankind; it robs people of their energy, their ability to enjoy life, and the capacity to make a living. Malaria is caused by protozoa called plasmodia, which are spread by the bites of mosquitoes. It is generally thought to be a disease of Africa, but it has flourished in the Middle East, China, and Europe well into modern times. In 2700 BCE, a Chinese medical classic dubbed the disease "mother of fevers" and accurately described the cycle of fever and chills and the enlarged spleen. The Sumerians in their cuneiform writings in 1600 BCE made it clear that malaria was a curse of the ancient world. Hippocrates (c. 460–c. 380 BCE) saw a link between swamps and

malaria but thought that drinking stagnant water caused the disease. Others believed the foul air from the swamps caused an illness called swamp fever, ague, or Roman fever (after the swamps around Rome). Some historians even traced the demise of the Greek and Roman civilizations to this disease.

The name *malaria* comes from two Italian words meaning "evil air." Horace Walpole, a British citizen visiting Rome, first used the term in a letter from Italy in 1740. He described a horrid disease called *mal'aria* that afflicts Rome every summer. Until the late nineteenth century, *malaria*, or "bad air," was used to mean the cause of the disease, not the disease itself.

Central America. Although these diseases may be treated with modern drugs, most are found in remote areas where medical assistance is not available, and people develop and carry the conditions for many years.

Toxoplasma gondii causes an infection called toxoplasmosis, or cat-scratch fever. Many people contract toxoplasmosis but do not show any symptoms, and severe illness generally develops only in fetuses and people with a weakened immune system. The parasite produces eggs only in the cells that line the intestine of cats, and the eggs may be eaten through soil or uncooked food contaminated with eggs from cats' feces. If a pregnant woman acquires the infection during pregnancy, she can transfer the infection to the fetus through the placenta. The result may be a miscarriage, stillbirth, or a baby born with congenital toxoplasmosis. These children may be severely ill and die shortly after birth, or they may have symptoms that include blindness, enlargement of the liver and spleen, jaundice, easy bruising, seizures, a large or small head, and mental retardation. Studies show that early detection and treatment can prevent such tragedies. Screening is advised for all pregnant women during prenatal visits and for all newborns.

Roundworms

Also called nematodes, roundworms are a group of invertebrates (animals without a backbone) with a wormlike body. Many are not harmful to humans, but some can cause a variety of infections in humans and

animals. The most common parasitic roundworms in humans are *Ascaris*, hookworms, threadworms, whipworms, pinworms, *Trichina*, and filarial worms.

Ascaris lumbricoides causes the most common roundworm infection in people, ascariasis. Over one billion people worldwide have the condition, and it persists in areas where people live in unsanitary conditions. Infection begins when the person swallows food contaminated with worm eggs, which are hardy and survive in the soil for years. Once ingested, the eggs hatch and release larvae (immature forms) in the intestine, which then migrate through the walls of the small intestine and travel through the lymph vessels to the lungs. From the respiratory tract, the larvae are coughed up and swallowed; they mature and live in the small intestine. Adult worms range from 6 to 20 inches (15–50 cm) in length. Common symptoms are coughing and pains in the abdominal area. The diagnostic findings may include presence of eggs or worms in the stool or in vomit. Left untreated, complications include a blocked intestine or problems with the liver or pancreas. Preventive measures includes adequate sanitation and avoiding uncooked foods. Drugs such as mebendazole treat the condition.

Two intestinal roundworms cause hookworm infection: *Ancylostoma duodenale*, which is referred to as Old World hookworm, affects people living in India, China, Japan, and the Mediterranean; and *Necantor americanus*, which is found in Africa, Asia, and the southern part of the United States. Warm, moist climates are ideal for hookworm development. About one billion people are infected with hookworms. Hookworm larvae enter the body through the skin—especially the feet—or mouth, and pass into the bloodstream. The larvae then travel through the bloodstream to the lungs. Larvae in secretions from the lungs are coughed up, swallowed, and passed into the stomach. The larvae then migrate to the intestines, where they mature. The head of the adult has sharp, curved plates that cling to the wall of the intestines. The difference between hookworms and *Ascaris* is implied in the name. Hookworms actually attach to, or bite into, the walls of the intestines; *Ascaris* just float freely. The female hookworms lay eggs that pass into the feces. If feces land in the soil, the eggs hatch into larvae, and the cycle is repeated. Symptoms include abdominal pain, anemia, heart problems, and retarded growth. Diagnosis is made by finding the eggs in the stool; treatments include taking the drug mebendazole. Preventive measures include the use of sanitary facilities and not walking barefoot on soil or wet ground likely be infested with hookworm larvae.

Threadworms (*Strongyloides stercoralis*) are found in contaminated soil in the southern part of the United States. They penetrate the skin and can produce pain in the pit of the stomach and cause diarrhea. Larvae may be seen in stools. Whipworms (*Trichocephalus trichiura*) are not common in the United States but can cause the same symptoms, and the eggs are seen in the stools. Both of these worms may cause dysentery (bloody diarrhea) or acute appendicitis. The lower bowel area may collapse in untreated children.

The pinworm (*Enterobius vermicularis*) infests the intestines. This worm is the most common flatworm in children in the United States. Infestation begins when a child ingests pinworm eggs that have been transferred from the area around the anus of an infected indiviudual to clothing, bedding, or toys. Eggs can live outside the body for as long as three weeks at normal temperature. After swallowing, the eggs hatch in the intestine, and young worms migrate to the intestinal and rectal areas. Usually at night, the female migrates to the area around the anus to lay her eggs in a sticky gelatinous material that causes

A photomicrograph reveals the structure of the head of a tapeworm, Taenia solium, *in a human intestine. The tapeworm attaches to the intestine wall with four suckers and two rows of hooks located in its head region, or scolex.*

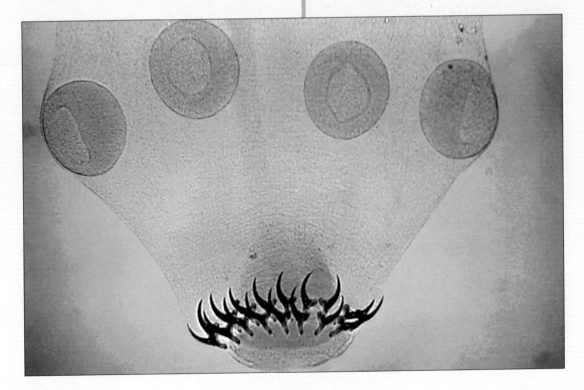

itching. Children may reinfect themselves by transferring the eggs to their mouths, thus making pinworms difficult to conquer. Thumbsuckers are at increased risk of infection.

Finding the white, hair-thin worms or their eggs is evidence of pinworms. Patting the sticky side of tape to the anal area after the child goes to bed may help the doctor find the worms to examine under the microscope. Treatment includes drugs such as mebendazole. Often, the whole family must be treated. The entire environment must be cleaned; yet the infection may still recur. Pinworms may occur even with high levels of sanitation.

The roundworm *Trichinella spiralis* causes the infection trichinosis. The larvae of the worm live in the muscle tissue of animals, typically pigs, wild bears, horses, and many carnivores. People get trichinosis by eating uncooked or poorly cooked meat from an animal that carries the parasite. At one time, human infections came from regions where pigs were fed uncooked meat scraps and garbage. Now the condition is rare in the United States. The life cycle begins when a person eats meat containing live cysts of the worm. Digestive enzymes break through the wall of the cyst and release larvae, which then mature and travel to the intestine. Females burrow into the intestinal wall and on the seventh day begin to produce larvae for a period of four to six weeks before dying. Larvae move to the muscles, where they remain and produce cysts. In the process, they cause inflammation. Muscles around the eyes, in the tongue, and between the ribs are most often infected. The symptoms vary depending on the number of invading larvae. The main symptoms are muscle pain, weakness, fever, muscle soreness, and swelling of the upper eyelids. Unlike most parasites, trichinella cannot be diagnosed by examination of the stools; blood tests or a biopsy of the infected muscle must be carried out. Drugs are generally effective against the parasite.

Filariasis is a group of diseases in tropical and subtropical countries caused by parasitic worms and their larvae. Certain species of mosquitoes spread the infection by biting victims and introducing the larvae into the host. The adult form lives in the lymphatic system and releases larval forms called microfilariae into the bloodstream, usually at night. If the person is bitten again, the insect ingests the new larvae and transmits them to a new host. A serious condition called elephantiasis—massive swelling—may affect the legs or scrotum area.

Blackflies infected with *Onchocerca volvulus*, found in remote African rural agricultural villages near rapidly flowing streams, spread worm larvae by biting the skin of humans. The larvae, called microfilariae, can migrate to the eye to cause onchocerciasis, also called river blindness.

Parasitic skin infections

Three kinds of parasitic skin infections have plagued mankind throughout the ages. Lice infestation, or pediculosis, has been linked to the historic plagues of epidemic typhus and typhoid fever. Pediculosis is a condition in which parasitic insects called lice infest the body and clothing or bedding. Found worldwide, lice affect people who are in close contact and spread quickly if not checked. There are three types of lice: head, body, and pubic lice. Head lice are transmitted through personal contact. They live on the scalp, eyebrows, eyelashes, and beard. Outbreaks of head lice are common among schoolchildren; they are not a result of a lack of hygiene. Body lice, uncommon in good hygiene conditions, cause a great amount of itching. Pubic lice affect the genital area and are usually transmitted through sexual contact.

Three forms of the lice exist: the egg (sometimes called a nit), the nymph, and the adult. Nits are white to yellow and attach themselves to hair. Nits of head lice may be seen around the hairline at the nape of the neck. The adult is about the size of a sesame seed, has six legs, and is tan to grayish white. Effective treatment is usually rapid with special shampoos and body lotions containing 1 percent hexachloride. Treatment must be repeated after 10 days to destroy any nits that survived.

A mite (insectlike animal) called *Sarcoptes scabiei* causes scabies. The female mite burrows into the skin and deposits eggs along the tunnel. When the larvae hatch, they congregate around hair follicles, and the person develops pruritis, or severe itching. If the individual has severely scratched the area, the burrow usually cannot be seen. Microscopic examination of scrapings from the area usually reveals the cause. Treatment with medications containing 1 percent gamma benzene hexachloride is generally effective.

CYCLOSPORA: A CONTAMINANT OF FRUITS, VEGETABLES, AND WATER

In the past several years, outbreaks of explosive diarrhea have connected *Cyclospora cayetanensis* to raspberries imported from Guatemala and Chile. The outbreaks began in 1995, and within the next two years, 90 outbreaks occurred in five states. Because the parasite can infect various types of fresh produce, finding the source of the infection is like looking for a needle in a haystack: symptoms of diarrhea, vomiting, fatigue, and muscle aches may not occur until a week after the event, when people have forgotten what they ate and where they ate it. The most recent notorious outbreak was on June 10, 2000, when 83 guests at a catered wedding reception in Philadelphia, Pennsylvania, became ill a week later. The health authorities were notified that many guests had a gastrointestinal illness, and stool samples revealed *Cyclospora*. The wedding cake had a cream filling with raspberries, and the leftover cake was positive for *Cyclospora* DNA. Other cases of cyclosporiasis have been reported in California, Florida, Nevada, New York, and Texas.

In order to prevent this illness it is best to avoid eating raw or undercooked foods or drinking untreated water. Cooking can kill *Cyclospora*, but a general food safety measure is to thoroughly wash all fresh produce before cooking or eating it.

Creeping eruption, or cutaneous larva migrans, is caused by the larvae of the dog and cat hookworm. The infested animals excrete feces and worm eggs in the soil or sandbox in which children play. The eggs hatch into larvae that penetrate the feet or other body part that touches the soil. The worm cannot get into the bloodstream of humans but stays on the skin area and burrows a path around the area of infection. Itching and scratching are common, and the area may become secondarily infected with bacteria. Creeping eruption can be treated with oral and topical medicines.

Tapeworms

Four kinds of tapeworms infect humans: the dwarf tapeworm (*Hymenolepsis nana*), the beef tapeworm (*Taenia saginata*), the pork tapeworm (*Taenia solium*), and the fish tapeworm (*Diphylobothrium latum*). Tapeworms are large, flat worms that live in the intestine and can grow up to 20 feet (6 m) long. The egg-bearing sections, or proglottids, are passed out of the body with the stool. If eggs are released into soil or water, pigs, cattle, or fish may ingest them and become intermediate hosts. The eggs hatch and the larvae penetrate the intestinal walls to lodge in the muscle as cysts. A human who eats inadequately cooked meat acquires the cysts, which hatch out and develop into adult worms that attach to the intestine wall. An infested person may have abdominal discomfort, lose weight, or have no symptoms. Noticing proglottids in the stool is usually the first indication of the worm.

One treatment of the drug praziquantel usually gets rid of the infestation. Inspecting meat and looking for visible cysts, as well as thoroughly cooking meat, prevent transmission of tapeworms.

Flukes

Flukes cause one of the most prevalent diseases in tropical regions of South America, Africa, and Asia, affecting over 200 million people. These parasites are rare in the United States and are usually seen in people who have visited the Far East. The most common fluke disease is schistosomiasis, also called bilharzia. Schistosomiasis is acquired by bathing or walking in water contaminated with schistosomes. The condition saps the energy of many inhabitants of the world. The fluke has an unusual way of reproducing. Schistosomes multiply inside specific types of water-dwelling snails. Fluke larvae are released into the water and swim freely. If they encounter a person's skin, they penetrate it and migrate through the bloodstream to the lungs, in which they mature into adult flukes. The adults pass through the bloodstream to their final home in the small veins in the bladder or intestine, where they remain for many years. Some of the adults travel through the bloodstream to the liver; some of the eggs then pass into the stool and urine; if they are passed back into the water, the cycle begins again. Another type of fluke—the liver fluke—infests the liver. Fluke infestations can be treated with drugs such as praziquantel.

Evelyn Kelly

Infections, viral

A wide variety of viruses can invade body cells. Viruses are infectious agents much smaller than bacteria or fungi. They attach themselves to cells, enter them, and then release genetic matter inside the cells to reproduce. Some viruses, such as cold viruses, are inhaled and infect cells in the upper respiratory tract, whereas others are transmitted in a variety of ways, such as by swallowing, during sexual contact, or by the bites of insects.

Viruses reproduce in unique ways. Although they are inert, once they enter a human cell, they use the cell's genes, take control, and force the cell to help them replicate. The cell usually dies, releasing new viruses that infect other cells. Occasionally a virus alters the cell's function, causing the normal cell to lose control and grow abnormally into a cancer. Other viruses enter the host's genetic material and live there for a while, before erupting years later.

Body defenses against viruses include physical barriers, such as the skin. If the virus gets into the body, the immune system responds. First the lymphocytes (types of white blood cells) attack to destroy the virus and the infected cells. Infected cells release interferons, substances that help other cells resist the attack of the viruses. If the body survives the virus, certain cells help remember the virus and respond more quickly to the next invasion of the same virus. Vaccines produce similar immunity.

Because viruses are so specific and replicate using a cell's machinery, antivirals—drugs against viruses—are hard to produce. Unlike bacteria, which are large and reproduce outside body cells, viruses present few targets for drugs to attack. Some antiviral drugs produce toxic reactions, and viruses can become resistant to them. Antiviral drugs include acyclovir, which targets the herpes virus and has few side effects; ganciclovir, which targets cytomegalovirus but affects white blood cells; and interferon-alpha, which targets hepatitis B and C viruses but causes flulike symptoms, bone marrow suppression, and depression.

Viruses usually infect specific cells. Many infect only plants; others infect specific animals, including humans. Because viruses can change their surface molecules and structure, an infinite number can exist. Familiar human viruses are influenza and cold viruses; hantavirus, which is spread by rodents; pox and measles viruses; the herpes family, which includes herpes simplex 1 and 2 viruses and cytomegalovirus (CMV); insect-borne viruses such as those that cause dengue fever and yellow fever; Epstein-Barr virus (EBV); hemorrhagic fever viruses, such as Ebola and Marburg fever viruses; severe acute respiratory syndrome (SARS) virus; and human

RELATED ARTICLES

VIRAL ATTACK

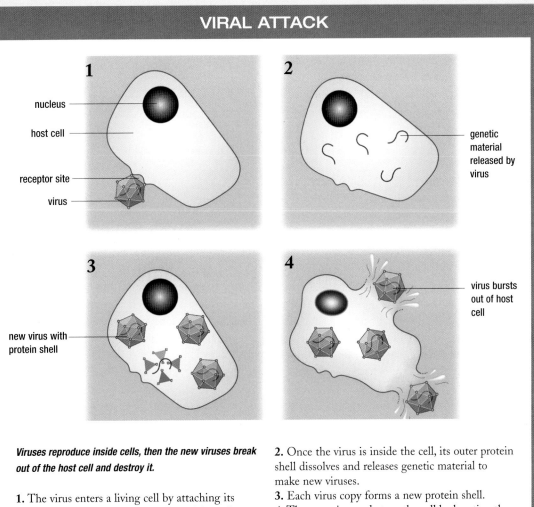

1
nucleus

host cell

receptor site

virus

2
genetic material released by virus

3
new virus with protein shell

4
virus bursts out of host cell

Viruses reproduce inside cells, then the new viruses break out of the host cell and destroy it.

1. The virus enters a living cell by attaching its protein shell to a site on the surface of the cell. The virus is absorbed into the cell membrane.

2. Once the virus is inside the cell, its outer protein shell dissolves and releases genetic material to make new viruses.

3. Each virus copy forms a new protein shell.

4. The new viruses destroy the cell by bursting the cell membrane, leaving to infect other cells.

immunodeficiency virus (HIV), which causes acquired immunodeficiency syndrome (AIDS).

Influenza and common cold viruses

Different viruses cause influenza (flu) and the common cold. The two conditions have many factors in common: they are both respiratory illnesses and produce a runny nose, sore throat, headache, muscle aches, and malaise. In general, symptoms of influenza are more intense than those of the common cold.

The structures in the nasal cavity trap particles. If cold viruses pass these structures, the viruses reach the back of the throat, where the adenoids—lymph nodes—are located. Once the virus reaches the back of the throat, symptoms, such as a runny nose, sneezing, and scratchy throat, develop 24 to 48 hours later. Symptoms are usually mild and last one to two weeks.

Colds are probably the most common illness known and are the leading cause of visits to the doctor and missed days from work or school. According to the Centers for Disease Control (CDC), the people of the United States suffer about 1 billion colds each year. Children have about 6 to 10 colds each year, probably because they are in contact with carriers in schools. Colds are transmitted when hands touch surfaces that have cold viruses on them, and then touch the eyes or nose. People can also become infected by inhaling drops of sneezed contaminated mucus from the air.

More than 200 different viruses cause colds. About 110 types of rhinoviruses (from the Greek *rhin*, meaning "nose") cause mild colds and are mainly active in fall, spring, and summer. Other viruses that cause more severe colds are parainfluenza virus, respiratory syncytial virus, coronaviruses, adenoviruses, Coxsackieviruses, echoviruses, orthomyxoviruses, and enteroviruses. These viruses are associated with more serious illness.

Influenza, a more severe disorder than colds, usually affects a deeper part of the respiratory system and can lead to complications such as pneumonia (inflammation of the lungs). Symptoms start 24 to 48 hours after infection and begin with chills and fever during the first few days. Body aches and headaches are common. At first, respiratory symptoms appear mild, with a simple scratchy throat and a dry cough, but later become severe as the person coughs up mucus. The severity of the illness, along with its high fever and body aches, distinguishes influenza from the common cold.

Influenza usually hits in epidemics and can travel around the world in a year or less. The symptoms last only about a week, but the infection may open the door for bacterial pneumonia, which can be fatal. In the 1980s, for example, influenza paired with pneumonia was one of the ten leading causes of death.

Influenza's origin is unknown. It was first mentioned in 1510. Several pandemics (widespread epidemics) occurred in the following centuries, but one of the most notorious was the epidemic of 1918. After World

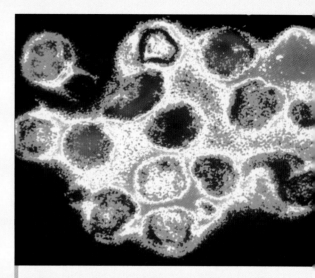

A colored electron micrograph shows the rubella virus. This is the virus that causes German measles; it can cause birth defects if a pregnant woman who has never had the disease is infected during pregnancy.

War I, a mild flu spread around the world, killing only a few, but it was different from previous epidemics in that many of the victims were young adults. However, in the fall of 1918, the virus changed and became more virulent and encouraged the growth of the secondary infection pneumonia. About ten months later, it had killed 550,000 people in the United States, about ten times more than had died in the war. Worldwide the number of deaths was estimated to be 30 million.

There are two types of influenza viruses: type A and type B, with many strains within each type. The strains are always changing, so that every year the influenza virus is a little different from the ones in previous years. Animals carry some strains that can infect humans; for example, avian, or bird, flu can cause serious disease in humans. Other types of influenzas, such as Hong Kong flu, are named after the place of origin of the strain of the virus.

Getting a vaccine containing inactivated or killed virus or pieces of the virus is the best way to avoid contracting influenza. Because the strains are forever changing, scientists must create the vaccine based on previous flu seasons. Antiviral drugs can be used to prevent infection with influenza viruses, especially in people recently exposed to infection who are at risk of complications, such as older people or those with

VIRUSES AND CANCER

When some viruses enter body cells, the viruses cause the cells to reproduce wildly, producing cancerous growths. At present only a few known viruses cause cancer or alter the growth of cells in an aberrant manner. The human papillomavirus (HPV) can cause cervical cancer. In people with AIDS, herpes virus B has been linked to Kaposi's syndrome and B cell lymphoma. Hepatitis B and C viruses are known to cause liver cancer. The Epstein-Barr virus is linked to homa, certain cancers of the nose and throat, and other lymphomas in people with AIDS.

chronic illnesses. Two new drugs, oseltamivir and zanamivir, can prevent infection with either virus type with minimal side effects.

In May 1993 an outbreak of an unknown pulmonary illness erupted in the southwestern United States in the Four Corners, an area shared by Arizona, New Mexico, Colorado, and Utah. A healthy Navajo man was the first victim of the outbreak, followed by his fiancée. Laboratory tests revealed no known disease, and authorities had a medical mystery on their hands. This area had been in a drought for several years, but the winter had brought snow and heavy rains that provided food for lots of plants and animals. Deer mice were especially prevalent that year, and laboratory analysis showed that these mice harbored hantavirus in their urine, saliva, and droppings. The virus causes hantavirus pulmonary syndrome (HPS), which can be fatal. HPS begins one to six weeks after inhaling aerosol-like dust containing the feces or urine of the mice. At first the symptoms are like a bad case of the flu, but then an infection of the lungs leaves the person short of breath. The virus does not spread from one person to another.

Indications are that HPS is not really a new disease. Past researchers had found lung samples of people who had died of an unexplained disease and called it *sin nombre*, meaning "no name." In 1959 a 38-year-old man in Utah died of the earliest known case of HPS. Navajo medical traditions recognize a similar disease and even correlated its occurrence with population bursts of mice. In other parts of the country, the cotton rat, rice rat, and the white-footed mouse can also carry hantavirus.

People risk exposure to the virus when they are cleaning areas such as barns or garages, where the mice live. When cleaning such buildings, the person should wear latex gloves and not sweep dust into the air. Recommended cleaning is to wet the area down with detergent or bleach, which kills the virus, and then sweep the wet materials carefully into bags. Workers, hikers, and outdoor campers must avoid coming into contact with rodent nests or burrows.

Viruses that cause pox and rashes

The variola virus caused one of the most dreaded of all plagues—smallpox. To differentiate between the great pox, or syphilis, the disease was dubbed smallpox.

The two kinds of smallpox viruses are variola major, which carried a death rate of about 30 percent, and variola minor, which claimed a death rate of about 1 percent. The virus spreads as people breathe contaminated air. People may also get the virus from bedding. Symptoms begin 12 to 14 days after infection, when the affected person develops fever, headache, and becomes extremely ill. After two to four days, a rash erupts that soon turns into blisters that become encrusted. People who survive have disfiguring scars.

Over 200 years ago, Edward Jenner developed the first vaccine for smallpox, and over the years the number of cases declined. The last case reported in the world was in Somalia in 1977. Samples of the virus are kept in two research facilities, one in the United States and one in Russia. Because the disease was eradicated, there was no need to vaccinate people. However, fears of bioterrorism after September 11, 2001, have made health professionals aware that an attack with the smallpox virus could find masses of people unprotected and result in a major epidemic.

The varicella zoster virus causes chicken pox, which occurs mainly in childhood but can be serious in adults. Contracted by breathing infected droplets, the patient develops a rash, about two weeks after exposure to the virus, that fills with a clear fluid then

A shingles rash around this person's nose and lips is caused by the varicella zoster virus, which infects the sensory nerves, causing an outbreak of blisters on the skin supplied by the nerve. Nerve damage causes severe pain.

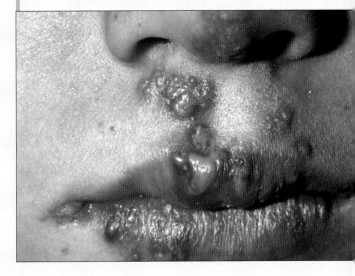

forms a crust. A pregnant woman who contracts the virus during the first or second trimester is in danger of having a newborn with a birth defect. The drug gammaglobulin may be given as a preventive measure to pregnant women.

When a person has chicken pox as a child, the varicella zoster virus spreads into the bloodstream and lives in the nerve cells. After years of dormancy, it may reactivate, travel down the nerve fibers to the skin, and cause a painful disease called shingles, which resembles chicken pox lesions. The condition usually occurs after the age of 50. The outbreak of the virus is usually limited to one side of the body. The blisters dry, scab over, and during this time can transmit the virus to susceptible people. One attack of shingles usually gives lifelong immunity from further attacks. Several antiviral drugs, such as famciclovir and acycloclovir, are available for relief.

Two kinds of viruses cause two kinds of measles—a medieval word for spots—which vary in severity and symptoms. The rubeola viruses that cause measles (red measles) are morbilliviruses that closely resemble those that cause distemper in dogs. Rubeola is most contagious before the lobster-red spots and other symptoms appear, making it difficult to avoid the disease. Often the victim has a high fever of about 104°F to 105°F (40°C–40.5°C) with a persistent cough, sneezing, and inflamed eyes. Complications can include pneumonia or encephalitis.

The rubella virus causes the second type of measles, also called German measles, with mild symptoms and a pink rash that appears on the face, trunk, neck, arms, and legs. In itself, rubella is mild, but if a woman becomes infected during pregnancy, her child is at risk of congenital cataracts, deafness, heart defects, and mental retardation. The MMR vaccine, routinely given to children, protects against measles, mumps, and rubella.

Herpes viruses

Herpes simplex viruses (HSV) produce small, painful, fluid-filled blisters on the skin or mucous membranes. Two types of the viruses are HSV-1, the usual cause of cold sores on the lips or infections of the eye, and HSV-2, which causes genital herpes. Cold sores begin with a tingling in the area, lasting from minutes to hours, followed by swelling and eruption of fluid-filled blisters that open and form sores. The virus then is dormant and resides in the nerves. The first bout of genital herpes is usually severe and painful, with multiple blisters in the genital area. Reactivation of latent oral or genital herpes may be triggered by a fever, menstruation, emotional stress, sunburn, or other trauma. HSV is very contagious, and contact with people with the virus should be avoided. Some treatments with antivirals, such as penciclovir and acyclovir, may help reduce discomfort if started early.

Cytomegalovirus (CMV) is a common herpes virus that causes disease in fetuses and in people with a weakened immune system. According to blood tests, about 60 to 90 percent of adults have had CMV at some time, without any symptoms. However, adolescents and young people may have an illness with fever and constant fatigue that is similar to symptoms of mononucleosis. In people with AIDS, infection with CMV is a common complication; it can infect the retina of the eye and cause blindness. In pregnant women, CMV can cause miscarriage, stillbirth, or even death of the newborn.

FIVE COLD MYTHS

Myth Feed a cold and starve a fever.
Fact This saying of unknown origin is certainly not based on scientific fact. However, eating may help the person with a cold feel better.
Myth Go to the doctor to get rid of the cold.
Fact There is no cure for the cold; the doctor will advise rest in bed, drinking plenty of fluids, gargling or using lozenges for a scratchy throat, and taking aspirin or acetaminophen for headache or fever.
Myth Drinking milk causes more mucus to develop.
Fact Milk is digested like other proteins and has nothing to do with nasal mucus.
Myth People with weakened immune systems get colds.
Fact Healthy people with strong immune systems also get colds once the virus reaches the back of the throat.
Myth Getting cold or chilled leads to catching a cold.
Fact Everyone becomes infected if the cold virus enters the nose, chilled or not.

Insect-borne viruses

A number of viruses are carried by flying insects in many parts of the world. Some of the most prominent include the viruses that cause West Nile fever, dengue fever, and yellow fever.

The *Aedes* mosquito carries a type 2 arbovirus that causes dengue fever. During the first few hours, the joints and legs ache so much that the infection was called "breakbone fever." Dengue fever is common in the tropics and subtropics, and cases have been known in south Texas and Florida. Eradication of the mosquito that carries the virus is the best prevention.

Mosquitoes also carry an arbovirus that causes yellow fever, so called because the skin turns yellow due to liver infection. Up to 50 percent of people with severe yellow fever die. In Africa the condition was considered just a childhood disease, but when it was brought to the New World, it affected many adults.

Hemorrhagic viruses

A number of viruses cause serious infections characterized by bleeding. Classified as filoviruses, Ebola and Marburg viruses are transmitted from person to person through infected blood or body tissues. Both infections are often fatal, with some strains of the Ebola virus causing 80 to 90 percent mortality. There is no specific treatment for this condition, so an infected person must be isolated to prevent further spread. Rodents transmit the arenavirus that causes Lassa fever and South American hemorrhagic fever. Drugs such as the antiviral ribavirin and vaccines are being investigated as potential treatments.

Other viruses

Epstein-Barr virus (EBV) causes a number of diseases, including mononucleosis, which is sometime called "kissing fever." In the United States, about 50 percent of all children more than five years and nearly 95 percent of adults have had EBV infections that resemble a common cold or mild flu. However, teenagers and young adults may develop more serious symptoms of mononucleosis. Depending on the strain of the virus, EBV produces a number of different symptoms. The most common is extreme fatigue, fever, sore throat, and swelling of the lymph nodes. The spleen is enlarged in more than 50 percent of affected people. Pain relievers are usually given to relieve discomfort.

THE YELLOW JACK

Although the African slave trade had been underway for more than a century, yellow fever, or the Yellow Jack, jumped the Atlantic in 1647 and caused great cities to quarantine their citizens to protect them from disease. At first, people thought the disease originated in filth and squalor. During the mid-nineteenth century, researchers looking for a germ decided that the culprit was an organism smaller than bacteria.

In 1899 Walter Reed was sent to Cuba to find the origin of yellow fever. He devised an experimental plan in which one group of volunteer soldiers was placed in a house, living with filthy blankets and clothing of yellow fever patients, but with insect screens. The other group lived in a clean cottage with no insect screens. The soldiers living in filth remained healthy, while those in the cottage with no screens contracted yellow fever. Combined with a vaccine developed in the 1930s and eradication of insect larvae by spraying, yellow fever is now restricted to its forest home, where it persists today with an occasional outbreak in small areas.

A new type of coronavirus causes severe acute respiratory syndrome, or SARS. First detected in the Guangdong province of China in late 2002, it spread to 17 countries, including Canada and the United States. SARS is relatively common in China, Hanoi, Vietnam, and Singapore. Transmission is usually by close contact with a person with the disease. Breathing difficulties may cause death.

Human immunodeficiency virus (HIV) causes acquired immunodeficiency syndrome (AIDS). The virus entered the United States in the late 1970s, although it is uncertain how it first infected humans. HIV enters the T-helper lymphocytes; when viruses burst out of the cells, they invade other cells and continue the cycle.

Most viral infections infect the nose, throat, and airways. A few, such as West Nile virus, rabies, and other encephalitis viruses, infect the brain and nervous system. A few may originate in the skin, causing warts. Antiviral drugs are constantly being developed, but the changing nature of viruses presents a challenge.

Evelyn Kelly

Infertility

Infertility is the inability to produce children. About 10 to 15 percent of couples are diagnosed with infertility, defined as one year of unprotected sexual intercourse without conception. The problem may lie with the faulty reproductive system of either the man or the woman, or from a combination of problems with both of them. The causes of infertility are discussed here, along with the tests that doctors can use to diagnose these problems, treatments for infertility, and the stress associated with this disorder.

A man's semen consists of sperm and seminal fluid (which helps sustain and protect the sperm), produced within his genital tract. The most important test to diagnose male factor infertility is a semen analysis, which counts the number of sperm in a man's ejaculate and analyzes their morphology (shape) and motility (ability to swim forward quickly). If the semen analysis is abnormal, the test should be repeated with an evaluation by a physician specializing in male infertility. A common cause of male factor infertility is a disorder called varicocele. A varicocele is a mass of enlarged veins near the testis, which may cause the temperature of the affected testis to be too warm for optimal sperm production, or may allow a high concentration of adrenal hormones or other substances that may inhibit normal sperm production. A varicocele may be corrected through surgery or treatment of the affected blood vessels; the efficacy of the treatment is under question and should be discussed with a fertility specialist.

Less common causes of male factor infertility include hormonal imbalances, sex chromosomal disorders, infection, obstruction, and immunological infertility. If a man has low levels of follicular stimulating hormone (FSH), the hormone that sends a signal to the testes to produce sperm, treatment with hormonal drugs may be effective. Some men have hormonal imbalances as a result of having an extra X chromosome, a condition called Klinefelter's syndrome. Chronic genital-tract inflammation or infection may contribute to male factor infertility;

it can be treated using appropriate anti-inflammatory medications and antibiotics. Obstruction occurs when the seminal ducts, through which sperm and seminal fluid pass, become blocked, so that sperm cannot get into the semen. For these patients, sperm may be surgically retrieved directly from the testis and then used in a procedure called intracytoplasmic sperm injection (ICSI). Men with this disorder should be evaluated for cystic fibrosis before pregnancy is attempted. After a vasectomy or severe testicular injury, a man's immune system may produce antibodies to his own sperm. Before considering a vasectomy, the man can be tested for reversal antibodies. If antibodies are present, in vitro fertilization with ICSI can overcome this problem.

Infertility treatments for men

In intrauterine insemination (IUI), semen from the man's ejaculate is processed and placed directly in the woman's uterus, using a narrow catheter. IUI improves pregnancy rates achieved with fertility drugs by decreasing the distance sperm have to swim to reach the fallopian tubes and egg, as well as by increasing the number of sperm in close proximity to the tubes and egg. The success rate depends on the sperm and if fertility drugs are used with this treatment.

RELATED ARTICLES

HEALTHY FORM AND FUNCTION

For conception to occur, a man's sperm must fertilize a woman's egg, or ovum, which then implants itself in the lining of the uterus, where it forms an embryo. The embryo contains genetic material from both the man and woman. This is the beginning of a healthy pregnancy; the embryo grows to become a fetus and, later on, a baby.

During sexual intercourse, a man ejaculates semen, which contains hundreds of millions of sperm, into a woman's vagina. These sperm swim from the vagina through the cervix into the uterus, and then into the fallopian tubes, where an egg may be present. A woman typically releases only one egg each month, during ovulation. After being released from the ovary, the egg enters a fallopian tube, where it remains for several days. If the egg does not meet a sperm in the fallopian tube, it is reabsorbed or passed out of the body and there will not be another egg until the following month.

Infertility can be equally attributed to reproductive problems with the man or woman (about 40 percent each). Sometimes it is as a result of mutual incompatibility.

In about 10 percent of infertile couples both partners contribute to the infertility (combined infertility). Up to 20 percent of couples have unexplained infertility in which, despite an evaluation, no cause can be found.

For in vitro fertilization (IVF), hormones are given to stimulate the development of multiple eggs within the ovary. These eggs are harvested using a needle and catheter in a minor surgical procedure. Depending on the age and health of the woman, typically about 10 eggs are retrieved, although up to 50 or more eggs can be obtained on any one cycle of treatment. These eggs are combined with the man's sperm in vitro (outside the body). The embryos are nurtured under carefully controlled conditions and develop into embryos. After two to six days, the healthiest-appearing embryos are selected for transfer; they are placed into the woman's uterus through a catheter, often under ultrasound guidance (allowing visualization of the uterus to ensure that the transfer catheter is correctly positioned). Transferring more embryos increases the likelihood that any one embryo will undergo implantation and result in a pregnancy. However, the trade-off is an increased risk of multiple gestations, in which the woman has twins, triplets, or even quadruplets. These multiple pregnancies are considered the major complication of IVF because of increased risks to both maternal and fetal health, so the goal of IVF is to achieve an excellent pregnancy rate with a low multiple gestation rate. IVF is helpful for almost any cause of infertility, including male factor, female factor, combined, and unexplained infertility. Success rates vary by patient age, diagnosis, and clinic but are roughly 25 to 35 percent for each course of treatment.

Intracytoplasmic sperm injection (ICSI) is a technique in which a single sperm is directly injected into an individual egg during IVF. ICSI is used in a number of male conditions to fertilize the eggs; otherwise, about 100,000 sperm are included with the egg.

Female factor infertility

There are numerous tests to evaluate a woman's eggs, fallopian tubes, and uterus. Blood tests or simply questioning a woman about her menstrual cycle can determine if she is ovulating. A hysterosalpingogram (HSG) is an X-ray during which a contrast dye is injected into the uterus; the dye can be seen filling the uterus and fallopian tubes and then spilling out of the tubes if they are open. A sonohysterogram is an ultrasound that permits an evaluation of the uterine cavity by separating the inner walls with fluid.

Ovulation disorders affect more than one-quarter of infertile women and are the most common cause of female infertility. These disorders usually result from a hormonal imbalance and are manifested by menstrual cycle irregularities such as oligomenorrhea (infrequent or light menstrual cycles) or amenorrhea (lack of menstrual cycles). Ovulatory dysfunction is often the result of polycystic ovarian syndrome but may also be due to premature ovarian failure (when a woman enters menopause earlier than expected). Measuring hormone levels is important in the evaluation of ovulatory dysfunction.

The two most common initial drugs for women with ovulatory dysfunction are clomiphene citrate and metformin. Although the majority of women will ovulate when taking these drugs, less than half will conceive. Treatment for women with premature ovarian failure is difficult. Their best chance of success is to undergo IVF using donor eggs from a young woman with more fertile eggs.

About one-fifth of women with infertility have problems with their fallopian tubes. A doctor may suspect tubal infertility in a woman who has an abnormal HSG, a history of pelvic inflammatory disease (a bacterial infection of the reproductive organs that causes inflammation and scarring), symptoms of endometriosis, or prior pelvic surgeries that could lead to scarring and adhesions (tissue or organs being abnormally fixed to each other).

If blocked fallopian tubes are suspected, a doctor may use laparoscopy (endoscopic surgery performed using a telescope connected to a camera) to diagnose and treat any damage in the pelvis. The success rates of these techniques range from 15 to 85 percent, but women with severe tubal infertility typically undergo IVF.

A false-color hysterosalpingogram of the abdomen of a woman reveals blocked fallopian tubes. Hysterosalpingography is an X-ray technique that uses a contrast medium to show the uterus and fallopian tubes—colored in this picture in pink and orange.

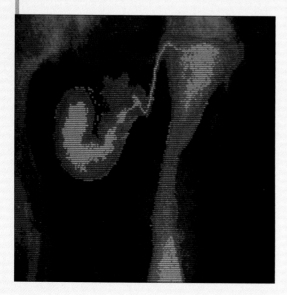

Other causes of female factor infertility

Endometriosis, the presence of endometrial (uterine lining) tissue outside the uterus, is a common cause of female factor infertility. The exact mechanism by which endometriosis causes infertility is unknown. Endometriosis may be treated surgically or with drugs, but infertile women with endometriosis often undergo fertility therapy such as IVF. Fibroids are noncancerous tumors in the walls of the uterus that can cause heavy menstrual flow and can contribute to infertility. There is no permanent treatment for fibroids, and their surgical removal is required if continued fertility is desired.

Less commonly, anomalies in the structure of the uterus may cause female infertility. Depending on the anomaly, surgical correction may be possible. Rarely, a woman with an uncorrectable uterine anomaly undergoes IVF and has her embryos transferred to the normal uterus of another woman (a surrogate) who carries the pregnancy for her.

Unexplained infertility

If all the tests for male and female factor infertility are normal, a couple is said to have unexplained infertility. The options for treatment are similar to those for people with a known cause: IVF and fertility drugs with IUI. Adoption is a well-accepted option to attain parenthood for couples who do not conceive with therapy or choose not to pursue treatment.

Infertility and psychosocial issues

Infertility is a medical condition that can be very stressful. Couples with infertility may experience depression and anxiety, reduced self-esteem, and strains on interpersonal relationships. Women tend to suffer more depression than men and blame themselves more for their infertility. Men and women use different coping mechanisms for the stress of infertility, which sometimes leads to difficulties in communication, further increasing their stress levels. It is important for practitioners engaged in infertility treatment to be closely attuned to the psychosocial impact this condition may have on their patients. Psychological counseling and support reduce anxiety and depressive symptoms, and it is critical that supportive resources be made available and offered to all appropriate patients.

Heidi Brown and Gary Frishman

Influenza

A severe viral respiratory infection, commonly called flu, that spreads rapidly from person to person and affects millions of Americans every year. During pandemics (worldwide epidemics), influenza may infect more than 50 percent of the human population. The complications that sometimes arise from flu can be life threatening in high-risk groups of people, including the very young or old and those with preexisting chronic illness.

Every year the flu strikes, causing thousands of deaths and hospitalizing more than 200,000 Americans. The viruses that cause flu in humans have the ability to mutate; that is, they change their genetic material and produce new strains. Public health officials try to stay one step ahead of annual flu outbreaks by producing vaccines tailored to the particular flu strains projected to be circulating. However, the resultant "best guess" vaccine may or may not be a good match. Beyond the minor, continual changes in genetic material, there are major changes leading to drastically different flu viruses to which the human immune system has no resistance. These changes are responsible for the massive pandemics that periodically march through the world's population, taking millions of lives in the process.

Causes

There are three types of flu viruses: A, B, and C. Both A and B cause the flu in humans. Type A is the greatest threat to health; it causes a more severe illness and easily mutates, which makes it easier to infect a human host.

Risk factors

Flu is a highly contagious illness that can be spread by infectious droplets produced by coughs or sneezes. If a person breathes in these infectious droplets, he or she can become ill with influenza.

Flu can also be spread by touch, for example if influenza-infected secretions are picked up on the fingers and then conveyed to the mouth. Anyone infected with the influenza virus is infectious to others from one day before symptoms develop through five days after symptoms first appear.

People with underlying chronic medical illnesses, those living in communities like nursing homes or other chronic care facilities, and those at the extremes of age are more susceptible to the flu and its complications. Also, those who have not received the annual flu vaccine are at greater risk of infection.

Symptoms and signs

Flu symptoms appear suddenly and include fever, cough, headache, weakness, and muscle aches, and sometimes a sore throat. Gastrointestinal symptoms

---

KEY FACTS

Description
Acute viral respiratory illness.

Cause
Infection by influenza A or B viruses.

Risk factors
Most likely to cause serious illness in people who are very young or old, those with preexisting chronic medical disorders, those who live in nursing homes or other care facilities, or those who have not received an annual influenza vaccine.

Symptoms
Abrupt onset of fever, cough, sore throat, muscle aches, weakness, and headache. Very young children may have nausea, vomiting, and diarrhea.

Diagnosis
Rapid diagnostic tests of nasal or other respiratory secretions; culture of the virus; blood test to check for antibodies.

Treatments
Two classes of antiviral medicines are available, but resistance is increasing to the older class of drugs. Antibiotics are useful only if bacterial complications develop.

Pathogenesis
Contact with secretions infected with influenza. The virus enters cells of the respiratory tract lining, where it multiplies, infecting other cells and ultimately spreading from person to person.

Prevention
Annual influenza vaccine can provide protection from influenza.

Epidemiology
Yearly outbreaks result in more than 200,000 hospitalizations and about 36,000 deaths among United States residents.

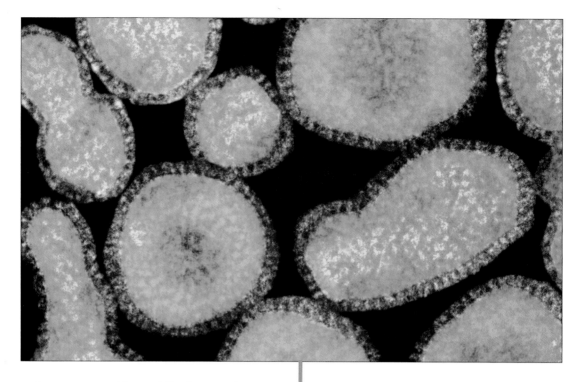

A colored electron micrograph depicts greatly magnified human influenza A viruses. This type of flu virus is one of the most virulent; it readily mutates and therefore it easily infects people who usually do not have immunity to it, causing severe illness.

such as nausea, vomiting, and diarrhea may also occur; however, those are more common in children. Flu lasts a few days to a week, although the fatigue that commonly accompanies the illness may continue for weeks afterward, when all other symptoms have cleared up.

There is a possibility of complications, the most common being pneumonia. Pneumonia can arise from the influenza virus itself or from a secondary bacterial infection. Common symptoms of pneumonia are high fever and shortness of breath that, if it worsens, can lead to respiratory failure and death. People with underlying chronic disorders can find that their existing symptoms worsen when they are in the throes of illness from influenza. Dehydration is a potential complication among all age groups with flu, but is more likely in those with gastrointestinal symptoms. In children, a dangerous illness called Reye's syndrome has been associated with the use of aspirin to relieve symptoms of viral infections such as flu (see box, p. 486). This syndrome is more often seen with influenza B infections and is marked by nausea and vomiting, followed by central nervous system complications that can lead to seizures, coma, and death.

Diagnosis and treatment

During a community outbreak of influenza, some physicians may make the diagnosis of flu based on symptoms common among a population. Rapid diagnostic tests using nasal and respiratory secretions to detect the presence of the flu virus are available for same-day diagnosis. Swabs of the throat, nasal washings, or sputum can be checked for the influenza virus or viral antigens (proteins). Viral cultures in which the organism is grown in nutrient gel can be performed. Cultures take up to 48 to 72 hours to produce results, but they are of value in determining the particular types of viruses that are circulating in a community. Blood testing is also available to look for raised levels of antibodies produced by the immune system to combat influenza; however, these tests will not show results until a person has had the infection for some days.

Two types of antiviral drugs are available for combating the enzymes found on the surface of the flu virus: M2 ion channel blockers (amantadine and rimantadine) and neuraminidase (NA) inhibitors (zanamivir and oseltamivir). Amantadine and rimantadine are effective against influenza A only. Over time, flu viruses have acquired increasing rates of resistance to these drugs. There is less resistance of flu viruses to NA inhibitors, and these medicines are effective against both influenza A and B. Relief of symptoms may include rest, taking acetaminophen for headache and muscle aches, and drinking plenty of fluids. Antibiotics are not effective against viral illnesses such as influenza and can only treat complications caused by bacteria.

Pathogenesis

In addition to humans, influenza A can infect other species such as birds, pigs, sea mammals, and horses. The virus is maintained naturally in the environment by aquatic birds. Various subtypes of this virus exist, identified by the different forms of proteins on the surface of the virus; these proteins are hemagglutinin A (HA) and NA. HA permits the virus to enter host cells. Inside the cells, the virus replicates itself and the new viruses break out (a function facilitated by NA) to infect more cells and ultimately to be passed from person to person. There are 16 subtypes of HA (H1 through H16); and there are nine subtypes of NA (N1 through N9). A specific virus is named for its HA and NA components, for example H1N1.

H1 through H3 viruses have been circulating in the human population for at least a century and were responsible for pandemics in 1918, 1957, 1968, and 1977. By far the most severe pandemic was in 1918.

H5 virus is not recognized by the human immune system, making it a major pandemic threat. The flu strain H5N1, first identified in Hong Kong in 1997, has caused worldwide concern. This strain is responsible for widespread infection in birds, can be transmitted from birds to humans, and has become increasingly resistant to the older class of antiviral drugs. Public health officials are aware that H5N1 may at some point undergo a mutation that will eventually allow it to be transmitted from human to human. Previous pandemics were the result of viruses crossing the species barrier, jumping from an animal host to a human. So far H5N1 meets two of the three criteria that make viruses risk factors for a pandemic: it is a new virus subtype and it can replicate in humans to produce severe illness. At present the virus is not passed easily from person to person.

Small mutations in genetic material, called antigenic drift, continually occur among influenza viruses, especially those of type A. Major changes in the genetic makeup, called antigenic shift, are less common but are more deadly since they lead to epidemics and pandemics. In antigenic shift, a virus evolves for which humans have little or no immunity because the body's defense mechanisms are unable to recognize the new virus. A process termed *reassortment* can likewise

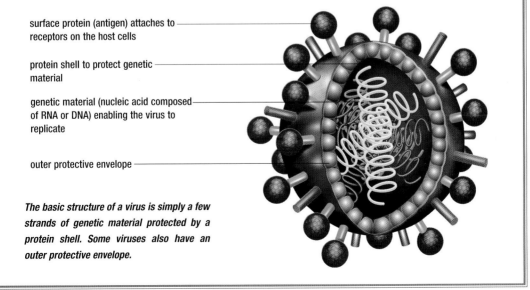

STRUCTURE OF A VIRUS

Viruses are the smallest infective organisms. They cannot exist separately, but they take over a human cell so that they can multiply. Viruses all have the same basic structure: a core of genetic material (RNA or DNA) surrounded by a protein shell. Proteins on the surface of the virus attach to specific receptor cells on the host.

surface protein (antigen) attaches to receptors on the host cells

protein shell to protect genetic material

genetic material (nucleic acid composed of RNA or DNA) enabling the virus to replicate

outer protective envelope

The basic structure of a virus is simply a few strands of genetic material protected by a protein shell. Some viruses also have an outer protective envelope.

REYE'S SYNDROME

Children 18 years of age or less should not be given aspirin when they have an viral illness like influenza, chicken pox, or the common cold, because of the risk of developing Reye's syndrome. This dangerous disorder, while rare, is associated with aspirin therapy in children who have acute viral infection. Reye's syndrome causes complications affecting the liver, blood, and brain that can lead to seizures, coma, and death. In children who develop the syndrome, symptoms appear about one week after the viral illness, with sudden and persistent nausea and vomiting. Symptoms can rapidly progress, leading to death in only four or five days. Management in an intensive care unit is required. If recognized and treated early, the child usually recovers without serious consequences, although serious brain injury can result. Since 1980, the incidence of Reye's syndrome has declined, possibly because of increased awareness of its links to aspirin and viral infection. However, the exact cause of the illness is not fully understood.

It is important to check the list of ingredients in over-the-counter medicines since aspirin may be present, particularly in remedies designed to treat a variety of symptoms. Some acceptable alternatives to aspirin include acetaminophen and ibuprofen. An additional preventive measure is for children to receive varicella (chicken pox) and influenza vaccines to reduce the risk of developing these viral illnesses.

produce a virus that is novel to the human immune system. Here, genetic material from one virus combines with that from a second virus. An example would be infection of a pig with both a human virus and an avian flu virus, which then exchange genetic material while in this host. The resultant influenza virus would be very different from others in circulation, making the human population exceptionally vulnerable to widespread infection.

Flu viruses can also be categorized by their pathogenicity, that is, their ability to produce disease in a host. Low-pathogenicity viruses cause mild respiratory symptoms, whereas high-pathogenicity viruses cause more severe illness.

Prevention

One type of antiviral drug used for the treatment of influenza, the NA inhibitor oseltamivir, is also approved for the prevention of flu, but antiviral medicines are not substitutes for the flu vaccine. An annual flu vaccine is available in the form of an inactivated vaccine given as a shot, or a live weakened virus given as a nasal spray. The flu shot is effective only against A and B strains of flu. The Centers for Disease Control collects data on flu strains throughout the world and decides every year which three subtypes of virus are most likely to be in circulation for the upcoming year. If estimates about which flu strains to include in the annual vaccine are accurate, the vaccine provides 50 to 80 percent protection rates. Outbreaks of flu occur during winter months in the Northern and Southern hemispheres, and thus the vaccine should be given in the fall. It takes about two weeks after vaccination for the immune system to produce antibodies against flu viruses.

While all people are encouraged to receive flu vaccine unless there are medical reasons to the contrary, vaccination is recommended for certain high risk groups, including children between the ages of 6 and 23 months; people aged 50 or older; residents of nursing homes and other long-term care institutions; those who have chronic medical conditions such as diabetes, or heart or lung disease; children between the ages of six months and 18 years who are on long-term aspirin therapy (see box, above); women who will be in their second or third trimester of pregnancy during the flu season; and health care workers, who could transmit flu to high-risk, susceptible populations. The nasal spray flu vaccine is approved only for healthy people between ages 5 to 49, and is not given to pregnant women.

Flu vaccine is made from viruses grown in eggs, and people with severe egg allergies should not receive the vaccine. Influenza viruses H5 and H7 are lethal to chick embryos and therefore cannot be grown in substantial quantities, so these viruses remain a serious threat. Flu vaccine should not be given to anyone who has been affected by Guillain-Barré syndrome within the previous six months. Babies aged less than six months and anyone who currently has a moderate or severe illness should not receive the vaccine. For people at high risk of complications from influenza but for whom vaccination is not recommended, antiviral medicines may be considered as a preventive measure.

Rita Washko

See also
- Avian influenza • Infections, animal-to-human • Infections, viral • Pneumonia
- Respiratory system disorders

Intersexuality

Intersexuality (also called disorders of sexual development) is a generic term for a wide spectrum of conditions characterized by abnormal development of the reproductive organs and genitalia. Intersex disorders can be broadly divided into four main categories: female psuedohermaphroditism, male psuedohermaphroditism, gonadal dysgenesis, and true hermaphroditism.

Although an in-depth knowledge of human development is not necessary to understand intersex disorders, a few basic concepts are helpful. First, every cell in every human being contains a blueprint for its function and for the function of the body as a whole, known as deoxyribonucleic acid (DNA). This blueprint functions in the same way as the software for a computer. It is this blueprint that makes people human; it also creates individual, unique characteristics. A component of DNA, the sex chromosomes, contains the program for development and function of sexual characteristics. For simplification, these sex chromosomes are given the letters X or Y. Normal males have one X and one Y, and normal females have two X chromosomes. Every person is born with two gonads. Gonads are groups of cells and structures from where future reproductive cells (sperm and eggs) mature and are stored. In men, the gonads are testes, and nearly every man is born with two. Similarly, normal women are born with two ovaries.

Sexual differences

Normal sexual differentiation is composed of three elements: genetic composition, gonadal differentiation, and genital expression. Whether someone has two X chromosomes or an X and a Y is that person's genetic composition. It is determined the moment that an egg and sperm fuse. One of the main reasons that intersexuality comprises a range of diseases is that more than 50 different parts of each sex chromosome play a role in normal sexual differentiation. All of these parts or genes are complexly intertwined, producing a variety of appearances and functions when components are not programmed correctly.

Gonadal differentiation refers to the early development of certain cells in an embryo (developing human)

into either ovaries or testes and is dependent on the program in the sex chromosomes. Genital expression is the formation of normal external genitalia as well as internal reproductive organs and is also dependent on genetic composition and correct gonad formation. If any of these elements do not occur in a strictly male or female pattern, a child is said to have an intersex disorder.

KEY FACTS

Description

Intersexuality is a generic term for a wide spectrum of conditions characterized by abnormal development of the reproductive organs and genitalia. There are four main categories of intersex disorders: female psuedohermaphroditism, male psuedohermaphroditism, gonadal dysgenesis, and true hermaphroditism.

Causes

Several possible causes, but generally they are chromosomal, hormonal, or environmental. In 25 percent of cases, the cause is unknown.

Risk factors

Exposure before birth to androgens is a risk factor for a female baby. In Klinefelter's syndrome, the older the mother, the higher the risk of her baby developing the syndrome.

Symptoms and signs

Noticeably atypical or unusual genitalia.

Diagnosis

Physical examination of newborn's genitalia, followed by chromosomal analysis.

Treatment

Involves determining if the child should be raised as a boy or a girl; possible reconstructive surgery; removal of gonads that may become cancerous; and hormonal treatment.

Pathogenesis

People with intersex disorders can live long, healthy lives, and some are even able to have normal children of their own.

Prevention

If a fetus is female (XX), there should be no exposure in utero to androgens.

Epidemiology

About 1 in 1,500 to 2,000 births have atypical genitalia. About 1 in 13,000 births will have congenital adrenal hyperplasia. However, some variations of sex anatomy are less obvious and do not show up until later in life.

Female pseudohermaphroditism

In female pseudohermaphroditism the internal female reproductive organs and gonads are normal, but the external genitalia appear ambiguous: they do not resemble either a normal vagina or penis and scrotum. For example, the external genitalia in female pseudohermaphroditism appear more masculine than feminine.

The most common cause of female pseudohermaphroditism is congenital adrenal hyperplasia (CAH), which is also the most common intersex disorder. CAH represents 80 percent of all intersex disorders. In CAH, a developing fetus is exposed to too much of the male hormone testosterone. The disorder takes its name because excess testosterone is most often due to an overproduction by the adrenal glands. The appearance of the external genitalia is determined by the timing and amount of testosterone exposure. These defects can range from mild to severe. In boys with CAH (not a part of female pseudohermaphroditism), the penis and scrotum have a normal appearance, but puberty will often begin earlier than normal.

Male pseudohermaphroditism

Similarly, in male pseudohermaphroditism the testicles and internal male structures develop normally, but the external genitalia may appear ambiguous or even have a normal female appearance. Men with androgen insensitivity syndrome, a form of male pseudohermaphroditism, have a vagina that appears normal, but they also have normal testicles, which are hidden inside the abdomen. Not infrequently, they are raised as females and only find out that they do not have normal internal female structures when puberty and menses do not begin at the appropriate time.

Gonadal dysgenesis

In people with gonadal dysgenesis, the gonads are termed dysgenetic, because of the abnormal genetic makeup of the gonad. In other cases, the genetic makeup of these abnormal gonads is a mix of XX and XY. As a result, the external genitalia and internal structures can vary widely in appearance and development, thus gonadal dysgenesis is a spectrum of conditions.

The most common gonadal dysgenetic makeup is a mixture of cells with just one X chromosome per cell in Turner's syndrome. Girls with Turner's syndrome may have short stature, widely spaced nipples, a webbed neck, and an abnormal aorta. Because the gonads in certain patients with gonadal dysgenesis can carry a risk of cancer known as gonadoblastoma when the child gets older, it is important as a preventive measure that these gonads are removed early in life.

Klinefelter's syndrome occurs in about 1 in 1,666 births. This is a chromosomal abnormality in which a male child has one or two extra X chromosomes. The condition may not be recognized until puberty, when breasts develop, but the testes do not enlarge.

True hermaphroditism

True hermaphrodites (TH) have both normal testes and ovaries. TH is distinctly different from psuedohermaphroditisms, in which only one type of gonad is present. Not surprisingly, TH is very rare. Sometimes there will be one testis and one ovary; in other cases a gonad contains both testicular and ovarian tissues, and is termed an *ovotestes*. The appearance of the external genitalia is dependent on the amount of male hormones produced by the gonads and is frequently ambiguous. Because the development of internal reproductive organs is dependent on the type of gonad on a particular side of the body, most individuals with TH will have both male and female internal organs.

Treatments

Treating people with intersex disorders is often challenging. When a child with an intersex disorder is born, health care professionals from a variety of different disciplines combine their expertise to find an acceptable, healthy outcome. A key component of that process involves deciding whether to raise the child as a boy or a girl. This decision is based on the appearance of the genitals, the sex chromosomes present, the internal reproductive organs, and the fertility potential. Parents may find it difficult to accept that their newborn is not normal, and it is not always clear whether the child is male or female. Surgeons may evaluate if and what type of reconstructive surgery may be needed. Removal of gonads with a potential for cancer can be performed at the same time.

However, current thinking suggests that the choice regarding sex and rearing should be delayed. These complex decisions are best made with input from numerous expert sources rather than for social expediency. People with disorders of sexual development can live long, healthy lives, and some are even able to have normal children of their own.

Kenneth Jacobsohn and Run Wang

See also
• Adrenal disorders • Genetic disorders
• Prevention • Sexual and gender identity disorders

Irritable bowel syndrome

Irritable bowel syndrome (IBS) is a chronic condition defined by abdominal discomfort or pain that is associated with changes in bowel frequency or appearance of feces. IBS is termed a functional gastrointestinal disorder, because standard medical evaluations of these symptoms fail to identify any laboratory or pathological foundation for the symptoms.

In addition to abdominal pain and changes in bowel patterns, other symptoms of IBS may include bloating, straining, or passage of mucus with bowel movements. People with IBS may also report some pain relief after defecation. Notably, those with IBS typically lack "red flag" symptoms such as blood in their stool, anemia, or weight loss, any of which should alert a physician to the possibility of another diagnosis.

The underlying causes of IBS are not fully understood. Food intolerances, allergies, stress, infection, or overcolonization of the small intestine have all been proposed as factors. However, these may account for symptoms in only some people with IBS, as these factors are not found in all patients with this condition.

For unclear reasons, women report symptoms of IBS more commonly than men. People with anxiety disorders or depression are also more likely to experience IBS. Stress may aggravate symptoms. IBS may be more common following gastroenteritis. Having other family members with IBS may also be a minor risk factor for the development of IBS.

Diagnosis, treatments, and prevention

A detailed account of the patient's bowel symptoms is necessary to make a diagnosis of IBS. The symptoms experienced in IBS are chronic (present for at least 12 weeks). In cases of IBS, previously performed clinical examinations, including laboratory testing, imaging (CT scanning or abdominal X-rays), or colonoscopy, should have ruled out other explanations.

The treatment of IBS depends on which bowel patterns predominate—constipation, diarrhea, or both—and the severity of pain. Dietary fiber supplementation is often used initially and may improve stool consistency and ease of passage. If diarrhea is a major complaint, antidiarrheal drugs can be prescribed. Similarly, if constipation is a predominant symptom, laxatives or newer agents that stimulate colon contractions can be used. Treating constipation or diarrhea often also improves IBS pain. When pain still persists, tricyclic antidepressants may help reduce bowel pain. Psychotherapy and efforts to reduce stressors may also be helpful if psychological factors contribute to symptoms. Avoidance of foods identified by the patient as triggers of symptoms is worthwhile, and minimizing life stressors is often beneficial.

Gregory Sayuk

KEY FACTS

Description

Abdominal discomfort or pain that is associated with changes in bowel frequency or form.

Symptoms and signs

Abdominal pain, changes in bowel patterns, straining, or passage of mucus with bowel movements.

Causes

Theories include intolerances or allergies, stress, and bacterial infection or overcolonization of the small intestine.

Risk factors

Women are more at risk, as are people with anxiety disorders or depression, recent gastroenteritis, or other family members with IBS.

Diagnosis

A detailed account of the patient's chronic bowel symptoms consistent with the syndrome.

Treatments

Dependent on bowel patterns; options include dietary fiber, antidiarrheal medications, laxatives, antidepressants.

Pathogenesis

Not well established; gut motility, intestinal sensitivity, and bowel inflammation are possible outcomes.

Prevention

Avoidance of foods that precipitate symptoms; minimizing stress.

Epidemiology

Affects 10 to 20 percent of adults, onset from adolescence through 50s, more common in women.

See also
- Allergy and sensitivity • Anxiety disorders
- Depressive disorders • Food intolerance
- Gastroenteritis • Infections, bacterial

Kidney disorders

A wide variety of disorders can affect the kidneys, from infections, kidney stones, and cancer to inherited diseases that affect the ability of the kidney to remove appropriate waste materials. Disorders of the kidney can range from those that are relatively uncomplicated and reversible to those that become chronic medical conditions requiring long-term medical care. People can survive with only one kidney, if the single kidney is healthy.

The urinary system is comprised of two kidneys, two ureters, the bladder, and the urethra. The kidneys are bean-shaped organs about the size of a human fist located in the middle of the back.

In adults, each kidney measures about 4 to 5 inches (10 to 12 cm) long, 3 inches (7.5 cm) wide, and 2 inches (5 cm) thick and weighs about 10 to 12 ounces (280 to 340 g). The kidneys generate urine, which removes water and waste products from the blood as byproducts of the body's normal processing of food. The kidneys also function to regulate the body's osmolarity and acidity, thereby maintaining homeostasis. Urine consists mainly of water, salts, and urea, which is a waste product of protein-containing foods (meat, poultry, and some vegetables).

Each kidney is comprised of about a million filtering units called nephrons. In each unit is a glomerulus, made up of a specialized network of blood capillaries, followed by a series of specialized cell-lined tubules that collectively function to produce urine. The formation of urine starts when blood enters the kidney, passes through the glomerular capillary network, filters urea and other waste products, but retains blood particles and proteins. This urinary filtrate then continues through the nephron.

Approximately 190 quarts (180 liters) of blood is filtered daily through the kidney, but only 2 to 4 pints (1 to 2 liters) of urine is produced daily. Thus, the vast majority of fluid filtered at the glomerulus must be reabsorbed during transit through the tubules. The kidney tubules possess specialized channels, which function to transport water, electrolytes, and other small molecules back into the bloodstream, effectively reabsorbing the vast majority of fluid initially filtered and helping to maintain body homeostasis. Wastes and excess fluid exit the kidney into the ureters as final urine. Once leaving the kidneys, no further processing of urine occurs. The ureters function as a conduit between the kidney and the bladder, a muscular organ that stores urine until the body is ready to empty. Normal human bladders can comfortably hold 2 cups (474 ml) of urine.

Assessment of kidney function and detection of a kidney disorder

Disorders of the kidney system vary widely and range from diseases affecting the ability of the kidneys to properly excrete waste products to infections and other disorders of the ureters and bladder that may cause pain and bloody urine. Symptoms vary and may include back pain, swelling of the body, elevated blood pressure, and protein or blood in the urine. Many patients have no symptoms and are often diagnosed during routine physical and laboratory examinations by their physicians.

RELATED ARTICLES

A mainstay test for the diagnosis of the presence of a kidney disorder is urinalysis (see box, page 492). Under normal conditions, urine is sterile and free of cells and proteins. Urinalysis can detect abnormalities, including presence of proteinuria (protein in the urine), hematuria (blood in the urine), and pyuria (leukocytes in the urine). Imaging techniques can visualize the urinary system and assess blood flow to the kidneys. Finally, blood tests, including serum creatinine, which is frequently used as a measure of kidney function, and blood electrolyes, may suggest the presence of an acid-base imbalance, and aid in the detection of a disorder. Urine cultures can determine the organism and guide treatment in cases of urinary tract infections.

Some kidney disorders may require diagnosis by renal biopsy, in which a small piece of kidney tissue is obtained, usually by a needle approach from the back. Renal biopsy allows structural and histological analysis of kidney tissue, but it is a more invasive diagnostic procedure. Disorders of the kidneys are generally divided into prerenal, intrarenal, and postrenal diseases, depending on the region involved.

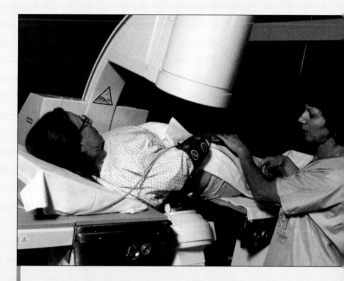

A therapy radiologist is giving a woman treatment for kidney stones. The therapy is called extracorporeal shock wave lithotripsy and the aim is to break up the kidney stone into small enough pieces to wash out in the urine flow.

Prerenal disorders

Prerenal kidney disorders refer to disorders resulting from reduced blood flow to the kidney and usually manifest with low blood pressure and a rise in serum creatinine. Disorders that result in blood volume depletion include bleeding, gastrointestinal, urinary, or cutaneous fluid losses in addition to any disorder causing relative hypotension, such as heart failure, shock, or liver cirrhosis, which can all lead to prerenal kidney disease. Volume depletion is generally managed with fluid replacement. Disorders leading to relative hypotension tend to involve more complex treatments. Regardless of etiology, early management usually results in reversal of kidney dysfunction without long-term effects.

Renal disorders

Renal disorders involve any process that affects the structure or function of the kidney. They are divided into vascular, glomerular, and tubulointerstitial disorders.

Vascular diseases encompass disorders affecting the arteries and veins supplying blood to the kidney. Common vascular disorders include hypertensive nephrosclerosis, renal artery stenosis (blockage of an

artery to the kidney), renal vein thrombosis (clot formation within the renal vein), atheroembolic disease (release of atherosclerotic cholesterol fragments that then migrate to the smaller arteries of the kidneys causing blockage), and vasculitis (inflammation of the blood vessels).

Hypertensive nephrosclerosis (HN) occurs as a consequence of chronic high blood pressure (hypertension) that results in narrowing of the smaller arteries and arterioles supplying the kidney. As a result, chronic glomerular ischemia and kidney dysfunction ensue. According to 2003 U.S. data, HN accounts for one-quarter of new cases of end-stage renal disease (ESRD). In Caucasians, ESRD from HN is second only to diabetes as the leading cause of ESRD. In the African American population, where hypertension is much more prevalent, HN is the leading cause of ESRD.

Renal artery stenosis (RAS) is a narrowing of the artery supplying the kidney. Around 80 to 90 percent of cases are caused by atherosclerosis, a buildup of plaque composed of fatty substances, cholesterol, and calcium along the inner wall of the arterial vessel. RAS is more common in older patients and often accompanies difficulty in controlling hypertension. Over time, this can lead to deterioration of kidney

URINALYSIS

Urinalysis (UA) is a relatively simple and noninvasive tool frequently used to diagnose some glomerular diseases, cancers, infections, and stones. Urinalysis refers to the analysis of urine, both grossly and microscopically, and is usually the first mainstay test done in most initial workups of kidney disorders. It is simple to learn and can be performed by nephrologists and urologists as well as primary care physicians. Specialized colorimetric dipsticks are available that provide information about the presence of glucose, protein, blood, bilirubin, and leukocytes, as well as urine pH and specific gravity. To perform a dipstick, a reagent strip is dipped into a fresh sample of urine obtained within 30 to 60 minutes of voiding. Colorimetric results are available within 2 minutes. For microscopic analysis, 10 milliliters of urine is spun at 3000 revolutions per minute for three to five minutes. The supernatant is poured off and the pelleted sediment resuspended. One drop of resuspended urine is placed on a microscopic slide and examined under a microscope for the presence of red and white blood cells and tubular casts, which may indicate a glomerular disease. The presence of certain types of urine crystals may be useful in the analysis of kidney stones.

function. Management involves aggressive treatment of blood pressure. Surgical interventions aimed at relieving the stenosis and increasing blood flow to the kidney are available treatment options; however, these interventions are fraught with complications and do not in all cases reverse the hypertension or renal dysfunction.

Glomerular diseases

Glomerular diseases usually present with high blood pressure, proteinuria, and hematuria. Glomerular diseases are generally categorized as having nephritic or nephrotic patterns. Nephritic renal diseases involve inflammation of the glomerulus with red and white blood cells in the urine and can result in a rapid decline in kidney function. Nephrotic renal diseases tend to be more insidious and are associated with large amounts of proteinuria. Diagnosis is by biopsy.

The etiology of most primary glomerular diseases is unknown. Depending on the disease, some patients respond to treatment with a combination of steroid and immunosuppressive medications. A primary goal of therapy is reduction in the amount of proteinuria lost by the kidneys. Patients are typically treated with medications to reduce the glomerular capillary blood pressure within the kidney thus decreasing the proteinuria.

Diabetic nephropathy (DN) is a complication of diabetes usually caused by uncontrolled blood sugar. Patients with DN often develop deterioration of kidney function and end-stage renal disease (ESRD). In the United States, DN is the leading cause of ESRD,

accounting for over 40 percent of incident cases of ESRD. Aggressive treatment of hypertension and blood sugar control can help retard progression to ESRD.

Tubulointerstitial diseases

Tubulointerstitial diseases are disorders affecting the tubules or the cells between the tubules of the kidney. Drugs and infections mainly cause this disorder.

Acute tubular necrosis, or ATN, refers to loss of intact kidney tubular cells and occlusion of the tubular lumen by cellular debris. Half of all cases of acute renal failure are caused by ATN, which is characterized by a rising serum creatinine, reduced or normal urine volume, and granular casts seen on urinalysis. Hospitalized patients are at risk for developing ATN, usually resulting from low blood pressure, radiocontrast agents, antibiotics, and a variety of other nephrotoxic drugs. Mortality rates range from 7 to 80 percent, depending on the underlying illness. Treatment is supportive and involves removal of offending drugs, and instituting temporary dialysis if necessary. ATN usually resolves within days to weeks after injury.

Pyelonephritis refers to an infection of the kidney, usually caused by bacteria that have migrated from the bladder. Risk factors include prostate enlargement, kidney stones, and chronic reflux of urine from the bladder, among others. Symptoms may include back and groin pain, nausea, vomiting, and fever. Antibiotics are used to treat underlying infection, and treatment of risk factors for pyelonephritis will prevent recurrence. Chronic pyelonephritis can lead to progressive scarring and fibrosis of the kidney.

KIDNEY CALCULUS

A kidney stone, or calculus, is formed from crystalline substances in the urine. If the stone obstructs the flow of urine, the result may be severe infection and kidney damage.

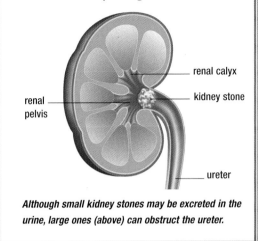

renal calyx

kidney stone

renal pelvis

ureter

Although small kidney stones may be excreted in the urine, large ones (above) can obstruct the ureter.

Acute interstitial nephritis (AIN) is associated with edema and an interstitial lymphocytic infiltrate (buildup of white cells in the spaces between tissues in the kidney). Drug toxicities, particularly from nonsteroidal anti-inflammatory drugs and antibiotics, cause the majority of cases of AIN. Treatment involves removal of the offending agent and prognosis is generally good.

Postrenal disorders

Postrenal diseases are disorders causing obstruction to the flow of urine anywhere along the urinary system and are termed *postobstructive uropathy*. Obstruction results in backflow of urine into the kidneys that over time can damage kidney tissue. Common causes of obstruction include prostate disease, cancers, and kidney stones.

Serum creatinine is elevated only when bilateral obstruction is present, since creatinine remains relatively stable when one kidney is healthy and functioning properly.

Genetic disorders

Monogenetic kidney disorders in which a mutation in one gene results in kidney disease are relatively rare compared with the preceding diseases. The most common genetic disorder affecting the kidneys is polycystic kidney disease (PKD). The hallmark of PKD is multiple cyst formation. As cysts continue to form and expand, the kidneys can grow to a massive size, and it is not uncommon for kidneys to grow to the size of a football or even larger. Most cases of PKD are autosomal dominant and affect 1 in 400 to 500 adults, making PKD the most common genetic life-threatening disease. PKD affects more than 600,000 Americans and an estimated 12.5 million people worldwide. More than 60 percent of affected patients develop ESRD. Current research has focused on treatment to halt cyst growth and slow progression to ESRD.

Renal tubular acidoses

The kidneys function to maintain the body's acid-base balance by reabsorbing filtered bicarbonate and excreting the daily acid load derived from the metabolism of sulfur-containing amino acids. Failure to properly excrete the daily acid load results in a renal tubular acidosis (RTA). RTA is a disorder caused by a defect in the ability of the kidney tubules to effectively reabsorb bicarbonate. RTAs are generally characterized by metabolic acidosis and disturbances in potassium levels in the body. Several subtypes have been characterized, each distinct by the location of the tubular defect and the ion transport process affected. The main goal of treatment is to prevent complications that typically affect the kidneys and bones.

Renal (kidney) failure

The term *renal failure* is used when the kidneys are unable to adequately remove water and waste products from the bloodstream. Acute renal failure is the sudden onset of kidney failure; it may be treatable and reversible. Chronic kidney disease leads to a gradual deterioration of kidney function that may become irreversible and lead to ESRD.

Signs or symptoms may not manifest until significant kidney scarring has occurred. Treatment options for ESRD include: hemodialysis, a procedure in which blood is removed from the body and sent to an artificial kidney filter, which removes wastes and water; and peritoneal dialysis, a procedure in which the abdominal membrane is used to remove water and waste products. Kidney transplantation is a treatment that may have a better long-term outcome.

Manakan Srichai and Matthew Breyer

Kidney stone

Kidney stones, also called renal calculi, are a common health problem affecting about 5 percent of the population. Kidney stones represent a significant U.S. health problem, and an estimated $2 billion is spent on treatment yearly. Effective medical and surgical treatments are available to manage stones and prevent recurrence.

A kidney stone is a solid piece of material composed of mineral crystals, which form on the inner surfaces of the kidney by precipitation of dissolved substances in the urine. Kidney stones usually form when certain substances in the urine are present at higher than normal concentrations. These substances can precipitate and crystallize, become anchored in the kidney, and increase in size to form a stone. Stone composition can vary, and although stones can form from any material that precipitates in the urine, 80 percent of all stones are composed of calcium. Other common stone compositions include uric acid, struvite (magnesium ammonium phosphate), and cystine.

Although several risk factors for developing stones have been identified, a personal history of kidney stones is the highest risk factor. Other risk factors for stone development include metabolic disorders (gout, gastrointestinal, endocrine, or other kidney problems), genetic disorders (cystinuria, primary hyperoxaluria, renal tubular acidosis), and dietary habits (diets high in green vegetables, fat, dairy products, salt and brewed tea, reduced water intake and dehydration, excess intake of vitamins C and D, and excessive alcohol consumption). Certain medications (especially diuretics or calcium-based antacids), recurrent urinary tract infections, and a family history of kidney stones are also risk factors for the formation of stones.

Symptoms and signs

Symptoms are usually caused by the migration and passage of stones from the kidney into the ureter. Many patients have no symptoms, and stones are detected during diagnosis of other medical conditions.

Pain is the most common symptom and can be intense enough to require hospitalization. The pain associated with stones is termed *renal colic* and usually occurs in paroxysms for up to an hour. Persons may present with lower back pain on the same side of the stone, but may also present with lower abdominal and groin pain, depending on the location of the stone.

Blood in the urine is commonly seen in patients with kidney stones. Urine may be visibly red; however, sometimes blood can be seen only microscopically. Other symptoms include nausea, vomiting, painful urination, and a frequent sensation of needing to urinate. Occasionally patients may pass visible gravel or small stones, but if stones become impacted within the ureter, accompanying fevers and chills can result from subsequent infection of the urinary tract.

Diagnosis and treatments

Diagnosis of kidney stones can be based on clinical presentation and laboratory and radiological examina-

---

KEY FACTS

Description
Mineral stones that form in the kidneys.

Causes
High concentrations of certain substances, such as calcium and uric acid, in the urine.

Risk factors
Personal or family history of kidney stones; cetain metabolic disorders, genetic disorders, and dietary habits; recurrent urinary tract infections.

Symptoms and signs
Often no symptoms; pain; blood in the urine; pain on urination; frequent need to urinate; nausea and vomiting.

Diagnosis
From clinical symptoms; radiological imaging, such as CT scanning, or ultrasound.

Treatments
Pain relief; shock wave lithotripsy; removal using endoscope or through the skin.

Pathogenesis
Left untreated can lead to obstruction, infection, and kidney malfunction.

Prevention
Medications; diet changes; drinking lots of fluids.

Epidemiology
Affects about 5 percent of the U.S. population. Generally more common in older people and men. Caucasians are more commonly affected than African Americans.

tions. Classic signs and symptoms, particularly if one has passed a stone, are all useful for the diagnosis of stones. A number of radiological examinations are available, although the gold standard for diagnosis is computed tomography (CT) scanning. Other radiological modalities include plain abdominal films and intravenous pyelogram, which involves injection of contrast dye and provides visualization of the urinary collecting system. Each of these diagnostic procedures involves exposure to radiation; for the pregnant patient in whom avoidance of radiation is desired, ultrasonography is the safest choice.

Most small stones up to 7 millimeters pass spontaneously; treatment is supportive and aimed at pain management and intravenous hydration to increase urine flow and subsequent stone passage. Nonsteroidal anti-inflammatory drugs (NSAIDs) are effective, but occasionally narcotics are required for effective pain control. Patients can usually be managed at home, but if signs suggest infection as a result of an obstructing stone, hospitalization for intravenous antibiotics may be required. Affected patients should strain their urine to collect any passed stones.

Larger stones more than 7 millimeters require removal. The treatment of choice is shock wave lithotripsy, which directs a high energy shock wave toward the stone, to help break it. Other treatment options include removal through the skin (for larger stones that cannot be broken) and telescopic removal of stones by use of a cystoureteroscope. These procedures are performed by interventional radiologists and urologists, respectively. Once a diagnosis of stones is made, further evaluation identifies risk factors. Urine should be examined for blood and crystals, and collected stones should be sent for analysis to determine their composition (calcium, uric acid, or struvite). Blood and urine tests should be done to rule out metabolic abnormalities, which are key to deciding on therapy aimed at preventing recurrence.

Acute stone disease can lead to obstruction and systemic infection if urinary flow is blocked. Struvite stones can grow rapidly over weeks or months, resulting in chronic obstruction, which, if left untreated, can lead to deterioration of kidney function. Recurrence of kidney stones is relatively high. For those who have been affected with one stone, the likelihood of forming a second stone is about 15 percent at one year, 35 to 40 percent at 5 years, and 80 percent at 10 years.

Recurrent stone formers should collect any passed stones, which can be analyzed. Depending on the stone type, medications are available that may help prevent recurrence. Dietary restrictions eliminate

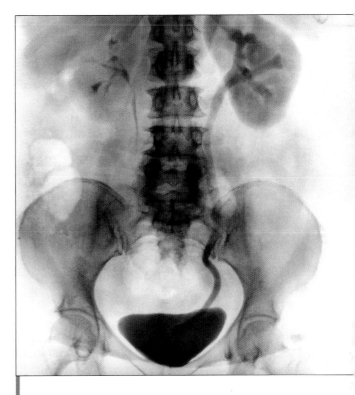

A colored urogram shows a ureter blocked by a kidney stone. The ureter at the right (red) is wide and the renal pelvis that collects the urine is enlarged (red) as a result of urine pooling, unable to pass to the bladder (black).

foods and alter food habits. If the stone type is unknown, it is probably calcium. Regardless of the stone type, patients should be encouraged to drink at least 4 to 6 pints (2 to 3 l) of fluid daily to achieve high urine volume flow. Any infections of the urinary tract should be treated with antibiotics to prevent complications.

The prevalence of stone disease is about 5 percent of the general population, and about 1 in 272 people are newly diagnosed yearly. Kidney stones affect men two to four times more often than women. However, struvite stones, which are typically associated with urinary tract infection, are more common in women. Kidney stones are more common in middle-aged people, and an estimated 12 percent of all men and 5 percent of all women will develop a kidney stone by age 70 years. Caucasians are more commonly affected than African Americans.

Betsy Manakan Srichai and Matthew Breyer

See also
• Genetic disorders • Infections • Kidney disorders • Metabolic disorders

Kwashiorkor

Kwashiorkor is a type of malnutrition caused by severe protein deficiency in the diet. It is a serious problem commonly seen in the underdeveloped countries of Africa, Central America, South America, and South Asia. Kwashiorkor occurs when famine, drought, or political unrest lead to food shortages. Children from infancy to about 5 years old are most at risk due to their increased dietary needs. The incidence of kwashiorkor in children in the United States is extremely low and is only rarely seen in isolated cases of neglect or child abuse.

Kwashiorkor in children was first described in 1935 by the British pediatrician Cicely D. Williams, writing in the medical journal *The Lancet*. The name of the disorder comes from one of the Kwa languages of coastal Ghana and means "deposed child," in the sense that a young child stops receiving its mother's milk when a newborn sibling arrives. In another African dialect, *kwashiorkor* means "red boy," from the discoloration of the hair that is a sign of the disease.

When a child is nursing, it receives certain amino acids that are essential for growth from the mother's milk. During weaning—if the diet that replaces the mother's milk is high in carbohydrates such as starches but deficient in protein—the child may develop kwashiorkor.

Symptoms and signs

Early symptoms of malnutrition include fatigue, irritability, and lethargy. As protein deficiency continues, growth failure, loss of muscle mass, generalized swelling, decreased immunity, and fatty infiltration of the liver occurs. Other commonly seen symptoms and signs include dry skin, change in pigmentation, a swollen belly (potbelly), thinning hair, anemia, and diarrhea. Late symptoms of kwashiorkor can include shock and coma.

Risk Factors

Living in impoverished countries, nations in political turmoil, and countries affected by drought, famine, or natural disasters are all risk factors for kwashiorkor. These conditions may directly or indirectly affect the food resources, leading to widespread malnutrition in children. Other causes of kwashiorkor include poor intestinal absorption (malabsorption), long-term alcoholism, kidney disease, infections, large burns, and other trauma that result in the abnormal loss of protein from the body.

KEY FACTS

Description

Medical name for malnutrition caused by severe protein deficiency.

Causes

A diet that is high in carbohydrates, such as starches, with deficient amounts of protein.

Risk factors

Food shortage in an area due to famine, political turmoil, or natural disasters such as droughts. In industrialized countries like the United States, it may be seen in cases of neglect or abuse.

Symptoms and signs

Common characteristics are indifference or apathy, swollen belly, change in hair and skin color, fatigue, irritability, and diarrhea. In severe cases, stunted growth, mental retardation, and physical disabilities may occur.

Diagnosis

Physical examination; growth measurements; laboratory tests; dietary and medical history.

Treatments

In early stage of the disease, food should be introduced slowly. Carbohydrates are given first, followed by protein-rich foods.

Pathogenesis

A diet lacking in proteins, which are necessary for amino acids—the building blocks for growth.

Prevention

Diet with sufficient amounts of carbohydrates, fats, and protein.

Epidemiology

In impoverished parts of the world, kwashiorkor is the leading cause of death in children under 5 years old. The number of cases in the United States is extremely low, although estimates show that 50 percent of the elderly in nursing homes suffer from this disease. Occurs in developed countries secondary to nutritional ignorance rather than food deprivation.

Treatments and prevention

Treatment of kwashiorkor depends on the severity of the condition but usually begins with rehydration. If shock is present, it requires immediate treatment with restoration of blood volume and maintenance of blood pressure. Calories are given first in the form of carbohydrates, simple sugars, and fats. Proteins are started after other caloric sources have already provided increased energy. Vitamin and mineral supplements are essential, too.

Because a person with kwashiorkor has been without food for a long time, the onset of oral feedings can present problems, especially if the caloric density of the food is initially too high. Therefore, food is reintroduced slowly: carbohydrates first to supply energy, followed by protein.

Many children with kwashiorkor will develop intolerance to milk sugar (lactose) and may need supplements with lactase enzyme in order to benefit from milk products. The consumption of dried milk-based formula has proved effective in treating kwashiorkor.

Treatment early in the course of kwashiorkor can lead to regression of symptoms with good results. Without treatment or if treatment is given too late, this condition is fatal. Many children treated too late are left with permanent physical and intellectual disabilities. There is good statistical evidence that malnutrition early in life permanently decreases intelligence quotient (IQ).

Physical examination may show hepatomegaly (enlarged liver) and generalized edema (swelling). Decreased kidney function is evident by changes in urine content and levels of the mineral potassium in blood serum. Anemia is seen on the CBC (complete blood-cell count). A diet composed of the appropriate amounts of carbohydrates, fat (minimum of 10 percent of total calories), and protein (12 percent of total calories) will prevent kwashiorkor.

Epidemiology

Kwashiorkor is prevalent in overpopulated and impoverished regions of the world, in particular in South Asia, Africa, and Central and South America. This type of malnutrition occurs usually in the midst of drought or political turmoil.

In the United States, the incidence of kwashiorkor in children is extremely low, with isolated cases rarely seen. When the disorder occurs in a child less than the age of 5 years in a developed country, child abuse or neglect is suspected. The disorder may also be found in geriatric and hospitalized patients in Western nations,

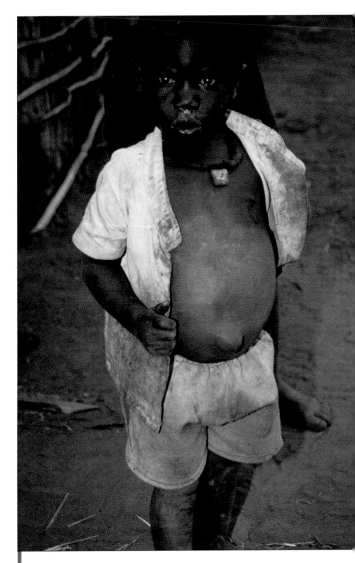

This young boy from Tanzania has the typical symptom of the severe form of malnutrition called kwashiorkor—a swollen belly. In addition, most likely as a result of his malnutrition, the boy is mentally retarded.

particularly if their appetite is greatly diminished and protein intake is negligible. One government estimate suggests that as many as 50 percent of the elderly people in nursing homes in the United States may suffer from protein malnutrition.

Isaac Grate

See also

- Anemia • Coma • Diarrhea and dysentery
- Kidney disorders • Mental retardation
- Nutritional disorders • Shock

Language and speech disorders

Language and speech disorders are difficulties in communication experienced by children and adults. People with language and speech disorders can have difficulty expressing themselves or understanding others. These difficulties significantly interfere with academic achievement or daily activities that require communication skills. The causes of language and speech disorders can be related to hearing, nerve or muscle disorders, head injury, viral diseases, or physical abnormalities.

Children who have language or speech disorders have difficulty achieving milestones of language development related to expression or comprehension, or both. Verbal communication is vital; if it is delayed, learning difficulties can ensue.

Types of language and speech disorders

There are four main types of language and speech disorders: expressive language disorder, mixed receptive-expressive language disorder, phonological disorder, and stuttering. Standardized tests will usually reveal deficits associated with the area of difficulty. People with language or speech disorders typically have average or above average intelligence.

Expressive language disorder occurs when people have problems expressing themselves using spoken language. Typically, individuals with expressive language disorders have below expected levels in vocabulary, as well as difficulties with the use of tense or production of complex sentences. Language development is usually retarded, and the vocabulary or structure of sentences is limited and simple. Language comprehension in individuals with expressive language disorder is intact.

Individuals with mixed receptive-expressive disorders often have problems expressing themselves using spoken language, and also have problems understanding what people say to them; that is, they have difficulty with language comprehension. This lack of comprehension may result in inappropriate responses, misunderstandings, or failure to follow directions. A child with mixed receptive-expressive disorder often appears to be deaf, but the child does in fact hear.

Individuals with phonological disorders have problems with creating speech at a level expected of their age group because of an inability to form the necessary sounds. The level of severity can range from speech that is completely incomprehensible to speech that can

be understood, but in which some sounds are slightly mispronounced.

Stuttering is typically described as a blockage, discoordination, or fragmentations of the flow of speech. Stuttering is often characterized by specific types of disruptions in fluency, such as repetitions of sounds and syllables, prolongation of sounds, and blockages of air flow. Individuals who stutter often show negative reactions to the stuttering, which can make the disorder more severe and difficult.

Causes and risk factors

The brain is divided into various sections that govern different behaviors. Some parts of the brain control the ability to speak, while others control the ability to understand the spoken word or to recognize what words and numbers mean. In people with language disorders, one or more of these areas may not function normally. More specifically, language disorders may be a result of neurological abnormalities that produce impairments in the regions of the brain that control visual and language processing.

Some language disorders may be genetically linked because a person can inherit abnormal brain structure or function. Children from families with a history of language disorders are more likely to develop disorders themselves. Left-handedness appears to increase the risk for expressive language disorder, although the exact reason is unknown.

Structural problems or abnormalities in the areas necessary for speech sound production, such as the tongue or roof of the mouth, can lead to phonological disorders. Neurological problems in which the muscles of the mouth do not work properly can also contribute to phonological disorders.

Finally, in addition to other potential causes, stuttering is often affected by the level of stress present in the environment. An environment that is overly stressful or demanding may cause children to have difficulties developing fluent speech.

Symptoms

In general, the symptoms of language and speech disorders impair an individual's ability to comprehend and produce language, thus making communication with others difficult. The symptoms often vary greatly from one person to the next, but in many cases, individuals are aware of their difficulties in communicating, which can make the disorder even more frustrating and difficult. The presence of language and speech disorders can affect both academic performance and social competence.

Symptoms of expressive language disorders include difficulty in putting sentences together coherently, using proper grammar, recalling the appropriate words to use, and other problems in piecing together conversations. Individuals with expressive language disorder are often not able to communicate their thoughts, needs, or wants at the same level as their peers. Their vocabulary and general sentence structure is generally much more basic and limited than their peers. Individuals with expressive language disorder do, however, understand the material they are trying to communicate to others.

Symptoms of mixed receptive-expressive disorder include those of expressive language disorder. Individuals have difficulty with both producing and understanding spoken language. In addition to problems in expressing language, individuals with mixed receptive disorder also have difficulty understanding what people are saying to them. These individuals may also have difficulty understanding abstract concepts or complex sentences. In addition, individuals with mixed receptive-expressive disorder are more likely to develop other learning disorders, such as reading disorders, so early detection is important.

Individuals with phonological disorders develop speech sounds in the same sequence as their peers, but at a slower rate. Some common mistakes that individuals with phonological disorders will make include omitting sounds (often at the ends of words), distorting sounds, or substituting one sound for another, usually with a sound that is more easily produced.

The primary symptoms of stuttering include excessive problems with fluency in speech, repeating sounds and syllables, and prolonging sounds. Symptoms also include the negative behaviors associated with stuttering that may make stuttering worse.

KEY FACTS

Description
A disorder that involves problems with language expression, comprehension, or a combination of the two.

Causes and risk factors
Thought to involve anomalies in brain structure and function, with various origins. May be also genetically linked or related to different medical conditions. Structural abnormalities related to speech or hearing may also be related.

Symptoms
Diagnosed when performance on standardized tests that measure receptive or expressive language development or sound production is significantly lower than expected for the individual's age, schooling, and level of intelligence.

Diagnosis
After ruling out other medical conditions that may affect performance, such as hearing problems, a series of educational and psychological tests are administered to determine whether achievement is below educational capacity. Diagnosed when a significant discrepancy between standardized scores on expressive or receptive language, or both, and measures on nonverbal intellectual capacity or expected age-appropriate behavior is observed.

Treatments
Usually consists of behaviorally reinforced exercises in practicing basic communication skills, such as vocabulary, sentence construction, sound production, or a combination of all of these necessary skills.

Pathogenesis
Symptoms of language and speech disorders can be present during early childhood. At this time, language develops at a rapid rate, and children with language or speech disorders will appear to fall behind in their development.

Prevention
Because the causes of most language and speech disorders are unclear, there is no obvious way to prevent them.

Epidemiology
For either receptive or expressive language disorders, approximately 1 to 13 percent of school-aged children are affected. Phonological disorders can affect 10 percent of children below 8 years of age and 5 percent of children older than 8 years of age. In the United States the prevalence of stuttering is about 1 percent of the general population, that is, around 3 million people. In all cases, males are almost 4 times more likely to be affected than females.

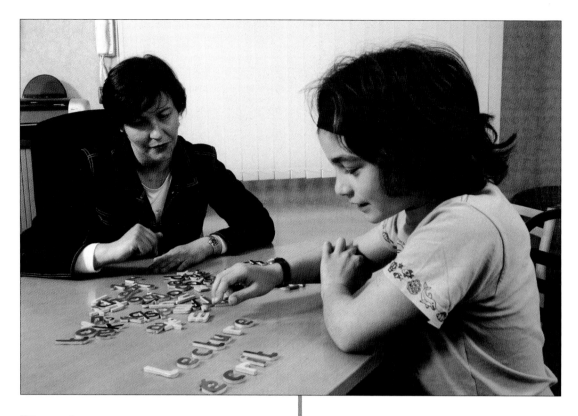

Children who have language and speech disorders can be helped by a speech therapist, who will devise appropriate exercises and games that include naming or verbal description. For children, early treatment is important because language and speech disorders prevent children from relating to other people and can impinge on learning skills.

Diagnosis

In order for expressive, mixed receptive-expressive, or phonological disorder to be diagnosed, individuals must be performing or developing at a level below their peers at tasks that require communication. This can be difficult because sometimes an individual may understand the material in a test but have difficulty expressing comprehension. Typically, nonverbal tests are used in addition to tests that require spoken answers. In all cases, hearing should be evaluated.

In order for any of the language disorders to be diagnosed definitively, the communication problems have to create difficulties for the individual in daily life. Finally, when diagnosing stuttering, a speech pathologist will usually collect speech samples from a variety of situations to determine the normal fluency of the individual.

Treatments

Once a language disorder has been diagnosed, one-on-one therapy is usually the preferred treatment. Typically during therapy, the individual will practice basic communication skills repeatedly to develop fluency. For phonological disorders, individuals will practice forming sounds during therapy. Sometimes the individual is shown the physical way the sound is

made, for example, by showing how to form the lips. In all cases, treatment involves practicing the basic skills necessary for communication (sentence construction, language comprehension, sound production) and also creating an environment at both school and home that is conducive to learning and fluency. This can be done by attempting to minimize stress and being patient with individuals as they learn.

Pathogenesis

Generally, the rapidity and degree of recovery depends on the severity of the disorder, the motivation of the individual to participate in the necessary components of therapy, and how quickly speech and language interventions began. When intervention occurs early, it can sometimes be discontinued by the end of high school. If, however, symptoms are not identified early enough, preferably before school age, or the symptoms are severe, interventions may be necessary into the high school years. With early diagnosis and intervention, the prognosis is usually good, but mild symptoms of language disorders may persist into adult life.

Expressive disorders usually become apparent during early adolescence, when language becomes more complex. By the age of four, most children with expressive language disorder speak in short sentences, but may forget old words or phrases as they learn new ones. With appropriate interventions, however, most children develop normal or nearly normal language skills by high school. In some cases, minor problems with expressive language may never resolve.

With mixed receptive-expressive disorders, the receptive components of the disorder may be apparent between the ages of four and seven. The expressive symptoms may be obvious later as the development of language becomes more complex. If mixed disorder is diagnosed early, it is usually severe in form and will affect the individual throughout life. If the symptoms of the mixed receptive-expressive disorder are milder, the disorder may go undiagnosed for some time, delaying immediate intervention. During this time, other learning disorders may develop, such as reading disorders, which may make the language disorder more obvious but may also hinder intervention.

Phonological disorders are typically diagnosed between the ages of three and six, when speech is developing quickly. Recovery is often spontaneous; those individuals who do not recover before the age of eight will often go on to develop other language and speech problems.

Stuttering usually develops before the age of 12 and peaks during the preschool years when individuals are learning to speak, and later during the elementary school years. During adolescence, stuttering can persist, but usually occurs in response to specific situations, such as reading out loud in class, speaking to strangers, or using the telephone. Fifty to 80 percent of children who stutter will spontaneously recover, but stuttering can continue throughout adult life.

Prevention

There are no known ways of preventing many of the language disorders. In the case of disorders that are caused by damage to the brain, any attempts to avoid any kind of injury could help prevent that type of disorder. In addition, a healthy diet during pregnancy may help prevent neurological or structural problems that can result in a disorder.

Finally, limiting stress during language development may prevent exacerbating already existing disorders and may also encourage development of fluency during therapy for language disorders.

Epidemiology

Language and speech disorders can be relatively common in school-age children and can also be difficult to diagnose. Expressive language disorder is a relatively common childhood disorder, affecting 10 to 15 percent of children under the age of three, and 3 to 7 percent of school-age children. Expressive language disorder is more common in boys than in girls, occurring between two to five times more often.

Mixed receptive-expressive disorder is diagnosed in about 5 percent of preschool-age children and 3 percent of school-age children. It is less common, but more severe, than expressive language disorder. In addition, individuals with mixed receptive-expressive language disorder are more likely to have other types of learning disorders. For example, between 40 to 60 percent of preschool children who have mixed receptive-expressive disorder also have phonological disorder. As many as half of these children may also have some type of reading disorder. They may also be more susceptible to psychiatric disorders, such as attention-deficit hyperactivity disorder (ADHD).

It has been estimated that about 7 to 8 percent of school-age children have phonological disorder. Like the other language disorders, phonological disorders are more common in boys than in girls. Estimates show that boys are up to four times as likely to develop phonological disorders than girls. Children who develop phonological disorders are also more likely to develop some other language problems or disorders.

Stuttering is a relatively low-prevalence disorder. Roughly 1 percent of the general population currently has a stuttering disorder. However, this number differs from the number of individuals who have been diagnosed with stuttering at some point in their lives, which approaches 5 percent. This difference suggests that a significant number of people who develop stuttering problems will often grow out of the problem.

Stuttering is approximately three times more likely in men than in women. This ratio is somewhat lower in childhood, which suggests that females are more likely than men to recover from stuttering problems during childhood.

Lori M. Lieving and Oleg V. Tcheremissine

See also
- Brain disorders • Childhood disorders
- Deafness • Genetic disorders

Lassa fever

A viral infection, largely confined to West Africa, that is transmitted to humans by rodents. In many cases, the Lassa fever virus does not cause illness. However, some infected people develop serious and widespread symptoms, including inflammation, hemorrhaging (abnormal bleeding) from mucous membranes throughout the body, and seizures.

Lassa fever is a potentially fatal hemorrhagic disease caused by the Lassa virus, which infects hundreds of thousands and kills as many as five thousand each year. Although Lassa fever is known primarily from West Africa, the disease has been found in North America and Europe in persons who have traveled to Africa, or in their close contacts.

Causes and risk factors

Rats of the genus *Mastomys*, which are common household pests in West Africa, are the natural carriers of the Lassa virus. Infected rats show no signs of illness, but they shed the virus in their urine and feces. Humans typically become infected by direct contact with rat excreta. The disease is also transmitted through exposure to the excreta, blood, or other bodily fluids of an infected individual.

Symptoms

Most infections are mild or produce no symptoms at all. However, in 20 percent of cases, the onset of Lassa fever is characterized by a gradual accumulation of symptoms, such as fever, weakness, and general feelings of illness. Days after the initial symptoms begin, a host of other symptoms may follow, including: headache, sore throat, pain, nausea, vomiting, and diarrhea. In severe cases, there may be inflammation, such as of the face; fluid buildup in the lungs; hemorrhaging from mucous membranes in the mouth, nose, genitals, or gastrointestinal tract; low blood pressure from fluid loss; and excess protein in the urine. Lassa fever can also affect the nervous system, causing symptoms ranging from deafness and seizures to coma.

Treatment and prevention

If given early enough after the onset of symptoms, antiviral drug treatment may be effective. Management of symptoms and supportive care, such as the replenishment of bodily fluids and electrolytes (sodium, potassium, chloride, and bicarbonate), is vital. There is no vaccine for Lassa fever. The only way to prevent the disease is to eliminate or reduce rat populations and maintain a clean environment.

David Lawrence

KEY FACTS

Description
A viral hemorrhagic fever that may affect many systems of the body.

Causes
Infection by the Lassa virus.

Risk factors
Exposure to rats of the genus *Mastomys*, which commonly live in or near human dwellings in West Africa, where the disease originates.

Symptoms
In 80 percent of infections, no symptoms occur. There may be fever, headache, sore throat, pain, and digestive disturbances (including nausea, vomiting, and diarrhea). Severe cases may feature inflammation, fluid buildup, hemorrhage (abnormal bleeding), low blood pressure, and nervous system disorders.

Diagnosis
Diagnosis is confirmed by tests for the presence of the Lassa fever virus in the blood.

Treatments
Antiviral drugs can be effective if given early enough. Symptoms are managed as they occur.

Pathogenesis
Infected rats shed the virus in their urine or feces. Contact with rat excreta transmits the virus to humans. The infection can also be spread from human to human.

Prevention
Control of the rat population and maintaining a clean environment.

Epidemiology
Between 300,000 and 500,000 cases are reported from West Africa each year. About 5,000 deaths occur annually.

See also
- Ebola fever • Infections, animal-to-human
- Infections, viral

Lazy eye

A visual condition in which the vision in one eye is weaker than the other because the affected eye and the brain are not working together properly. The medical term for lazy eye is *amblyopia*. Lazy eye is mainly a developmental disorder that affects children from birth to about age seven. The disorder affects between 2 and 3 percent of all children.

Amblyopia is the medical condition in which the brain and the eye, which normally work together to produce vision, have been compromised in their function. Normal vision develops with regular, equal use of both eyes. Amblyopia, commonly called lazy eye, usually occurs when one eye is not used enough for the visual system in the brain to develop properly. The brain ignores the images from the weak eye and uses only those from the stronger eye, leading to deteriorating vision in the weaker eye. Both eyes typically appear normal, but one does not see as well as the other. Amblyopia usually affects only one eye but may occur in both. Children can develop amblyopia during the first decade of life, typically between birth until about the age of seven.

Causes and risk factors

Amblyopia may be caused by any condition that affects normal visual development or use of the eyes. Amblyopia can be caused by strabismus, an imbalance in the positioning of the two eyes. Strabismus can cause the eyes to cross in (esotropia) or turn out (exotropia). Amblyopia may be caused when one eye is more nearsighted (myopic), farsighted (hypermetropic), or astigmatic than the other eye. Occasionally, amblyopia is caused by other eye conditions, such as cataract. Other risk factors include family history, premature birth, and low birth weight.

Signs and symptoms

Some children may appear to have an eye that wanders or does not move with the other eye. In most cases, however, amblyopia is hard to detect. Other symptoms of amblyopia include eyes that do not move in the same direction or fix on the same point, crying or complaining when one eye is covered, squinting or tilting the head to look at something, or an upper eyelid that droops.

Diagnosis and treatment

Treating amblyopia involves making the child use the eye with reduced vision. Current treatment includes atropine drops and patching of the stronger eye. Atropine causes the stronger eye's vision to temporarily blur, forcing the child to use the weaker eye. In patching, an opaque, adhesive patch is worn over the stronger eye intermittently for weeks to months; this forces the child to use the eye with amblyopia. Both methods force use of the weaker eye and help the part of the brain that manages vision to develop more completely.

Rashmi Nemade

KEY FACTS

Description
Also known as amblyopia, a condition in which one eye has reduced vision.

Causes
Any circumstance that affects normal visual development.

Risk factors
Family history of amblyopia or strabismus, being more nearsighted, farsighted, or astigmatic in one eye than the other, or having strabismus.

Symptoms
Wandering eye, reduced vision, and eyes that do not move in the same direction or fix on the same point.

Diagnosis
Eye exam.

Treatment
Patching of the stronger eye or atropine drops in the stronger eye to force more use of the eye with amblyopia.

Pathogenesis
Eye and brain do not work together properly; cannot be remedied after the age of eight years.

Epidemiology
Amblyopia is the most common cause of visual impairment in childhood. The condition affects approximately 2 to 3 out of every 100 children.

Prevention
Patching and atropine of stronger eye can prevent permanent damage to vision in young children.

See also
- Astigmatism • Cataract • Eye disorders
- Myopia and hypermetropia •

Learning disorders

Learning disorders are learning difficulties experienced by children and adults of average to above-average intelligence. People with learning disorders have difficulty with reading, writing, or mathematics, or any combination of the three subjects. These difficulties significantly interfere with academic achievement or the ability to carry out daily activities that require any of these three skills.

People with learning disorders have problems collecting new information, remembering and processing that information, and acting on verbal and nonverbal information. The three main types of learning disorders are reading disorders, mathematics disorders, and writing disorders. Standardized tests usually reveal deficits associated with the area of difficulty. Difficulties are due to neurological differences in brain structure or functioning. By definition, people with learning disorders have average or above average intelligence. Thus, they may score poorly on tests, but the low scores are due to a problem with learning, not low intelligence.

Reading disorders

Disorders concerned with reading are the most common type of learning disorder. Individuals with reading disorders have difficulty recognizing letters and words and remembering what they mean (dyslexia). They find it difficult to understand the sounds and letter groups that make up words. Because of these problems, individuals with reading disorders often have impaired performance in reading comprehension.

Mathematic disorders

Individuals with mathematic disorders have problems recognizing numbers (dyscalculia), doing calculations, or understanding abstract mathematical concepts. For example, they may not remember how to use numbers in counting. They have trouble understanding how numbers can apply to everyday situations. A mathematics disorder is present in one of every five cases of a learning disorder. Those with mathematic disorders often have reading or writing disorders as well, or both.

Writing disorders

Individuals with writing disorders have problems with the basic skills of writing, such as spelling, punctuation, and grammar. They have problems with handwriting or with creating sentences that make sense to others. They often have one other type of learning disorder as well.

Causes

The brain is divided into various sections that control different behaviors. Some parts of the brain control the ability to speak, whereas others control the ability to understand the spoken word or to recognize what words and numbers mean. In people with learning disorders, one or more of these sections may not function normally. Thus, learning disorders may be due to neurological abnormalities that produce impairments in the regions of the brain that control visual and language processing, attention, and planning.

Risk factors

Some learning disorders may have a genetic factor because a person can inherit abnormal brain structure or function. Children from families with a history of learning disorders are more likely to develop disorders themselves. Environmental risk factors for learning disorders include prenatal exposure to a maternal infectious illness, extremely low birth weight, premature birth, birth trauma or distress, or any other factor that can affect the uterine environment, which is so important for healthy brain development. Several factors in early childhood also can contribute to delayed brain development, including neonatal seizures, a poor learning environment, developmental trauma, toxins in the environment, or poor nutrition.

Symptoms

Some individuals earn high scores on intelligence tests, suggesting that they should do well in school, but the grades they receive may be far below what those tests predict. This mismatch may be a sign of a learning disorder. Aside from academic underachievement, other warnings signs that a person may have a learning disorder include overall lack of organization, forgetfulness, and taking unusually long amounts of time to complete assignments. In the classroom, teachers may observe one or more of the following characteristics: difficulty paying attention, unusual sloppiness and disorganization, social withdrawal, difficulty working independently, and problems switching from one activity to another. In addition to these signs related to school and schoolwork, certain general behavioral and emotional features often accompany learning disorders. These include impulsiveness, restlessness, distractibility, poor physical coordination, low tolerance for frustration, low self-esteem, daydreaming, inattentiveness, and anger or sadness.

Symptoms of a reading disorder include difficulty identifying groups of letters, failure to correctly identify the sounds different letters make, reversals and other errors involving letter position, chaotic spelling, difficulty with breaking words into syllables, failure to recognize words, hesitant reading aloud, and word-by-word reading rather than contextual reading.

Symptoms of a writing disorder may often be seen in the kind of written work someone produces. Symptoms include problems with letter formation and writing layout on the page, repetitions and omissions, punctuation and capitalization errors, "mirror writing" (writing right to left), and a variety of spelling problems. Individuals with writing disorders typically take much longer to complete written work than other individuals, often only to produce writing that is large in size and filled with errors.

Individuals with mathematical disorders often cannot count in the correct sequence. They may not be able to name numbers and perform mathematical operations, such as addition and subtraction. Individuals with mathematical disorders may have spatial problems and difficulty aligning numbers into proper columns. They may have difficulty with the abstract concepts of time and direction. For example, they may become confused about the sequences of past or future events. Interestingly, it is common for individuals with mathematical disorders to have normal or accelerated language acquisition, such as verbal skills, reading, writing, and good visual memory for the printed word. They are typically good in the areas of science (until higher-level mathematical skills are needed), geometry (figures with logic, not formulas), and creative arts.

Diagnosis

The first step in diagnosing a learning disorder is conducting a complete medical, psychological, and educational examination. The purpose of this examination is to rule out other conditions with symptoms similar to

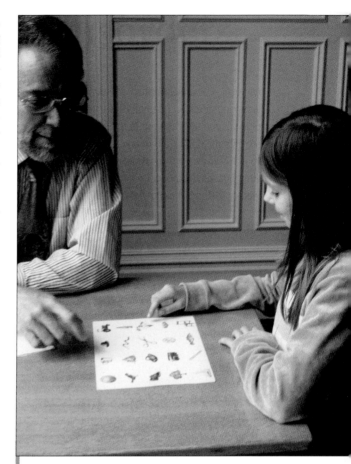

A girl is assessed for dyslexia by an educational psychologist. She is asked to perform a variety of tasks involving words, numbers, and symbols. From her response, the psychologist is able to produce a profile, a unique pattern of strengths and weaknesses, which is then analyzed for evidence of dyslexia.

those of learning disorders. For example, a child with mental retardation, attention-deficit hyperactivity disorder, or an unusually poor educational background may show the symptoms of a learning disorder. These conditions are different from a learning disorder and need to be treated differently. If no medical problems are found, a series of psychological and educational tests is completed. Some of the tests commonly used include the Wechsler Intelligence Scale for Children, the Woodcock-Johnson Psychoeducational Battery, and the Peabody Individual Achievement Test-Revised. These tests measure intelligence and mental achievement. Performance on the standardized tests is compared to actual academic performance. When a significant discrepancy between the two is observed, a specific learning disorder is diagnosed.

Treatments

Once a learning disorder has been diagnosed, special education must be planned, which involves identifying what the individual can and cannot do. After a systematic analysis of learning strengths and weaknesses, an individualized education plan (IEP) is developed that outlines the specific skills that need to be developed. Most effective learning strategies use multiple skills and senses. IEPs may involve special instruction within a regular classroom or assignment to a special-education class. All IEPs also provide for annual retesting to measure the child's progress.

An IEP for an individual with a reading disorder may focus on increasing recognition of the sounds and meanings of letters and words (or phonics training). As training progresses, instruction shifts to improving the ability to understand words and sentences, to remember what has been read, and to learn how to study more efficiently.

Students with writing disorders are often encouraged to keep a daily record of their activities. They often find it easier to express their thoughts by using a computer rather than a paper and pencil. Individuals with mathematical disorders are often given number problems from everyday life. For example, they are taught how to balance a checkbook or compare prices on a shopping trip.

Pathogenesis

In general, although the symptoms of learning disorders may be present before reaching school age, they are seldom recognized or diagnosed prior to the first years of school, when formal education and testing occur. More specifically, the symptoms of a reading disorder may occur as early as kindergarten, but they are seldom diagnosed before the end of kindergarten or the beginning of first grade because formal reading instruction usually does not begin until this point in most schools.

Particularly when associated with high intelligence, individuals may function at or near grade level in the early grades, and reading disorders may not be fully apparent until the fourth grade or later. When intervention occurs early, it can sometimes be discontinued by the end of first or second grade. If, however, symptoms are not identified early enough or the symptoms are severe, interventions may be necessary into high-school years. With early diagnosis and intervention, the prognosis is usually good, but reading disorders may persist into adult life.

Mathematical disorders usually become apparent during second or third grade, or by the age of 8 years. Since the developmental progress of mathematical disorders has yet to be well studied, it is estimated that the symptoms can be diagnosed even into and beyond fifth grade (the age of 10 and later).

KEY FACTS

Description

A developmental disorder that involves problems with reading, writing, mathematics, or a combination of these three disciplines.

Causes and risk factors

Thought to involve anomalies in brain structure and function, with various origins. May be also genetically linked or related to different medical conditions. Toxins *in utero* or in a person's early environment can also cause learning disabilities.

Symptoms

Diagnosed when performance on standardized tests in reading, mathematics, or writing is significantly lower than expected for the individual's age, schooling, and general level of intelligence.

Diagnosis

After ruling out other medical conditions that may affect academic performance, a series of educational and psychological tests are administered to determine whether achievement is below educational capacity. Diagnosed when a significant discrepancy between standardized scores and academic performance is observed.

Treatments

Based on psychoeducational testing, individual education plans (IEPs) are developed that include basic-skill training in the deficient areas, which can be built upon to reach mastery of reading, mathematics, or writing.

Pathogenesis

Symptoms of learning disorders may be present at an early age, but are usually not recognized until individuals reach school age. Typically, reading and mathematical disorders will be recognized before writing disorders.

Prevention

Early intervention may allow prevention of prolonged academic difficulties that may adversely affect family relationships and occupational outcomes.

Epidemiology

Learning disorders affect about 2 million children between the ages of 6 and 17, and one in every seven people in the United States. The male to female ratio for learning disorders is about 5:1. Reading disorders represent four out of every five cases of a learning disorder.

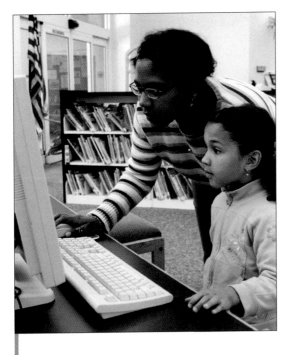

Children who have writing disorders often find that using a computer is easier than writing on paper. They record daily activities to help improve their writing skills.

Because individuals usually learn to speak and read well before writing well, reading disorders are usually diagnosed first, and writing disorders are diagnosed last. Thus, writing disorders are usually apparent by the age of 7 but may not be recognized until the age of 10 or later, with the more severe cases being identified earlier.

As with most other learning disorders, early discovery and intervention is of the utmost importance. Writing disorders may occasionally be seen in older children or adults, but little is known about their long-term prognosis.

Prognosis

The outlook is good for individuals who are diagnosed with learning disorders early in their school years. Early diagnosis allows the development of individualized education plans that will help affected people overcome their disorders. Learning disorders continue into adulthood, but most people who receive proper educational and vocational training can complete college and find a satisfying job.

Studies of the occupational choices of adults with dyslexia indicate that they do particularly well in people-oriented professions and occupations, such as nursing and sales.

Prevention

Although there may be no way to completely prevent the occurrence of a learning disorder, it is important to prevent the symptoms of learning disorders from going undiagnosed. The high school dropout rate for individuals with learning disorders is almost 40 percent. Many of these individuals are never properly diagnosed or given appropriate instruction. As a result, they never become fully literate.

In addition, 10 to 25 percent of individuals with learning disorders also meet criteria for other disorders, such as conduct disorder, oppositional-defiant disorder, attention-deficit hyperactivity disorder, major depressive disorder, or dysthymic disorder.

Learning disorders can lead to other problems. Individuals may become frustrated and discouraged. They may not learn how to get along with other people and become aggressive and troublesome. In addition, learning problems may be stressful for family members and subsequently strain family relationships.

Epidemiology

One in every seven people in the United States has a learning disorder. Learning disorders affect about 2 million children between the ages of 6 and 17, or about 5 percent of schoolchildren. The male to female ratio for learning disorders is about 5:1. More specifically, reading disorders represent four out of every five cases of a learning disorder. Research shows that 60 to 80 percent of individuals with a reading disorder are males. However, the rate of reading disorders in boys may be inflated; boys' reading disorders are usually noticed because of behavioral difficulties in the classroom. As individuals with reading disorders become adults, the sex differences are no longer present.

The prevalence of mathematical disorders has not yet been well established, but is estimated to be about 5 percent. There is an expectation that mathematical disorders are more likely in girls than boys. Similarly, while the prevalence of writing disorders is not well established, it has been estimated to be present in about 3 to 10 percent of schoolchildren.

Oleg Tcheremissine and Lori Lieving

See also
- Brain disorders • Childhood disorders
- Deafness • Diagnosis • Disabilities
- Ear disorders • Environmental disorders
- Genetic disorders • Language and speech disorders • Mental retardation • Nutritional disorders • Prevention

Legionnaires' disease

Legionnaires' disease is infection with *Legionella* bacteria, which may cause pneumonia (inflammation of the lungs). Members of the American Legion at a convention in Philadelphia in 1976 suffered an outbreak of a short-term, feverish respiratory illness, which led to the discovery of the disease.

The incidence of Legionnaires' disease depends on the degree of contamination of water reservoirs with *Legionella* bacteria, the susceptibility of the host, and the extent of the exposure to that water. The infection is thought to be contracted through airborne transmission of contaminated water from heat-exchange systems, respiratory therapy devices, whirlpools, shower stalls, and humidifiers. Person-to-person transmission has not been found to occur.

Those at risk for this disease are people who live or work near construction sites, those with long-term lung disease or diabetes, alcoholics, smokers, people with HIV infection, and victims of trauma. Legionnaires' disease can occur at any age.

Symptoms and signs

Legionnaires' disease has two forms: Pontiac fever and *Legionella* pneumonia. Pontiac fever has a one- to two-day incubation period, followed by flulike symptoms of fever, chills, muscle aches, and headaches. This form is usually of brief duration, with full recovery in one week and a low mortality rate. No pneumonia occurs, although there may be a cough and chest pain.

The incubation period for *Legionella* pneumonia is 2 to 10 days. Those affected have fever, chills, headache, malaise, dry cough, and shortness of breath. Half of the patients will have gut symptoms of no appetite, diarrhea, nausea or vomiting, and possibly chest pain and coughing up streaks of blood. The patient looks ill, with rapid breathing patterns and a slow heart rate. Mental status can range from confusion to coma. Complications cam include respiratory failure, shock, coma, and heart problems.

Diagnosis, treatments, and prevention

In infected people, blood tests show a high white blood cell (WBC) count. Blood levels of sodium and phosphorus may be checked because they are commonly low in infected people. Examination of sputum typically shows numerous WBCs with few or no *Legionella* cells.

Most infected people show improvement in 12 to 48 hours after starting antibiotics such as azithromycin. If the source of the disease is the hospital water supply, prevention of hospital-acquired disease is possible. Using monochloramine to disinfect community water supplies has decreased the risk of infection.

Epidemiology

In the United States, between 8,000 and 18,000 people are hospitalized each year with Legionnaires' disease, about 15 percent of whom die from its effects. *Legionella* is more frequent in hospitalized patients, especially those in intensive care units.

Isaac Grate

KEY FACTS

Description
A type of pneumonia.

Causes
Legionella bacteria.

Risk factors
Working or living near construction sites; having lung disease, diabetes, alcoholism, HIV infection, or an injury; smoking.

Symptoms and signs
Fever, headache, malaise, cough, nausea, chest pain, vomiting, diarrhea, blood-streaked sputum.

Diagnosis
Exam of sputum; blood tests.

Treatments
Azithromycin is the drug of choice.

Pathogenesis
People in good health can recover in 2 to 3 weeks; anyone with weakened immunity may die.

Prevention
Monochloramine disinfecting of communities' water supplies has decreased the risk of *Legionella* infection.

Epidemiology
The disease accounts for 2 to 9 percent of community-acquired pneumonia and has a fatality rate of 15 percent.

See also
- Infections, bacterial • Pleurisy
- Pneumonia • Respiratory system disorders

Leishmaniasis

Leishmaniasis is a disease caused by protozoan parasites of the genus *Leishmania* that is found in localized areas throughout tropical and subtropical regions. The disease is transmitted by small biting flies called sand flies.

Several species of *Leishmania* can infect humans. In most cases, humans are incidental hosts of the parasites, and other mammals are the reservoir hosts. The various species of *Leishmania* have different geographical ranges. In general, each species of *Leishmania* causes a particular type of disease, which can range from a self-healing skin lesion to a disfiguring lesion of the skin and mucous membranes, such as the lining of the nasal passages, called mucocutaneous leishmaniasis or a disease of the internal organs (visceral leishmaniasis). About 12 million people have leishmaniasis, with an estimated 1.5 to 2 million new clinical cases diagnosed each year.

Pathogenesis and symptoms

The infection is acquired when a person is bitten by an infected sand fly. The parasite is taken up by white blood cells called macrophages and then replicates within the macrophages. Parasites are released from the host macrophage and are taken up by other macrophages and continue this replication cycle. This usually results in an ulcerated skin lesion at the site of the original sand fly bite. With time the host's immune response will eliminate the parasites and the lesion will heal, perhaps leaving a scar.

Occasionally the infected macrophages will spread from the original site and cause secondary skin lesions or invade mucosal tissue—especially around the mouth and nose. The invasion of the mucosa results in a disfiguring disease in which the cartilage of the nose and surrounding tissue is destroyed. This mucocutaneous form of the disease is difficult to treat and does not readily cure itself.

In some species of *Leishmania* the infected macrophages do not remain in the skin but migrate to the bone marrow, liver, and spleen and cause a systemic infection known as visceral leishmaniasis. Symptoms of visceral leishmaniasis include fever and enlarged liver, spleen, and lymph nodes. As the disease progresses, patients often exhibit a wasting syndrome, characterized by weight loss and failure to thrive, despite good appetite. Visceral leishmaniasis is usually fatal if not treated.

Diagnosis, treatments, and prevention

Leishmaniasis is diagnosed by immunological tests or by looking for parasites in tissue samples. Drugs called pentavalent antimonials are used to kill the parasites. Personal preventive activities should include measures that avoid sand fly bites such as protective clothing, insect repellants, bed nets, and insecticides.

Mark Wiser

KEY FACTS

Description

A chronic disease characterized by either skin lesions or a systemic (visceral) infection.

Causes

Protozoa of the genus *Leishmania*.

Risk factors

Being bitten by infected sand flies.

Symptoms

The cutaneous disease is characterized by chronic skin lesions that are slow to heal. The visceral disease is characterized by a wasting syndrome.

Diagnosis

Detecting the parasite in scrapings from skin lesions or in bone marrow samples from systemic infections. Immunological tests are also available.

Treatments

Pentavalent antimonial drugs.

Pathogenesis

Parasites transmitted by sand fly bites invade macrophages and may spread to other cells and tissues.

Epidemiology

About 12 million people are infected, with an estimated 1.5 to 2 million new clinical cases each year.

Prevention

Protective clothing, bed nets, insect repellants, and insecticides.

See also
- Immune system disorders • Infections, animal-to-human • Infections, parasitic

Leprosy

Leprosy is a chronic bacterial infection that is a worldwide health problem. Also called Hansen's disease, leprosy causes skin lesions and damages nerves, usually in the limbs and face. There has often been stigma associated with leprosy. Although many still remain afflicted, the prognosis of this condition has dramatically improved with appropriate therapy and continuing public health efforts.

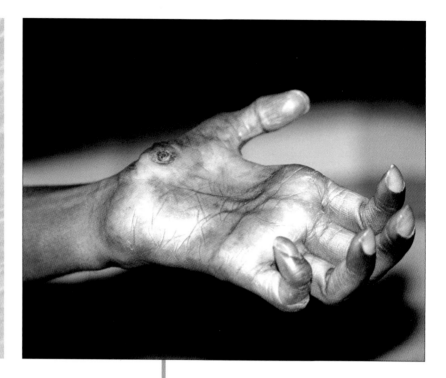

Leprosy is caused by the bacterium *Mycobacterium leprae*. It is a type of bacteria that replicates very slowly and grows best at temperatures of 27°C to 33°C (80.6°F–91.4°F). It is a hardy organism that can survive outside the body for several weeks. It grows well in cooler areas of the human body, such as skin, mucous membranes, and superficial nerves.

Risk factors

The strongest risk factor for leprosy is close contact with infected patients, because the bacterium can be transmitted through the respiratory route, by inhalation of infected nasal secretions. Advanced age and impaired immune function may predispose patients to leprosy. Various poorly defined genetic factors may also increase the risk of developing certain types of the disease. It does not appear that humans acquire leprosy through contact with animals.

Symptoms and signs

The clinical features vary widely. Because the organisms grow slowly, the incubation period ranges from several months to many years. In its earliest form, there may be a localized area of flat skin discoloration. In most people this resolves spontaneously without

Nerve damage, as a result of infection with Mycobacterium leprae, *causes numbness of the hands. The lack of feeling can lead to injury and sometimes loss of the fingers.*

therapy; however, it can progress to more severe disease in a minority of patients. The area of skin involvement may remain localized but can spread anywhere on the body and often progresses to elevated or nodular lesions. The color of these lesions is usually red, but sometimes they lack pigment. Invasion of the nasal and laryngeal mucosa may also occur, resulting in cartilage erosion and perforation. Another common feature of the bacterium is its ability to infect nerves, typically those closer to the surface of the skin. The affected nerves often enlarge and can be palpated. As a result, there may be progressive impairment in sensation and motor strength, depending on the site of involvement. In severe cases, the organism may infect the nerves of the eyes and lead to blindness. Leprosy is rarely fatal but is a chronic condition that can result in severe disfigurement and disability.

Diagnosis and treatments

The diagnosis of leprosy requires observation of one or more of the three cardinal signs: a characteristic skin patch with loss of sensation, thickened peripheral nerves, and the presence of the bacteria on skin smear or biopsy. The bacterium cannot be grown on laboratory media, and blood tests are not helpful in diagnosis.

There are several different antibiotics available, including rifampin, dapsone, clofazimine, and clarithromycin. A combination of these medications, also called multidrug therapy (MDT), taken over prolonged periods (6 to 12 months), is required for successful treatment. Patients should be monitored closely during therapy for any signs of nerve damage or adverse effects of treatment to try to prevent long-term disability. Treatment also involves an educational element regarding the nature of leprosy and the importance of adhering to prolonged courses of therapy.

Pathogenesis and prevention

The exact mode of transmission is unknown. However, the infection is most commonly spread from person to person through aerosol spread of nasal secretions and inhalation by the uninfected host. Once inside the body, bacteria can spread to distant sites. It grows best at superficial areas including skin and mucous membranes. The bacterium preferentially attacks cells of peripheral nerves. It replicates very slowly, which accounts for the chronicity of the disease. Host cells are damaged by invading bacteria but also by the inflammation that ensues as the human immune response attempts to contain the infection.

People should avoid close contact with leprosy patients until the patient has started on treatment. This includes household contacts. A key to preventing the spread of leprosy lies in early detection of the disease and prompt treatment. Once a person has taken MDT for several days, he or she is no longer infectious to others and does not need to be isolated from society. There is no vaccine that is approved for prevention of leprosy. A vaccine called BCG vaccine, commonly given outside the United States for possible protection against tuberculosis, may provide partial immunity.

Epidemiology

Leprosy is extremely uncommon in the United States and other developed nations. About 100 to 150 cases are reported in the United States annually, and most of these are diagnosed in immigrants. Most cases of leprosy are found in developing countries, particularly in areas of poverty and overcrowding. Leprosy most commonly occurs in tropical and warm temperate areas such as Africa, Asia, and Central America. In 1985, about 12 million people were afflicted with leprosy. The World Health Organization (WHO) has launched a campaign aimed toward the elimination of leprosy. Since that time, the number of leprosy patients has fallen to around 600,000 worldwide. Efforts toward complete elimination are ongoing but unlikely to be achieved in the near future.

Joseph M. Fritz and Nigar Kirmani

KEY FACTS

Description

A chronic bacterial infection that most commonly causes skin lesions and nerve damage.

Causes

Mycobacterium leprae, an organism that can survive outside the body for several weeks.

Risk factors

Close contact with those infected. Age, poor immune function, and genetic factors may also predispose people to develop leprosy.

Symptoms and signs

Typically starts as a localized area of skin discoloration. The skin lesions may progress and can spread anywhere on the body with widely varying appearances. The infection spreads to nerves, and damage results in both motor and sensory impairments. Disfigurement and disability commonly occur with advanced disease.

Diagnosis

Characteristic skin lesions with loss of sensation, thickened peripheral nerves, and identification of typical bacteria in skin biopsy.

Treatments

Multiple antibiotics available. Multidrug therapy (MDT) is required for at least 6 to 12 months.

Pathogenesis

Bacteria living in secretions of those infected spread via aerosol route to susceptible patients and enter new host through respiratory tract. Bacteria most commonly infiltrate cells in skin and nerves.

Prevention

Avoidance of those infected until therapy has been started. Early recognition and treatment of disease also helps prevent spread to others. No vaccine available specifically for leprosy.

Epidemiology

In 2002, about 600,000 patients worldwide. Most cases in tropical and warm temperate areas. Only 100 to 150 cases per year in the United States.

See also
- Blindness • Immune system disorders
- Infections, bacterial • Nervous system disorders

Leukemia

Leukemia is the malignant growth of leukocytes (white blood cells). There are four main types of leukemias: acute lymphocytic leukemia (ALL), acute myelogenous leukemia (AML), chronic lymphocytic leukemia (CLL), and chronic myelogenous leukemia (CML). Leukemias are classified according to the particular type of cancerous cell and how quickly the cancer progresses. Current treatments have the potential to cure leukemia.

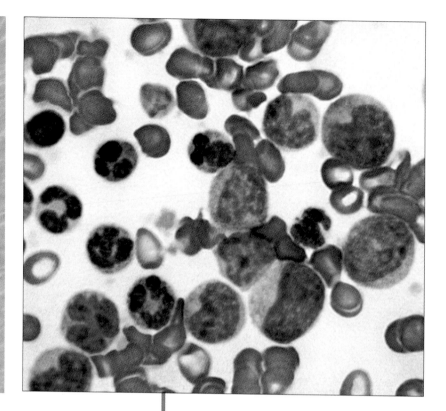

Leukemia is an acute or chronic disease in which there is an abnormal increase in white blood cells in the blood and tissues. The word *leukemia* is derived from the Greek *leuk*, meaning "white," and *emia*, meaning "blood."

There are three types of cells in blood: white blood cells (leukocytes), which fight infection and disease; red blood cells, which carry oxygen and carbon dioxide to and from the cells of the body; and platelets (also called thrombocytes), which help form blood clots to control bleeding. When there are genetic changes in the DNA of leukocytes that cause them to grow uncontrollably, the resulting cancer of these cells is called leukemia. Anyone can develop leukemia, and people of all ages and both sexes can be affected.

Blood cells are made in bone marrow, the soft, spongy substance in the middle part of bones. When leukemia develops, the production of white blood cells becomes so rapid that red blood cells and platelets are crowded out and become reduced in number. Impaired white blood cells can lead to serious and life-threatening infections; and fewer platelets can lead to bruising or bleeding. Low numbers of red blood cells (anemia)

A microscopic picture of blood cells shows a large increase in the number of abnormal white blood cells (purple). These cells do not function properly, and they crowd out the red blood cells (red) and prevent the formation of normal white blood cells. As a result, someone with leukemia is unable to fight off infection, bleeds easily, and tends to become anemic.

can cause weakness and fatigue. When cancerous white blood cells leave the bone marrow and travel through the bloodstream, the cancer may metastasize (spread) to other parts of the body such as the liver, spleen, lymph nodes, testes, and brain. Leukemia is related to lymphoma, which is the cancer of lymphocytes, the white blood cells that circulate in the lymphatic system.

There are two kinds of abnormal white blood cells that cause leukemia. If the cancerous changes have occurred in lymphocytes or in cells that normally produce lymphocytes, the disease is called lymphocytic leukemia. If the cancerous changes are in cells that normally produce neutrophils, basophils, eosinophils, and monocytes, the disease is called myelogenous leukemia. Leukemias may also be acute or chronic. In acute leukemia, cancer cells are blasts (immature cells) that grow quickly, whereas chronic leukemia cells are a combination of immature and mature cells and grow more slowly. There are six types of leukemias, which are identified according to the speed of growth and the type of cancer cell. Acute lymphocytic leukemia (ALL) is the most common leukemia found in children and in some cases adults over the age of 65. Acute myelogenous leukemia (AML) is a type of leukemia that almost always affects adults and is rarely seen in children. It is also called acute nonlymphocytic leukemia (ANLL). Chronic lymphocytic leukemia (CLL) usually affects adults over age 55 and sometimes is found in younger adults, but it almost never affects children. Chronic myelogenous leukemia (CML) is a type of leukemia that almost always affects adults and is extremely rare in children. Hairy cell leukemia and acute promyelocytic leukemia are two forms of leukemia that are extremely rare in both adults and children.

Causes and risk factors

The cause of leukemia is a change in the DNA of leukocytes that causes abnormalities and uncontrolled multiplication of these cells. The cause for this change in DNA is not known. However, there are several known risk factors such as family history, diseases present at birth, exposure to carcinogens, and infection by viruses. Chromosomal disorders present at birth, such as Down syndrome, are associated with a higher risk of leukemia. In addition, chronic and high exposure to industrial carcinogens such as benzene and toluene can lead to leukemia. Furthermore, certain viruses, such as human immunodeficiency virus (HIV, responsible for AIDS) or human T-lymphotropic viruses (HTLV-1 and HTLV-2), are linked to some forms of leukemia. Fanconi anemia, a rare genetic disease, is also a risk factor for developing leukemias.

Although researchers continue to investigate the causes of leukemia, what is already known is that leukemia is not contagious and cannot be transmitted from person to person.

Hematopoiesis is the term for the development of blood cells. Before birth, hematopoiesis occurs in the yolk sac, then the liver, and eventually in the bone marrow. In normal adults it occurs in bone marrow (myeloid tissue) and lymphatic tissues. All blood cells develop from pluripotential stem cells, which are undifferentiated cells that are able to divide and differentiate into other cell types. In other words, stem cells can produce offspring cells to become whatever kind of cell that its environment dictates. Stem cells are not committed to becoming any particular kind of cell, such as

liver or skin cells. Pluripotential hemopoietic stem cells are the precursor cells that give rise to all the blood cell types of both the myeloid and lymphoid lineages.

If a mutation occurs in the genes of hemopoietic stem cells, the result is usually uncontrollable growth of cells in that lineage. For example, a mutation in myeloid stem cells will probably lead to myelogenous leukemia. Leukemia cells ultimately live in the bone marrow, constantly making new cancer cells and suppressing the function of cells that develop into normal blood cells. By circulating in the blood, leukemia cells may also invade other organs, including the liver, spleen, lymph nodes, testes, and brain.

Symptoms and signs

Symptoms of leukemia are general and can sometimes be confused with other disorders or even ignored.

KEY FACTS

Description
Malignant, excessive growth of leukocytes (white blood cells).

Causes
Environmental carcinogens and heredity cause changes in leukocyte DNA that alter its ability to control growth.

Risk factors
Family history of cancer, Down syndrome, viral infection, and exposure to environmental carcinogens, such as benzene and toluene.

Symptoms
Fatigue, weakness, unexplained weight loss, shortness of breath, easy bruising and bleeding, persistent low-grade fever, bone pain, and abdominal pain.

Diagnosis
Examination of blood cells and bone marrow biopsy.

Treatment
Drug therapy or radiation, often in combination with bone marrow transplant.

Pathogenesis
Develops from mutations in stem cells of the bone marrow; likely progression not known.

Prevention
Reduction of contact with environmental carcinogens and in the case of family history, regular visits to the doctor for full physical examinations.

Epidemiology
About 35,000 people in the United States are diagnosed with one of the types of leukemias each year.

Feelings of chronic fatigue, weakness, and shortness of breath from anemia are some of the initial symptoms. Observation of enlarged lymph nodes, easy bruising and bleeding, pain in joints and bones, recurrent infections, abdominal pain due to an enlarged spleen or liver, and unexplained fever may cause a person to seek medical attention.

Diagnosis

At the present time, there is no definitive screening test for diagnosing leukemia. Routine blood tests such as those for employment, military service, pregnancy, and before surgery are typically the ways in which leukemias are discovered. One of these routine tests includes a complete blood count in which all the cells in blood are analyzed. This test provides information about the white blood cell, red blood cell, and platelet populations. This information includes the number, type, size, shape, and some of the physical characteristics of the cells.

If these results are abnormal, further testing of bone marrow or spinal fluid can be carried out to determine if leukemia cells are present and how far they may have spread. Imaging through X-rays or computed tomography (CT) scans of the chest, abdomen, and pelvis can show whether or not the disease has spread to these areas. Furthermore, chromosome analysis may show certain genetic changes that are associated with leukemia. Based on this combined information, the type of leukemia and the stage of the disease are determined.

Treatments

Treatments for leukemia may include drug therapy, radiation, or bone marrow or stem cell transplant. Both drug therapy (chemotherapeutic or immunological agents) and radiation can begin to kill or slow down cancerous cells, but these treatments rarely cure leukemia. The most effective strategy for curing leukemia involves using drug and radiation therapies in combination with bone marrow transplantation. In bone marrow transplantation, normal stem cells from blood or marrow from a matched donor are injected into the patient's blood. The stem cells enter the marrow and start producing normal blood cells. In some cases, the patient's own stem cells may be used.

The goal of treatment for leukemia is to bring about a complete remission. When a patient is in complete remission, it means that there is no evidence of the disease and the patient returns to good health with normal blood and marrow cells. However, sometimes a relapse can occur, indicating a return of the cancerous cells and the return of leukemia's associated signs and symptoms.

Pathogenesis

The outcome is unpredictable and varies from patient to patient. A patient suffering from chronic lymphocytic leukemia may live with the disease for many years and die from other causes. Alternatively, some people receive many forms of therapy and die of the disease within a few years.

Prevention

In most cases, nothing can be done to prevent leukemia from occurring. Small preventive measures can be taken by avoiding exposure to environmental carcinogens and viruses that are associated with leukemia. In the case of family history, regular visits to the doctor for full physical examinations can help detect early stages of leukemia and initiate treatment.

Epidemiology

In the early part of the twenty-first century, 198,257 people in the United States were living with leukemia, and it is estimated that almost 35,000 new cases of leukemia will be diagnosed yearly in the United States. Most cases of leukemia occur in older adults; more than half of all cases occur after age 67. The most common types of leukemias in adults are acute myelogenous leukemia (AML) and chronic lymphocytic leukemia (CLL).

In children 14 years old and younger, about 35 percent of all cancers are leukemia. The most common form of leukemia in children is acute lymphocytic leukemia (ALL). Nearly 62 percent of new cases of ALL occur among children.

Incidence rates for all types of leukemia are slightly higher among males than among females; in 2005, it was estimated that males accounted for 56 percent of the new cases of leukemia. Leukemia is also more common in Americans of European descent than among those of African descent.

Rashmi Nemade

See also
- Aging, disorders of • AIDS • Anemia
- Blood disorders • Bone and joint disorders
- Cancer • Diagnosis • Down syndrome
- Genetic disorders • Hodgkin's disease
- Infections, viral • Liver and spleen disorders • Lymphoma • Thalassemia

Leukodystrophy

The word *leukodystrophy* is derived from two Greek words; *leuko*, meaning "white," referring to the white matter of the brain, and *dystrophy*, meaning "abnormal growth" or development.

Leukodystrophy refers to a group of rare genetic disorders that result in progressive degeneration of the myelin, also known as the white matter of the brain. Myelin is a protective sheath composed of protein and lipids (fatty substances) that forms layers around the nerve fibers and acts as insulation. The nerve is similar to an electrical wire. The nerve fiber (axon) that transmits the nerve impulse resembles the wire, and the myelin sheath is like the insulation around the wire. The purpose of the myelin sheath is to allow rapid and efficient transmission of impulses along the nerve cells. If the myelin is damaged, the impulses are disrupted. A decrease in impulse transmission leads to a reduction in speed of impulses and inefficient functioning of the nervous system.

Currently there are more than 30 described leukodystrophies. Some of the more common leukodystrophies include: Canavan disease, X-linked adrenoleukodystrophy (ALD), Krabbe disease, metachromatic leukodystrophy, Alexander disease, and Pelizaeus Merzbacher disease. Although the prognosis varies based on the specific diagnosis, these disorders are progressive. Additionally, a younger age of onset typically implies a worse prognosis. None of the leukodystrophies can be cured, and effective treatments are limited.

Causes and risk factors

The leukodystrophies are caused by either an abnormality in one of the protein components of myelin, or by a defective or missing enzyme that assists in the production or normal breakdown of myelin. In addition to affecting the myelin sheath, a defective protein or enzyme may affect other parts of the body. For example, the defect in X-linked ALD results in an enzyme that fails to break down a chemical in the nervous system and the adrenal glands.

There are several different genes associated with the leukodystrophies. Some of the genes are responsible for making the protein components of myelin; a defect in any of these genes may lead to leukodystrophy. There are different types of inheritance patterns, depending on the type of leukodystrophy. For exam-

ple, Krabbe disease and Canavan disease are inherited in an autosomal recessive manner (usually both parents are carriers of the gene). Adult onset autosomal dominant leukodystrophy is inherited in an autosomal dominant manner (only one parent has the defective gene). Alexander disease is also considered to be an autosomal dominant disorder. However, most reported cases are thought to be due to a spontaneous new mutation; that is, the condition was not inherited from either parent. X-linked ALD and Pelizaeus-Merzbacher disease are both inherited in an X-linked recessive manner (the mother has a defect on one of her X chromosomes); therefore, typically only boys are affected (girls may be carriers).

People who have a family history of leukodystrophy may be at an increased risk to be affected with, or have a child with, leukodystrophy. This risk is dependent upon the specific diagnosis and the mode of inheritance. For some of the leukodystrophies, ethnic background may impact an individual's risk. For example, Krabbe disease is more common in individuals of Swedish ancestry, and Canavan disease is more common in individuals of Ashkenazi Jewish ancestry. In fact, approximately 1 in 40 Ashkenazi Jews is a carrier of the autosomal recessive Canavan disease.

Symptoms

Each leukodystrophy affects a different part of the myelin sheath, causing a range of symptoms and affecting different parts of the nervous system. In general, individuals affected with a leukodystrophy may have delays or regression of mental and physical development, decreased or increased muscle tone, impaired vision or hearing, speech difficulties, a lack of coordination, and behavior problems.

The symptoms and age of onset vary considerably, both within and between the different types of leukodystrophies. For example, children with the most common form of metachromatic leukodystrophy appear normal for the first several months of life. By six months to one year of age, affected children begin having problems with skills such as walking and speech. Once symptoms are noticed, they appear to progress rapidly over a period of several months. Eventually, the affected child becomes bedridden and is unable to speak or feed independently. Seizures may develop. The child may eventually become blind and unresponsive. For example, the average life expectancy of a child with Krabbe disease is two years.

There are variants of some of the leukodystrophies that have a later age of onset and a less progressive course. For example, in adrenomyeloneuropathy, the most common form of X-linked ALD, the symptoms typically begin in the twenties. The first symptoms noted may include stiffness or clumsiness in the legs, weight loss, nausea, and generalized weakness. Other major problems may include difficulty with walking, problems with urination, sexual dysfunction, cognitive defects, and depression. The disease tends to progress slowly, and within 5 to 15 years the individual will generally need the aid of a cane or wheelchair.

Diagnosis

The diagnosis of leukodystrophy is typically suspected based on physical and neurological findings. However, in some cases, if there is a family history of the disease, the diagnosis is suspected even before the symptoms become apparent.

Magnetic resonance imaging (MRI) is used to identify any abnormalities of the white matter of the brain. Biochemical testing to look for abnormal or absent enzymes that are associated with myelin can be used to help determine the specific type of leukodystrophy. Finally, for some of the leukodystrophies, genetic testing is available to identify the specific DNA change (mutation) responsible for the diagnosis. Once a mutation has been identified in a family, carrier testing and prenatal testing are available to help determine who is at risk for these conditions.

There is significant overlap in the clinical symptoms of the various leukodystrophies, so multiple tests may be needed to reach a diagnosis. In some cases, testing cannot determine a specific cause for the symptoms or for the MRI findings.

Treatments

For most of the leukodystrophies, treatment is aimed at reducing the symptoms for the comfort and well-being of the patient. These treatments may include medications and physical, occupational, and speech therapies. Dietary management has also been suggested as a treatment for leukodystrophies. Lorenzo's oil was created by the father of a boy with X-linked ALD. However, the oil has not been clinically proven to be

STRUCTURE OF A NEURON (NERVE CELL)

There are billions of neurons in the nervous system. Their function is to receive and transmit impulses or messages to and from the dendrites of other neurons, organs, and muscles. The nerve fibers or axons are insulated by a myelin sheath, which speeds up impulses. The nodes of Ranvier, which are at even gaps along the nerve fibers, also help speed up the impulses. At the nerve ending or synapse, chemicals called transmitters help send information from cell to cell.

A neuron consists of a cell body, from which nerve fibers or dendrites project. A single long fiber, an axon, joins to the cell body; the dendrites receive impulses from other neurons, while the axon takes impulses away.

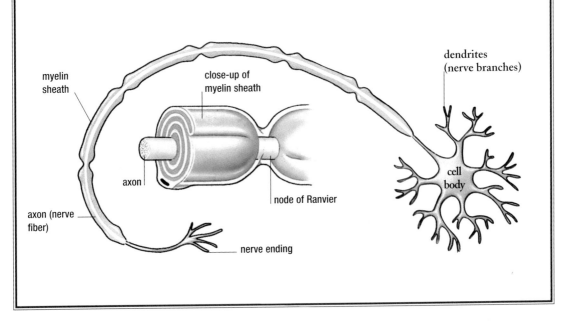

myelin sheath

close-up of myelin sheath

dendrites (nerve branches)

axon

node of Ranvier

cell body

axon (nerve fiber)

nerve ending

---

effective against the progression of the disease. Further studies are underway to determine if the oil may reduce the chances of developing symptoms if treatment is started before they begin.

Enzyme replacement therapy (ERT), in which the abnormal or decreased enzyme is replaced by normal enzyme, is problematic because of the difficulty of getting the replacement enzyme from the blood to the brain.

Bone marrow transplantation (BMT) has been successful in treating certain leukodystrophies. The best outcome is achieved if the BMT is performed before the patient develops symptoms. However, this treatment is somewhat controversial because the treatment itself has a significant risk of complications.

The use of stem cells from umbilical cord blood for transplantation has been shown to slow the course of the disease in some cases; however, the long-term outcome of individuals receiving stem cell transplantation is not known.

Additionally, research in the field of gene therapy is underway. This treatment involves inserting a "normal" gene inserted into an individual's DNA to replace an "abnormal," disease-causing gene.

Epidemiology

The incidence of leukodystrophy varies based on the specific diagnosis. For example, Canavan disease is the most common leukodystrophy and occurs among Ashkenazi Jews in about 1 in 8,000 births. X-linked ALD occurs in approximately 1 in 20,000 to 40,000 male births. Metachromatic leukodystrophy has an incidence of approximately 1 in 40,000 births, and Krabbe occurs in approximately 1 in 100,000 births.

Brian Brost

See also
- Blindness • Brain disorders • Deafness
- Genetic disorders • Multiple sclerosis
- Paralysis

Lice infestation

Lice infestations occur in every part of the world. Two genera of sucking lice, *Pediculus* and *Phthirus,* are parasitic for humans. *Pediculus humanus* var. *capitis* (head louse) and *Pediculus humanus* var. *corporis* (body louse) are similar flattened grayish insects, 2–4 millimeters in size. *Phthirus pubis* (pubic or crab louse) is round and 2–3 millimeters long.

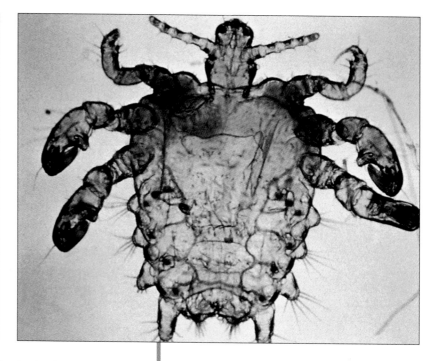

This is a greatly enlarged picture of Phthirus pubis, *the pubic or crab louse. The pubic louse is about 2 millimeters across. It is transmitted through sexual contact and infests the pubic region in adults and the eyelashes of affected children.*

Lice are small insects that live by feeding on human blood. They are wingless and spread by moving from person to person.

Pediculosis capitis

Head lice live on the scalp and can be transferred by close personal contact, as well as sharing of combs, hats, towels, and bed linen. Schoolchildren and their families are affected most often. Infestation is common, but it is not related to personal hygiene.

The adult female lays seven to ten eggs (nits) daily, which are firmly attached to the hair shaft of the scalp and occasionally to the beard. Nits hatch in one week and must feed on blood. Adult lice can survive for two days without a host. Inflammatory responses can cause intense itching of the scalp; a tickling feeling of movement and excoriations (abrasions) from scratching are additional clinical manifestations of infestation, although some children may be asymptomatic. Secondary bacterial infection and cervical lymphadenopathy (swollen glands in the neck) can occasionally occur.

The diagnosis of lice infestation is made by finding the louse or nits. Using a fine toothed nit comb is more effective than visual inspection. Nits that are attached to hairs close to the scalp indicate active infection.

Treatment with topical pediculicides (1 percent premethrin rinse, gamma benzene hexachloride shampoo, pyrethrins, and malathion) is effective in 95 percent of cases. However, resistance is emerging. Scalp application is repeated in one week because nits are more resistant to treatment than adult lice. Lindane shampoo is associated with neurotoxicity in rats and offers no advantage over other agents.

Nits should be removed by applying a solution of equal parts vinegar and water, then combing the hair with a fine-toothed comb soaked in a pediculicide. Taking oral ivermectin, 200 milligrams per kilogram of body weight as a single dose, with a repeat dose two weeks later, is an alternative to using topical agents.

The most common causes of treatment failure are lack of compliance and continued contact with infested individuals. On the other hand, "no-nit" policies in many school districts may be excessive, as many children with nits do not develop active infection.

To prevent reinfection, all clothing and bed linen must be washed in very hot water. To halt the spread of infestation, contacts of the people infected should be traced and alerted to the problem. If found to be infected, close contacts should be treated with a topical pediculicide, which is an agent that destroys lice.

Pediculosis corporis

Body lice are seen where overcrowding and poor sanitation exist, and they are a problem of homelessness and poverty. The body louse lays its nits on the seams of clothing, where they are viable for up to one month. Body lice are a vector for epidemic typhus, trench fever, and relapsing fever.

Itching is the chief complaint. Macules (patches of skin of a different color), papules (small elevations on the skin), and excoriations are seen on the trunk, often as a result of secondary bacterial infection. Generalized hyperpigmentation and thickening of the skin can occur with chronic infestation (vagabond's disease).

The patient should be bathed thoroughly. Clothing and linen should be discarded or laundered in very hot water and then ironed. A rinse of 1 percent premethrin or other pediculicide may be applied to the body if nits are found on body hair.

Phthirus pubis

The pubic (or crab) louse is transmitted by sexual or close body contact, but children can be affected by transmission of the lice from their parents. The life span of the female louse is three to four weeks, and she lays three eggs per day, which are cemented to the base of a hair and hatch after six to eight days. The pubic hair is generally infested, but armpits, chest hair, and eyebrows can also be affected by the lice.

Although some people are unaware of any symptoms, many people notice the signs of pubic lice. Sometimes they leave small spots or tiny specks of blood on the skin, and the brown eggs may also be noticed. However, the primary complaint is marked itching in the affected areas. Macules and papules may be seen but are less severe than in other forms of pediculosis. Small blue spots (maculae cerulae) are the result of injection of an anticoagulant saliva into the skin when the louse feeds. Infestation of the eyelashes causes crusting of the lids and an associated conjunctivitis.

Diagnosis is made by detection of the louse or nits. Evaluation for other sexually transmitted diseases is important, as coinfections are common.

Pubic lice can be treated with 1 percent permethrin cream rinse, 1 percent lindane shampoo, pyrethrins with piperonyl butoxide, or malathion. Ivermectin or 5 percent permethrin cream can be used for treatment

failure. It is important to treat all sexual contacts at the same time to prevent cross infection.

Bedding and clothing should be machine washed in water that is hotter than a temperature of 140°F (60°C) and dried in a hot dryer. Eyelid infestation can be treated by applying petrolatum for eight days, or by giving two doses of ivermectin one week apart.

Nigar Kirmani

KEY FACTS

Description

Infestation of the scalp (head lice), seams of clothing (body lice), or pubic hair (crab lice).

Causes

Pediculus humanus var. *capitis* (head louse), *Pediculus humanus* var. *corporis* (body louse), and *Phthirus pubis* (pubic or crab louse).

Symptoms and signs

Itching of the scalp, body, or genital area. Itching leads to macules, papules, and excoriations.

Diagnosis

Detection of the louse or nits.

Treatment

Application of topical pediculicides (1 percent premethrin rinse, pyrethrins, malathion) is used for head and pubic lice. Thorough bathing and washing of clothes and bedding is required for body lice.

Pathogenesis

The adult female lays eggs or nits, which are cemented to the hair shaft on the scalp, pubic hair, or seams of clothing. Nits hatch and must feed on blood to survive.

Prevention

Avoiding the sharing of combs and hats prevents head lice. Improved sanitation and attention to personal hygiene eliminates body lice. Avoidance of sexual or close body contact with infested individuals and treatment of sexual contacts eliminates pubic lice.

Epidemiology

Lice infestation occurs worldwide. Head lice occurs in persons from all socioeconomic backgrounds and is very frequent in school children. Overcrowding and poor personal hygiene lead to body lice. Pubic lice are transmitted by sexual or close body contact.

See also

• Environmental disorders • Immune system disorders • Infections • Infections, animal-to-human • Infections, bacterial • Infections, parasitic • Lyme disease

Listeria infection

Listeria infection is caused by bacteria that affect both animals and humans. Although there are several different strains of the bacterium, *Listeria monocytogenes* is the only strain that infects humans. It typically causes infections in patients with an impaired immune system.

Listeria monocytogenes can be found worldwide in soil and decaying vegetable matter. It also grows well at refrigeration temperatures. Because of this characteristic, many cases of infection (listeriosis) are food-borne, resulting from the ingestion of contaminated food products such as unpasteurized dairy products and undercooked or processed meats.

Listeria infection more commonly occurs in patients who have some impairment of their immune system. This includes people at extremes of age (newborns and the elderly), pregnant women (especially those in the third trimester), organ transplant recipients (especially kidney transplant), patients with human immunodeficiency virus (HIV), and those taking medications that weaken the immune system, such as corticosteroids. Less commonly, infection may occur in people with healthy immune systems.

Listeria can cause several different symptoms. If the bacterium is ingested, gastrointestinal infection (gastroenteritis) may occur and is associated with the acute onset of fevers, vomiting, abdominal pain, and diarrhea. The bacteria may also enter the bloodstream and cause infection of the central nervous system (meningitis). Patients with meningitis may experience fever, headaches, neck stiffness, confusion, and coma. The bacteria can also cause infections involving the respiratory tract, heart valves, skin, eyes, and joints.

The diagnosis of listeria infection can be made by performing cultures of infected body fluids, such as stool, blood, and cerebrospinal fluid. There are several antibiotics available for treatment, including ampicillin, penicillin, gentamicin, and trimethoprim-sulfamethoxazole. Resistance to these antibiotics is rare.

Most infections are thought to result from oral ingestion of the bacteria and invasion of the gastrointestinal tract. The organism may also gain access to the bloodstream and infect other areas of the body, such as the nervous system and lungs. Infection can occur in animals and humans and may be transmitted between the two species. This usually occurs through the accidental ingestion of foods contaminated by the feces of infected animals in areas of poor sanitation. Transmission between humans can occur similarly.

Prevention and epidemiology

There is no available vaccine to protect against listeria infection. The risk of infection can be decreased by proper hygiene, appropriate handling of food, and avoidance of foods that are likely to be contaminated, such as unpasteurized dairy products, raw meat, and other foods that may have been improperly cooked.

An estimated 2,500 cases occur annually in the United States, accounting for roughly 500 deaths. Outbreaks continue to occur and can sometimes be traced back to a causative food-borne source.

Joseph Fritz and Bernard Camins

KEY FACTS

Description
An infection that is usually food-borne.

Causes
The bacterium *Listeria monocytogenes*.

Risk factors
Eating certain foods. At risk are people with impaired immune systems: organ transplant recipients, newborns, the elderly, pregnant women, and patients on immunosuppressive drugs.

Symptoms
Most commonly infection of the gastrointestinal tract, central nervous system, and bloodstream.

Diagnosis
Growth of the bacteria from infected body fluids.

Treatment
Antibiotics.

Pathogenesis
It may lead to overwhelming infection that can be life threatening.

Prevention
Proper sanitation systems and habits; avoidance of improperly stored or undercooked foods.

Epidemiology
At least 2,500 infections and about 500 deaths yearly from listeriosis in the United States.

See also
• Food poisoning • Gastroenteritis
• Infections, bacterial • Meningitis

Liver and spleen disorders

The liver is the second largest organ in the body after the skin. It has a dual blood supply, receiving blood directly from the heart and also from the stomach and intestines. The liver plays a central role in the metabolism of fats, proteins, sugars, alcohol, and drugs, as well as in the synthesis of key blood proteins such a clotting factors and albumin. The liver is also the site of bile formation, which is secreted into the intestine and serves to help with absorption of fats and to remove potentially toxic substances from the body. The spleen is closely associated with the liver in that their blood supplies are connected. The spleen's functions are to store blood cells, destroy old red blood cells, and produce certain cells of the immune system. The spleen can be enlarged in certain liver diseases.

A careful medical history, physical examination, blood tests, and radiological tests are critical in evaluating disorders of the liver and spleen. Biopsy is sometimes necessary in diagnosing liver diseases. Many diseases can affect the liver and spleen. Excessive alcohol consumption and viruses can cause inflammation of the liver or hepatitis, which over time lead to scarring and abnormal regeneration called cirrhosis. Inherited and autoimmune diseases affect the liver. Obstruction of the bile ducts and tumors can also involve the liver. The spleen can be enlarged secondary to liver diseases, blood disorders, and types of leukemia. It sometimes has to be removed surgically if it is damaged, usually in an accident.

The liver lies in the upper right quadrant of the abdomen, mostly below the rib cage. It has a dual blood supply. The portal vein carries blood from the digestive system to the liver. For this reason, the liver acts as the first site of metabolism ("first pass" metabolism) for many nutrients, ingested drugs, and alcohol. Additionally, the liver receives blood from the hepatic artery, which delivers highly oxygenated blood directly from the heart. Blood leaves the liver via the hepatic vein, which drains into the inferior vena cava and then directly to the heart. Because the liver has a rich blood supply, liver infarction (obstruction) rarely occurs. A major branch of the portal vein is the splenic vein, which delivers blood to the spleen situated in the left upper part of the abdomen. The liver and spleen are thus connected in their blood supplies and, if blood has a difficult time passing through the liver for any reason, as most commonly occurs in cirrhosis, it can back up into the spleen, causing it to be enlarged.

The liver performs many functions that are critical for life. One cannot live without a functioning liver. Most of the liver's functions take place in the hepatocytes, the major cells. Some of the most important functions of the liver are: metabolism of fats, proteins, sugars, alcohol, drugs, environmental toxins, and some vitamins; secretion of substances, including bilirubin, into the bile; and synthesis and secretion of important proteins into the blood, including proteins involved in blood clotting and the protein albumin, the predominant protein in blood.

An important function of the liver that merits special mention is its role in the metabolism and secretion of bilirubin, a compound derived mostly from the breakdown of old red blood cells in the spleen. The liver's inability to secrete bilirubin into the bile is the most common cause of jaundice, a characteristic yellowing of the whites of the eyes and skin that can occur when the liver fails to function properly. Bilirubin must be eliminated from the body because it can be toxic, especially in babies during early brain

RELATED ARTICLES

development. In most adult-acquired liver diseases, such as cirrhosis, bilirubin accumulates in the blood mainly because it cannot be adequately secreted from the hepatocytes into the bile. In other conditions, overproduction of bilirubin, failure to efficiently chemically modify it in the liver, or inadequate uptake from the blood can lead to jaundice. Jaundice may also occur as a result of obstruction of the larger bile ducts within or outside the liver, which most often occurs as a result of gallstones or tumors.

Acute versus chronic liver disease

A important distinction when approaching a patient with liver disease is to determine if the disease is acute (of sudden onset) or chronic (long-standing). Liver diseases lasting longer than six months are considered chronic. Acute liver diseases can vary from mild to very severe. Severe acute liver failure with alteration in mental status, sometimes coma, is known as fulminant hepatic failure. There are three possible outcomes of acute liver disease: the patient dies of the acute disease or is saved by liver transplantation; the disease completely resolves; or the disease becomes chronic. The major concern about a chronic liver disease is that over time, usually many decades, it can cause cirrhosis. Cirrhosis is scarring accompanied by abnormal regeneration of liver cells. When advanced, cirrhosis can lead to an inability of the liver to carry out its metabolic, secretory, and synthetic functions. Cirrhosis can also cause blood flow through the liver to be impeded, resulting in several complications. These include varicose veins in the esophagus that can bleed extensively, abnormal fluid accumulation in the body, an enlarged spleen leading to a decrease in platelets involved in blood clotting, other abnormalities in blood clotting secondary to decreased synthesis of clotting factors, and mental status alterations known as hepatic encephalopathy. Some of these same symptoms can occur in severe acute liver disease, sometimes making it difficult for a doctor to determine if the condition is acute or chronic unless a very careful medical history is obtained.

When complications of cirrhosis do not respond to supportive medical therapy, or when the liver irreversibly fails in acute fulminant hepatic failure, liver transplantation is the only lifesaving option.

Not all patients with liver failure are candidates for liver transplantation. Evaluation for transplantation is a complex process that can only be carried out at centers where the procedure is performed. Transplantation can be from a cadaver or a piece of the liver from a living donor.

Evaluation of liver and spleen disorders

As with any medical condition, careful history and physical examination are the initial steps in evaluating a patient with suspected disease of the liver or spleen. Some symptoms and signs of liver disease include jaundice, abdominal swelling or swelling in the feet and ankles secondary to fluid retention, and easy bruising. Sometimes the spleen can be enlarged secondary to liver disease, but it can also be enlarged in other conditions.

Blood tests are important in the evaluation of a patient with liver or spleen disorders. The complete blood count may particularly show a decrease in platelets, or small blood cells involved in clotting, if the spleen is enlarged. Measuring the blood bilirubin concentration, albumin concentration, and prothrombin time (a test of blood clotting) can give clues as to how the liver is functioning. While none of these tests are specific for liver dysfunction, elevations in the blood bilirubin concentration, decreases in albumin concentration, and prolongation in the prothrombin time may occur when the liver is not functioning properly. Tests for the activities (a biochemical term roughly proportional to amounts) of certain enzymes in the blood, which are normally present in hepatocytes or bile duct cells, are also important in assessing the patient with liver disease. These blood enzyme activity tests are often erroneously referred to as "liver function tests." While these liver enzyme tests in fact do not tell anything about liver function, abnormal elevations suggest inflammation of the liver, liver cell destruction, or problems in bile flow. Many special blood tests are also used to help diagnose specific liver diseases.

Radiological tests are important for the evaluation of some patients with liver or spleen diseases. Tests such as ultrasound or computed tomography scans are used for assessing the size of the liver and spleen and for detecting the presence of tumors, some problems with blood flow, and bile duct obstruction. Scans do

LIVER AND SPLEEN STRUCTURE

The liver is the largest internal organ. The falciform ligament divides the liver into two lobes; the right lobe is larger than the left lobe. Each lobe has thousands of lobules, which contain cells that enable the liver to carry out its functions. The liver takes part in digestion; it secretes bile, which is stored in the gallbladder until required. The liver stores nutrients and releases them when they are needed; it also breaks down toxins, such as alcohol, so that they are less harmful to the body. The spleen, which is located in the top left part of the abdomen, removes damaged red blood cells and produces antibodies.

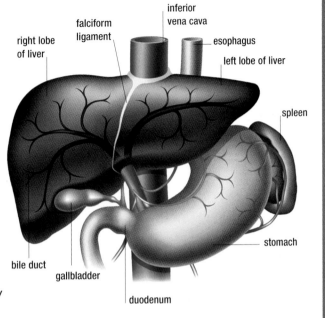

Breakdown products of blood waste and dietary fat drain out of the liver as bile.

not, however, provide information about liver function or the degree of liver inflammation or the presence of scar tissue. Radiological tests cannot always diagnose cirrhosis unless the liver is significantly damaged and shrunken.

Sometimes, biopsy is essential in the diagnosis of liver disease, especially chronic ones. Besides making or confirming a diagnosis, it is often the only way to assess the degree of inflammation and scar tissue in the liver. Liver biopsy is usually an outpatient procedure performed by sticking a small needle through the skin and into the liver and extracting a piece of tissue to examine under the microscope. It can also be performed in other ways, including a surgical procedure.

Alcoholic liver disease

Perhaps the function of the liver best known is its role in metabolizing alcohol. Most people also know that excessive alcohol consumption can lead to liver disease. However, the quantity of alcohol that an individual may drink before developing liver disease varies greatly from one person to another. In fact, most individuals who drink excessive quantities of

alcohol do not develop significant liver disease; however, it is not possible to predict those who will.

Excessive alcohol consumption can cause three different pathological conditions in the liver. However, there can be overlap, and more than one can be present at the same time. The first, and most benign, is fat accumulation in hepatocytes. This condition, known as fatty liver, will go away if the person stops drinking. The second is hepatitis or inflammation of the liver, which, when caused by alcohol, is called alcoholic hepatitis. Alcoholic hepatitis can vary from a fairly mild condition to a severe and life-threatening disease. It is also reversible if the patient abstains from drinking. Of note, fatty liver and a type of mild inflammation resembling alcoholic hepatitis, known as nonalcoholic steatohepatitis, can occur in individuals who do not drink extensively but are obese, are diabetic, or both. Finally, excessive alcohol consumption over long periods of time, generally decades, can lead to cirrhosis. In addition to affecting the liver, excessive alcohol consumption can cause many other medical problems. While various measures may be taken to relieve symptoms, the only definitive treatment of alcoholic liver disease is abstaining from alcohol. In addition to alcohol, many other drugs, including those prescribed by doctors to treat various conditions, can potentially cause liver damage, often only infrequently and in an unpredictable fashion.

Viral hepatitis

Infection by certain viruses can cause hepatitis. There are five major viruses that cause hepatitis: hepatitis A virus, hepatitis B virus, hepatitis C virus, hepatitis D virus, and hepatitis E virus. Hepatitis A and E viruses are transmitted primarily by contaminated food and water and cause only acute hepatitis, which usually resolves spontaneously but rarely can kill the patient or require emergent liver transplantation for survival. Hepatitis B and C virus infection cause either acute or chronic liver disease. They are transmitted by blood and blood products and, especially hepatitis B virus, by sex and from mother to infant. There are various treatments, including interferon-alpha, for chronic hepatitis B virus infection and hepatitis C virus infection that are successful in some cases. Hepatitis D virus can only infect patients who are also infected with the hepatitis B virus, as the presence of hepatitis B virus is needed for replication. There are effective vaccines to prevent hepatitis B and hepatitis A virus infections. Notably, there is no vaccine currently available to prevent infection with the hepatitis C virus.

Inherited diseases and the liver

The most common inherited disease that affects the liver is primary hemochromatosis, a disorder of iron metabolism. In hereditary hemochromatosis, high levels of iron accumulate in the liver, which can lead to cirrhosis. The abnormal iron accumulation can also cause diabetes, pituitary damage, and arthritis. Wilson disease is a rare genetic disorder of copper metabolism that can also lead to liver damage, as well as brain damage. The liver can also be affected by many other inherited diseases not covered in this article.

Autoimmune diseases

Autoimmune diseases are those in which the body's immune system abnormally attacks its own organs. Three liver diseases are thought to be of autoimmune etiology: primary biliary cirrhosis; primary sclerosing cholangitis; and autoimmune hepatitis. Primary biliary cirrhosis occurs 90 percent of the time in women and is characterized by inflammatory destruction of the small bile ducts within the liver that progresses slowly to cirrhosis. Primary sclerosing cholangitis occurs more commonly in men and is characterized by inflammation and scarring in the larger bile ducts within or outside the liver. Most patients also have ulcerative colitis, an inflammatory disease of the large intestine. Autoimmune hepatitis is inflammation attacking the hepatocytes and occurs more frequently in women. Autoimmune hepatitis can respond to treatment with immunosuppressive drugs such as corticosteroids.

Other liver diseases

Many other diseases can affect the liver; an exhaustive list is beyond the scope of this article. Importantly, bile ducts obstruction as a result of gallstones or tumors can cause liver damage and, if long-standing, cirrhosis. Obstruction of the bile ducts may have to be evaluated by radiological procedures, and sometimes by a procedure known as endoscopic retrograde cholangiopancreatography (ERCP), in which a tube is passed into the common bile duct and dye directly injected to take high-resolution X-ray images. The liver can also be infiltrated with tumors or bacterial infections such as tuberculosis. Tumors, both benign and malignant, can also arise in the liver. Primary hepatocyte cancer, known as hepatocellular carcinoma, most often occurs in subjects who have cirrhosis. Some specific liver diseases only affect certain individuals, such as pregnant women and newborn infants.

Disorders of the spleen

As discussed above, the spleen can often be enlarged secondary to liver disease, most often cirrhosis. Enlargement of the spleen can lead to a low platelet count and bleeding tendencies. There are disorders of the blood that may involve the spleen, and sometimes it is enlarged in lymphomas or leukemia.

A person can live without a spleen. Sometimes it is removed surgically because of irreparable damage, usually in accidental trauma. People who do not have a spleen are at increased risk for some types of bacterial infections but generally do well.

Howard J. Worman

Liver fluke

Liver flukes are flatworms that have a specific tendency to affect the liver and biliary system in mammals. The three major liver flukes that infect humans are oriental liver flukes (*Clonorchis sinensis, Opisthorchis species*), and *Fasciola hepatica*. In addition, *Metorchis conjunctus* is common in North America in raw, infected fish. These four liver flukes will be discussed here.

L iver flukes are flat and leaf-shaped, and measure a few millimeters (oriental liver flukes) or several centimeters (*Fasciola*). Each worm has both male and female sexual organs. They reproduce sexually in mammalian hosts, and asexually in freshwater. The adult liver flukes live in the biliary tract of mammals and produce minute eggs which pass out with bile into the feces. If these feces contaminate freshwater, the portion of the fluke's life cycle that occurs in water begins. The eggs hatch into first-stage larvae either before or after ingestion by specific snail species. They multiply within snails and develop into second-stage larvae. After development within the snail, which may take up to seven weeks, the mature larvae are released into surrounding freshwater. In case of *Fasciola*, they attach to various kinds of aquatic plants, and in the case of oriental liver flukes and Metorchis, they penetrate under the scales of certain freshwater fish and enter the muscle layers. These larvae develop cysts around them and are known as metacercariae. When fish-eating mammals such as dogs, cats, and occasionally humans eat the infested fish, the parasites enter the small intestine and travel to the liver through the biliary tract. Similar infestation occurs with *Fasciola* when herbivores (such as sheep and cattle) or humans eat the infested aquatic plants. Adult *Fasciola* worms live in human beings for up to 13 years, while the oriental liver flukes may live up to 30 years. The life span of adult worms of *Metorchis* in humans is unknown.

Symptoms and signs

Most people that are infected with liver flukes do not develop any symptoms. When the larvae travel from the small intestine to the liver through the bile ducts, symptoms such as fever, abdominal pain, jaundice, body aches, and itching may occur, along with painful enlargement of the liver. Even in heavily infected indi-

KEY FACTS

Description

Local or systemic infection. Not communicable. Acute or chronic and progressive.

Causes

Eating infected freshwater fish (*Clonorchis* and *Metorchis*) or eating infected aquatic vegetables such as watercress, alfalfa sprouts, or parsley (*Fasciola*).

Risk factors

Living in places with poor sanitation, especially sheep and cattle-raising areas (*Fasciola*); eating raw or inadequately cooked fish, such as sushi (for the other flukes).

Symptoms and signs

Mainly asymptomatic. Acute illness with fever, acute abdominal pain, enlarged liver. Cough, chest pain, and pleural effusion may occur. Chronic illness with abdominal pain and jaundice.

Diagnosis

Stool examination for eggs. Identifying adult worms on surgery or ERCP (endoscopic retrograde cholangiopancreatography). Ultrasound, CT, or MRI may identify masses of adult worms as well as dilatation and stricture of bile ducts. Serologic tests for fascioliasis.

Treatments

Antiparasitic drugs such as Praziquantel or albendazole for oriental liver flukes and *Metorchis*. Triclabendazole or Bithionol for *Fasciola*. Rarely, surgery is needed to remove the worms and relieve obstruction.

Pathogenesis

Larvae in contaminated food or water enter the small intestine and travel to the bile ducts. They mature into adult worms in four weeks and cause tissue damage and scarring in the liver. The adult worms may cause partial or complete blockage or inflammation, or both, and scarring of bile and pancreatic ducts, causing clinical symptoms.

Prevention

Boiling or purifying drinking water, avoiding raw or undercooked fish or salads made from fresh aquatic plants, and control or eradication of the snails in areas known to have disease due to liver flukes. There is no vaccine. Cooking or freezing fish kills the parasites.

Epidemiology

Fasciola occurs worldwide. *Metorchis* is common in Canada and the U.S. *Clonorchis* and *Opisthorchis* are common in the Far East, Southeast Asia, and Russia. In the U.S., *Clonorchis* may occur in those who eat raw imported fish.

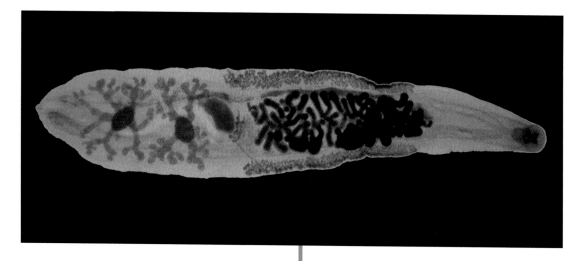

viduals, symptoms occur in only about 10 percent. Chronic disease may occur even up to 30 years after ingestion of contaminated food or water. *Metorchis* is an exception, as it is not known whether it causes chronic infection.

The symptoms and signs are due to injury, irritation, inflammation, and physical obstruction of the bile ducts by the adult flukes. Obstructive jaundice, liver abscess, pancreatitis, recurrent cholangitis, and cholecystitis may occur. Gallstones may develop.

The amount of liver damage is dependent on the number of parasites ingested. If the worms reach other organs like the lungs, heart, and the brain by accident, symptoms and signs related to the affected organs occur.

Diagnosis and treatments

Stool examination may reveal eggs that are typical. These patients often have increased eosinophils in blood as well as impaired liver function tests. Imaging such as ultrasound, computed tomography, or magnetic resonance imaging scans of the liver may show the adult worms as masses, gallstones, and areas of blockage and destruction in the liver and bile ducts. If ERCP is done, it may be possible to see or remove the adult worms from the bile ducts. Tests such as enzyme immunoassay or immunoblot assay in the serum can detect antibodies to *Fasciola*. Liver biopsy is rarely necessary.

Treatment with anti-parasitic drugs mostly results in complete cure. Praziquantel and albendazole are the first-line drugs for infection with oriental liver flukes and *Metorchis*. Triclabendazole, bithional, and nitazoxanide are effective against *Fasciola* infection. In acute severe illness, a short course of steroids may be given in addition to specific antiparasitic therapy. The prog-

nosis is good with light infections, but death occasionally occurs in long-standing heavy infections that are associated with complications. Patients with obstructive jaundice may require surgery aimed at relief of symptoms.

Antibiotics may also be needed to treat complications resulting from bacterial infections. When a diagnosis of fascioliasis is made in one member of a family, other family members at risk should also be evaluated. Asymptomatic cases should be treated to avoid the risk of future complications.

Epidemiology

About 7 million people are infected worldwide with *Clonorchis sinensis*. *Fasciola* has a worldwide distribution with an estimated 2.4 million infected people, in more than 60 countries. *Metorchis* is known to cause outbreaks in Canada and the United States. Surveys in the United States have suggested that up to 26 percent of Southeast Asian immigrants have an active liver fluke infection. Those who have never traveled to places with fluke infections can acquire infection by eating food imported from those places.

Pranavi Sreeramoju

Lou Gehrig's disease

Lou Gehrig's disease is an incurable, debilitating disease in which the nerve cells that control muscular movement die, leading to weakness, wasting and rigidity of muscles, and paralysis. The cause of Lou Gehrig's disease is unknown. One form of the disease is linked to a gene mutation that runs in families.

Lou Gehrig's disease (a type of motor neuron disease), also called amyotrophic lateral sclerosis, is named after the U.S. baseball player who died from the disease. *Amyotrophic* simply means that there is no muscle growth, *lateral* refers to the position in the spinal cord of nerve cells called motor neurons, and *sclerosis* indicates the hardening of tissues that results from cell death. Motor neurons normally control muscle activity. Lower motor neurons, which are found in the spinal cord, directly activate muscles; upper motor neurons, which occur in the front part of the brain, regulate the activity of spinal motor neurons and indirectly influence muscle function. In Lou Gehrig's disease, both types of motor neurons die, and the related muscles stop functioning and waste away.

Symptoms

The onset of Lou Gehrig's disease is gradual, and symptoms, which appear over months, are variable. In the early stages, a person may experience fatigue, muscle twitching, weakness of limb muscles, slurred speech, difficulty swallowing, or uncontrolled laughing and crying. Later symptoms include increasing weakness, rigidity, and wasting of muscles, followed by paralysis. Breathing difficulties can occur if the muscles that control respiration are affected. Some people deteriorate rapidly; in others, there is a spontaneous slowing, or arrest, of the disease. Lou Gehrig's disease does not usually affect the senses or mental faculties. Respiratory arrest or pneumonia are often the cause of death.

Diagnosis

There is no specific test; diagnosis involves tests to rule out other diseases. Comprehensive neurological exams are followed by electromyography, X-rays and MRIs (magnetic resonance imaging) of the brain and spinal cord, nerve conduction tests, testing of blood, urine, and hormones, and muscle and nerve biopsies.

Treatments and epidemiology

There is no cure for Lou Gehrig's disease. The only FDA-approved drug for treating the disease is Rilutek, which slightly slows the progression of the disease. Other drugs, including growth factors to stimulate cell formation, are currently being tested, as are stem cells and gene therapy. Research into genetic factors is underway. Lou Gehrig's disease is diagnosed in 5,600 Americans annually; 93 percent of those affected are of Caucasian origin.

Sonal Jhaveri

KEY FACTS

Description

Also called amyotrophic lateral sclerosis (ALS). The disease causes progressive muscle wasting and paralysis.

Causes

Unknown.

Risk factors

More likely to affect people above the age of 50, particularly men.

Symptoms

Rigidity, twitching, and weakness in limb muscles; slurred speech; tripping; fatigue; difficulty swallowing; trouble with daily activities; progressive paralysis.

Diagnosis

Tests include: neurological exams, electromyography, measuring nerve conduction, spine imaging, nerve and muscle biopsy, spinal tap, and tests of blood, urine, and hormones.

Treatments

Drug treatment with Rilutek provides some relief and slows the progression of the disease.

Pathogenesis

Ongoing degeneration of nerve cells.

Prevention

None. Genetic counseling is offered when Lou Gehrig's disease runs in families.

Epidemiology

About 30,000 people are affected in the United States, of whom 5–10 percent have a genetic form of the disease. Lou Gehrig's disease is 1½ times more common in men than in women.

See also
- Disabilities • Motor neuron disease
- Nervous system disorders • Spinal disorders

Lupus

Lupus is a chronic, complex systemic autoimmune disease that primarily affects young women of all ethnic backgrounds. The signs and symptoms of the disease are highly variable and can affect virtually any organ or tissue in the body. No two cases of lupus are alike, and the pattern of symptoms can change over time in a single individual. About 1 to 4 in every 1,000 women are affected by lupus; rates of the disease are about 10 times lower for men.

The immune system has evolved to eliminate infectious organisms, infected cells, and other abnormal cells from the body by first recognizing the unwanted substances as "foreign" to the body, then mounting an inflammatory attack to destroy the foreign cells. For reasons that remain unknown, the immune system in lupus patients begins to recognize normal, healthy cells and tissues as "foreign" and mounts an immune response against them. It is currently believed that lupus patients inherit genetic predisposition (probably a combination of multiple genes) toward developing the disease, but then another stimulus, likely environmental, triggers the onset of the disease itself. The influence of heredity can be seen in identical twin studies; the risk of developing lupus in an identical twin of an affected patient is nearly 50 percent. However, most cases of lupus occur in people without a family history of the disease. Some possible environmental triggers may include certain viruses like Epstein-Barr infection (which causes mononucleosis) and sunlight. Sex hormones have also been considered as a trigger; however, the exact causes of lupus remain unknown.

Symptoms and signs

Because lupus can affect almost any organ or tissue in the body, there are numerous symptoms that can be present, and these may change over time. Symptoms are generally the result of an inflammatory attack of the tissues. They may range from mild and barely noticeable to severe permanent organ damage or death. The most commonly affected tissues include the skin, joints, blood vessels, blood cells, and lining around the heart and lungs. Patients often experience rashes across the bridge of the nose, extreme sensitivity to the

sun, sores in the mouth, hair loss, and swelling in the joints. Chest pain when breathing deeply and a sensation of shortness of breath may occur if there is inflammation of the lining of the heart or lungs. In more severe cases, the immune response will be directed against the kidneys. Early symptoms may include swelling of the lower legs, headaches, and high blood pressure. When lupus is in remission or is mildly active, there may be no symptoms at all. Physicians rou-

KEY FACTS

Description

A chronic noninfectious autoimmune disease, in which the immune system attacks any variety of organs and tissues in the body.

Causes

Unknown.

Risk factors

Female gender, pregnancy, family members with lupus, and unknown environmental exposures (viruses, sunlight, and hormones).

Symptoms and signs

Rashes on the face and body, hair loss, swollen joints, and sores in the mouth.

Diagnosis

Examination by a specialist in rheumatology; careful assessment of symptoms and blood tests. The diagnosis can take many months to confirm.

Treatments

Many different medications that suppress the immune system can be used, depending on the organs involved.

Pathogenesis

Lupus is characterized by flare-ups and remissions and can range from very mild to more severe. Kidneys are the most common major organ to be affected. Before good treatments were available, kidney failure was very common.

Prevention

No known strategies to prevent the onset of lupus, but flares can be minimized by avoiding direct sun exposure, refraining from smoking, and taking medications as prescribed.

Epidemiology

Prevalence estimates range from 50 to 150 in 100,000 adults. Women are affected nine times more commonly than men. The most common ages at diagnosis are between 15 and 45. About 20 percent of lupus cases are diagnosed before the age of 20.

tinely check blood and urine tests in asymptomatic patients to detect and treat any indications of lupus activity before symptoms become apparent.

Diagnosis

There is no single test that can make a diagnosis of lupus. Experienced physicians rely on a series of 11 criteria, four of which must be present currently or in the past to make the diagnosis. The majority of these criteria are physical symptoms, and only a few are based solely upon laboratory tests. The most frequent screening test for lupus is the antinuclear antibody (ANA) level. This test detects the presence of antibodies (proteins that mark abnormal cells or particles as foreign and subject to attack) in the blood.

Although most people with lupus will have elevated ANA levels, a positive ANA test can be seen in numerous other diseases and in up to 10 percent of healthy people. Because many of the early symptoms can be vague (fatigue, fevers, and joint pains), a definitive diagnosis of lupus may take many months to years as specific signs and symptoms accrue. Additionally, other conditions that can cause similar symptoms, including thyroid problems, anemia, and infections, must be evaluated.

Treatments and prevention

There is no known cure for lupus. The goals of treatment are to relieve symptoms, prevent organ damage, and to restore normal functioning. Treatment for lupus is as varied as its symptoms. The majority of medications used to treat active lupus are immunosuppressive medications that reduce the overall immune system in the body. Steroids (like prednisone) are among the most common medications used to treat lupus, and the doses may range from very low (5 milligrams daily) to much higher (60 milligrams daily), depending on the severity of the lupus. Many lupus medications are the same as ones used after organ transplantation and those used to treat certain cancers.

Doses and types of medications are commonly adjusted depending on the degree of disease activity and the presence of side effects. Treating active inflammation must always be balanced against the risk of potential side effects from medicines, including weight gain, hair loss, abdominal pain, and diarrhea. Among the most serious potential side effect from lupus medications is the increased susceptibility to infections caused by suppressing the immune system. Other side effects of medications—and of lupus itself—are fatigue, depression, and change in physical appearance.

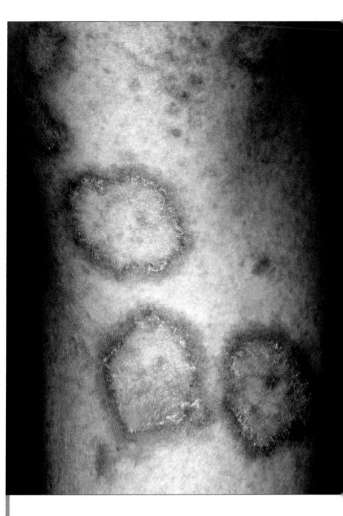

This blotchy red rash on a patient's leg is typical of lupus. It is caused by the immune system attacking connective tissue in the skin and producing inflammation.

These must all be addressed when caring for lupus patients. Another goal of treatment is the prevention of flare-ups. Although it cannot be predicted when flare-ups are going to occur, several factors have been shown to reduce the incidence of and severity of flare-ups, including regular use of sunscreen and sun-protective clothing (even when it is cloudy), adequate sleep, abstention from smoking, taking medications as instructed, and delaying pregnancy until the disease is in remission (quiet).

Eliza Chakravarty

See also
• Anemia • Epstein-Barr infection
• Immune system disorders • Kidney disorders • Pleurisy

Lyme disease

An inflammatory disease caused by the bacterium *Borrelia burgdorferi*, Lyme disease is transmitted to animals and humans through the bite of an infected tick. Lyme disease is the most common tick-borne disease in the United States.

Lyme disease was first reported in the United States in the town of Old Lyme, Connecticut, in 1975 and now is reported throughout the United States. Most cases occur in the Northeast (in the states of New York, Massachusetts, Connecticut, Rhode Island, and New Jersey), in the upper Midwest, and along the Pacific Coast. Lyme disease is also found in Europe, China, Japan, Australia, and across the former Soviet Union. There are more than 16,000 cases of Lyme disease each year in the United States.

Causes and risk factors

There are several types of ticks that cause Lyme disease: in the Northeast and Midwest, the deer tick (*Ixodes Dammini*); in the South, the black-legged tick (*Ixodes scapularis*); in the West, *Ixodes pacificus*, the Western black-legged tick. The lone star tick, or *Amblyomma americanum*, is found in several regions.

Risk factors include walking in high grass and heavily wooded areas in the spring, summer, and early fall; wearing shorts and short-sleeved tops; and having a pet that can carry ticks home.

Symptoms

In about 90 percent of cases of Lyme disease there is a characteristic red rash, called erythema migrans, usually occurring at the site of the bite within a few days to weeks, which generally looks like an expanding red ring with alternating light and dark rings. At the same time, flulike symptoms may appear with headache, sore throat, fever, muscle aches, stiff neck, fatigue, and general malaise. Some individuals develop the flulike symptoms without a rash. There may also be a flat or slightly raised lesion at the site of the bite.

If ignored, early symptoms of the disease disappear but are followed in months to years by the more serious complications of joint inflammation (arthritis), neurological symptoms, and sometimes heart, eye, respiratory, and gastrointestinal problems, which may be chronic or intermittent.

Diagnosis, treatments, and prevention

Diagnosis can be difficult because the symptoms can mimic other diseases, and the rash can be confused with that from poison ivy, spider or insect bites, or ringworm. If Lyme disease is suspected, a blood test may confirm the diagnosis, although it is not conclusive. Treated early, the disease can be cured with antibiotics. Recent studies suggest that a single dose of the antibiotic doxycycline after a tick bite can prevent the disease. If the disease remains untreated and complications develop, anti-inflammatory drugs may relieve joint pain and stiffness. Intravenous drugs may be used to treat persistent arthritis or severe heart or neurological symptoms that do not respond to oral antibiotics. For those in tick-infested areas, a vaccine is available that can prevent infection. Other preventive measures include clothing that covers the limbs, light clothing so ticks can easily be seen and removed, and repeated inspection of the body for ticks.

Isaac Grate

KEY FACTS

Description
Inflammatory disease caused by *Borrelia burgdorferi*.

Cause
A bite from an infected tick.

Risk factors
Walking in high grass and heavily wooded areas infected with ticks in spring, summer, and early fall; wearing shorts or short-sleeved tops outdoors.

Diagnosis
Characteristic rash; blood test.

Treatments
Oral antibiotics.

Pathogenesis
A bite from an infected tick releases bacteria into the bloodstream that spread throughout the body; if untreated, symptoms can develop years later.

Prevention
A vaccine helps prevent infection; keeping arms and legs covered; removal of ticks from the skin.

Epidemiology
The most common tick-borne infection in the United States; more than 16,000 cases each year.

See also

Arthritis • Infections, animal-to-human • Infections, bacterial

Lymphoma

Lymphoma is a general term for a group of cancers originating in lymphatic tissues. According to the Leukemia and Lymphoma Society, 56 percent of blood cancers diagnosed are lymphomas. Lymphomas are classified as Hodgkin's lymphoma, also known as Hodgkin's disease, and non-Hodgkin's lymphoma.

The main difference between Hodgkin's lymphoma and non-Hodgkin's lymphoma is the type of white cells involved in the cancer development. Under a microscope, the appearances of abnormal white cells in Hodgkin's lymphoma and non-Hodgkin's lymphoma are different, so doctors can differentiate the two types of diseases and make treatment plans accordingly. This article mainly focuses on non-Hodgkin's lymphoma. For information on Hodgkin's lymphoma, see Hodgkin's disease.

Causes and risk factors

The exact causes of non-Hodgkin's lymphoma are unknown. Possible risk factors for non-Hodgkin's disease, which might increase the chances of developing the disease, include age, sex, weakened immune system, genetics, and environmental factors.

The chance of developing non-Hodgkin's lymphoma increases as people get older, and the disease occurs more often in men, especially white men, than women. According to the American Cancer Society (ACS), in the United States about 58,870 people were diagnosed with non-Hodgkin's lymphoma in 2006; among those people, 30,680 were men and 28,190 were women.

Diseases or infections that weaken the immune system increase the incidence rates of non-Hodgkin's disease. Infection with HIV is a common cause of immune system deficiency and is a risk factor of developing certain types of non-Hodgkin's lymphoma. Infection with human T-cell leukemia or lymphoma virus (HTLV-1) is a risk factor of developing certain types of T-cell non-Hodgkin's lymphoma. According to the ACS, HTLV-1, like HIV, spreads through sexual intercourse and contaminated blood supply and can also be passed on to children through breast-feeding.

According to the ACS, some genetic diseases can cause children to be born with a deficient immune sys-

KEY FACTS

Description

A type of cancer that originates in lymphoid tissues.

Causes

The exact causes are unknown.

Risk factors

Age, sex, weakened immune system, genetics, and environmental factors.

Symptoms

Painless swelling in the lymph nodes, fever, night sweats, weight loss for unknown reason, tiredness, itchy skin or skin rash.

Diagnosis

Physical examination, blood test, biopsy, X-ray, and computed tomography (CT) scan.

Treatments

Radiation therapy, chemotherapy, biological therapy, and watchful waiting.

Pathogenesis

Lymphoma can spread to other parts of the body.

Prevention

Difficult to prevent the disease.

Epidemiology

Non-Hodgkin's disease affects men more than women. White people are more at risk of the disease than black people. In the U.S., however, black people between mid-20s and late 40s have higher risk of contracting non-Hodgkin's disease.

tem that could increase the risk of developing non-Hodgkin's disease. Environmental risk factors for the disease include radiation and chemicals. Studies have suggested that chemicals such as benzene and insecticides could increase the incidence rates of non-Hodgkin's lymphoma. Confirmational studies are still ongoing. According to the National Cancer Institute (NCI), taking immunosuppressant drugs, having a diet high in animal fat, and a previous treatment of Hodgkin's lymphoma can also increase the risk of developing non-Hodgkin's lymphoma.

Diagnosis and staging

Physical exam is generally the first step of the diagnosis of non-Hodgkin's lymphoma. Because other types of disease can also produce the same signs or symptoms as non-Hodgkin's lymphoma, further diagnosic methods, including imaging and biopsy, are used to confirm the disease. Imaging techniques such as computed tomography (CT), magnetic resonance imaging (MRI), or positron emission tomography (PET) scans are often used to look for enlarged lymph nodes; biopsy is often used to confirm non-Hodgkin's lymphoma. A small part of an enlarged lymph node or a small amount of tissue from the tumor is removed. The biopsy is examined and the type of non-Hodgkin's lymphoma is diagnosed. Once non-Hodgkin's lymphoma is diagnosed, further tests are needed to determine the stage of the disease. Common tests for staging the disease include further physical exam, blood test, imaging test, and sometimes bone marrow aspiration and lumbar puncture. Non-Hodgkin's lymphoma is generally classified into four stages according to the Ann Arbor staging system. In stage I, the lymphoma is found only in one lymph node or a few nodes in only one region. In stage II, the cancer extends from a single lymph node or a group of lymph nodes in one region to lymph nodes in other areas on the same side of the diaphragm. In stage III, the cancer may have extended to both sides of the diaphragm and even the nearby organs or spleen. In stage IV, the cancer has spread outside the lymph system. Depending on how fast the cancers grow and the locations of the affected lymph nodes, non-Hodgkin's lymphomas can also be classified into indolent lymphomas, aggressive lymphomas, contiguous lymphomas, and noncontiguous lymphomas. Indolent lymphomas tend to grow and spread slowly; aggressive lymphomas grow and spread very rapidly. Patients with aggressive lymphomas often have more severe symptoms than patients with indolent lymphomas. In contiguous lymphomas, the affected lymph nodes are next to each other, whereas in noncontiguous lymphomas, the lymph nodes with cancer cells are not.

Treatments

Depending on the type of lymphoma, the stage of the disease, age, and the general health condition of patients, different types of treatment can be used. Radiation therapy, chemotherapy, biological therapy, and watchful waiting are currently the four standard treatment options for non-Hodgkin's lymphoma. Unlike other kinds of cancer, surgery is rarely used as a therapeutic option for non-Hodgkin's lymphoma.

Radiation therapy uses high energy X-rays to kill cancer cells. Depending on whether the source of the X-rays is outside or inside the body, radiation therapy is referred to as external therapy and internal therapy. For external therapy, a machine outside the body pro-

duces high energy X-rays toward the area containing cancer cells. For internal radiation therapy, a radioactive seed, such as a wire or needle, is inserted into the affected area to directly kill the cancer cells. Chemotherapy uses chemical drugs to stop the growth of cancer cells, by killing the cells directly or preventing them from dividing. Chemotherapy is often classified into systemic chemotherapy and local chemotherapy, depending on whether the drug travels through the bloodstream or is placed in the affected area. Radiation therapy and chemotherapy are the most common treatments for non-Hodgkin's lymphoma, and they can be given alone or combined.

Biological therapy, also known as immunotherapy, uses materials made either by the body or in a laboratory to stimulate the body's immune system to fight the disease. Watchful waiting is closely monitoring the patient without giving any treatment and it is normally used at an early stage of non-Hodgkin's lymphoma or indolent lymphoma before symptoms appear.

The goal of surgery is to remove confined lymphoma tissues. Unlike chemotherapy and radiation therapy, surgery is rarely used as a therapeutic option for the treatment of non-Hodgkin's lymphoma. It is only used to remove confined cancer tissues unrelated to the lymph nodes, such as stomach tissues.

For some patients, especially those in whom non-Hodgkin's lymphoma has recurred, bone marrow transplantation may also be an option. This treatment provides the patients with stem cells, which are healthy immature cells that produce blood cells, to replace cells damaged during radiation therapy or chemotherapy. In addition to these treatments, new types of treatment for non-Hodgkin's disease, including vaccine therapy and high-dose chemotherapy with stem cell transplant, are currently testing in clinical studies.

Because the causes of non-Hodgkin's lymphoma are unknown and certain risk factors of the disease, including age and sex, cannot be avoided, it is difficult to prevent the disease.

Epidemiology

Around 67,000 people in the United States were diagnosed with lymphoma in 2006. Of these, about 8,000 cases were Hodgkin's lymphoma.

Y. Wang

See also
• AIDS • Cancer • Genetic disorders
• Hodgkin's disease • Immune system disorders

Macular degeneration

Macular degeneration is the breakdown or deterioration of the macula, the small, central area in the retina responsible for fine detail in the central vision. Damage to the macula may cause distorted or blurry vision, eventually leading to blank spots and severe vision loss. However, because macular degeneration affects only central vision, peripheral vision is retained, and the condition does not result in total blindness.

The most common form of macular degeneration is age-related macular degeneration (AMD). AMD occurs in two types: dry (atrophic) and wet (exudative). Dry AMD is much more common than wet AMD; it accounts for more than 85 percent of patients with AMD. Dry AMD is caused by the body's natural aging process and slow deterioration of macular tissue, resulting in a gradual loss of vision. Wet AMD is caused by the development of abnormal blood vessels under the retina, which leak blood and fluid, causing the central vision to blur. In wet AMD, vision loss occurs very rapidly.

Risk factors

Age and a family history of macular degeneration are the primary risk factors for developing macular degeneration. Other factors include smoking, obesity, and race (Caucasians have a greater chance of developing macular degeneration), sex (women are more likely to develop the condition), and low nutrient levels. Macular degeneration usually develops gradually and without pain. With dry AMD, early symptoms may include blurriness and the need for greater light. Gradually, a blind spot may begin to develop in the center of the field of vision. In wet AMD, early symptoms generally include a distortion of vision, such as lines appearing wavy or crooked and objects appearing closer or farther away than they should. The symptoms then progress rapidly and involve central vision loss.

Treatments

No treatments are available to reverse dry AMD. Wet AMD has no cure, but treatments are available to slow or possibly stop vision loss. Laser surgery is one option, in which a laser is used to slow or stop the blood vessels that are damaging the macula. Another option is photodynamic therapy, in which a cold laser is used with a drug, verteporfin, to seal off leaky blood vessels. Other emerging treatments are available, including anti-VEGF (vascular endothelial growth factor) therapy, in which drugs injected into the eye target proteins that induce abnormal growth and leakage of blood vessels, and angiostatic therapy, in which a steroid that stops growth of abnormal blood vessels is delivered into the back of the eye. Recent studies show that consumption of omega-3 fatty acids, such as are found in salmon and other fish, reduces the risk of developing AMD.

The number of people over the age of 60 is predicted by the United Nations to grow from 688 million in 2006 to 2 billion in 2050, so people suffering from macular degeneration is also expected to rise. According to the World Health Organization, macular degeneration is the third leading cause of blindness worldwide and the first leading cause in developed nations.

Josephine Everly and Herbert Kaufman

KEY FACTS

Description
Deterioration of the macula, an area in the retina.

Risk factors
Age, family history, race, sex, obesity, smoking, low nutrient levels.

Symptoms
Blurred or distorted vision.

Diagnosis
Eye exam by an ophthalmologist, visual acuity test (Amsler grid), fluorescein angiography.

Treatments
No treatment for dry AMD; laser surgery and photodynamic therapy, as well as some other emerging treatments, are available for wet AMD.

Pathogenesis
Deposits in the choroid area of the eye and growth of new blood vessels.

Prevention
Nutritionally balanced diet, supplemental vitamins, smoking cessation, regular eye exams.

Epidemiology
The third leading cause of blindness worldwide, but leading cause of blindness in developed countries due to the larger populations of elderly.

See also
• Eye disorders • Retinal disorders

Malaria

Malaria is one of the world's major infectious diseases, transmitted from human to human by mosquitoes. Each year, there are about 300 million to 500 million cases of malaria and between 1 million and 3 million human deaths, most of them children. Although various treatments and preventive measures are available to tackle the disease, these are often too expensive for developing countries, where malaria is most common.

Malaria has been eradicated from the United States and temperate regions of the world for several decades. Nevertheless, over 40 percent of the human population lives in areas where malaria is endemic (firmly established). In general, these are poor areas in tropical and subtropical regions. There, a number of factors are responsible for the continued presence of this illness, including climate changes, political unrest, and increased resistance of the parasite to drug therapies and of mosquitoes to insecticides.

Cause

Malaria is caused by single-celled protozoa belonging to the genus *Plasmodium*, often referred to collectively as the "malaria parasite." There are about 170 species of malaria parasite, able to infect many different types of vertebrates (backboned animals), but only four of these can cause infection in humans: *Plasmodium falciparum*, *P. ovale*, *P. vivax*, and *P. malariae*. *Plasmodium vivax* occurs in the Middle East, India, and Central America, while the other three species are found mainly in Africa. Of the four species, *Plasmodium falciparum* causes the most serious cases of illness and the majority of deaths.

Malaria parasites are carried from person to person by mosquitoes of the genus *Anopheles*. When an anopheles mosquito pierces the skin to suck blood, it may pick up the parasite from an infected person or, conversely, it may pass on the parasite to someone who is uninfected. It is always female mosquitoes that are involved, because males do not suck blood. Occasionally, a person can become infected with more than one species of malaria parasite at the same time.

Risk factors and epidemiology

Malaria is endemic in many subtropical and tropical regions of the world. Its absence from other regions may be because it has been eradicated but also because the malaria parasite, or the anopheles mosquitoes that transmit it, or both, cannot survive in colder regions.

Children under the age of five years, pregnant women, and travelers visiting regions with endemic malaria are at risk of having a more severe course of illness. In the case of travelers, the risk comes because they have not built up immunity after previous bouts

KEY FACTS

Description

A potentially fatal infectious disease involving the bloodstream and internal organs.

Cause

A single-celled parasite transmitted by the bite of infected *Anopheles* mosquitoes.

Risk factors

Children under the age of 5 years, pregnant women, and nonimmune travelers to areas where malaria is endemic are at greatest risk.

Symptoms

Recurrent attacks of flulike symptoms such as fever, chills, and body aches.

Diagnosis

Microscopic examination of blood smears.

Treatments

Various antimalarial drugs, although parasites are developing resistance to these.

Pathogenesis

The parasite's life cycle involves both humans and mosquitoes of the genus *Anopheles*; various stages of the malaria parasite's development occur in both of these hosts.

Prevention

Reducing contact with mosquitoes by using insect repellents and insecticide-treated bed nets. Taking preventive drugs before visiting areas where malaria is endemic.

Epidemiology

Malaria is endemic in many subtropical and tropical regions of the world. It can be spread elsewhere by travelers returning from these regions, at airports, or by infected mosquitoes "hitching a ride" on airplanes.

of malaria, as many local people will have done. About 30,000 people from developed countries contract malaria every year, after visiting regions where the disease is endemic. Pregnant women infected with *P. falciparum* are at higher risk of premature delivery and low birth weight in their offspring. Such infection can also lead to transmission of malaria to the child during pregnancy or delivery.

In endemic areas, risk of malaria decreases at altitudes above 6,560 feet (2,000 meters). The risk increases in the more rural areas. Transmission also varies by season, being highest at the end of the rainy season.

In nonendemic areas, malaria can be introduced, at least temporarily, as long as a mosquito capable of transmitting the disease also lives in the area. In the United States, two species of anopheles mosquitoes capable of transmitting this disease are still present. If, for example, a traveler returns to the United States after having been infected with malaria abroad and is bitten by a local anopheles mosquito on return, this infected mosquito can in turn bite and infect humans. Airport malaria, in which the infected mosquito arrives at an airport and transmits malaria there, can also occur. Of the thousand or so cases of malaria diagnosed each year in the United States, most are acquired outside the country and are referred to as "imported" malaria.

Malaria is not transmitted directly from person to person. It can, however, be acquired through blood transfusions, organ transplants from persons who have the infection, or by sharing needles with someone carrying the infection. Studies have shown that some genetic blood disorders, such as sickle-cell anemia, may actually help protect against malaria, because the alteration in the hemoglobin molecule hinders malarial growth and development.

Symptoms and pathogenesis

In a typical case of malaria, symptoms begin within 10 days to 4 weeks after a bite by an infected mosquito. Characteristic symptoms can be flulike and include fever, shaking chills, or "rigors," headache, and muscle aches. Nausea, vomiting, diarrhea, and jaundice, as well as severe fatigue, may also occur. The symptoms often appear regularly every other to every third day and last for several hours, although there is not always such a regular cycle. The liver and spleen may also become enlarged.

The symptoms of malaria can be related to the life cycle of the parasite (see diagram, p. 537). An infected mosquito releases sporozoites (a particular stage of the

MOSQUITOES AND MALARIA

There are about 430 species of anopheles mosquitoes worldwide, but only 30 to 50 can transmit malaria. In sub-Saharan Africa, the principal carrier of malaria is *Anopheles gambiae*, a mosquito that searches for its human blood meal between dusk and dawn, thus making the evening and night the times of greatest risk of infection.

When an anopheles mosquito infected with malaria parasites bites a human, it can release the parasites into the bloodstream while taking a blood meal.

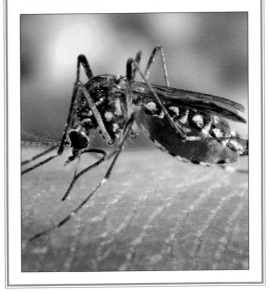

parasite's life cycle) into a person's bloodstream while taking its meal of blood. The sporozoites travel to the liver, where they invade the liver cells. There, they multiply asexually (without using sexual reproduction) by the thousands, developing into another stage called merozoites. A person does not usually show symptoms at this stage.

After a few days or weeks, the infected liver cells burst open and release the merozoites into the bloodstream, where they invade red blood cells and multiply further. Typically, infected blood cells tend to burst and release more parasites all at roughly the same time, either every two or every three days depending on the species of parasite. This cycle leads to the repeated flulike symptoms of malaria. Many parasites are released again from red blood cells in the form of more merozoites, ready to invade more red blood cells and continue the cycle of fever. Some parasites, though, are produced in a different form that is able to give rise to sex cells (gametes). If such potential sex cells are sucked up by a mosquito when it drinks an infected person's blood, the parasite undergoes sexual fertilization and multiplication in the mosquito's body until it is ready to be transmitted to another human victim, thus completing its life cycle.

Not all cases of malaria follow the pattern described above. For example, people who have already been infected by malaria before may show few symptoms when they are attacked once again. Where the infection is with *P. ovale* or *P. vivax*, the parasites can remain dormant (inactive) in the human liver and only cause obvious disease at a future date, sometimes as long as several years later. The species *P. malariae* can, in rare cases, remain in the human host for many years without producing symptoms.

An attack of malaria can cause various complications. All four species sometimes cause imbalances in the blood, with lowered blood sugar and increased acidity. Parasites also deform the outer membranes of red blood cells, making the cells more likely to be taken out of circulation by the spleen, further complicating the anemia caused by the bursting of parasite-infested cells. Organ failure involving the respiratory system or heart can occur, as can kidney failure. Dark pigments in the blood resulting from the destruction of large numbers of red blood cells can spill over into the urine, a condition called by the common name *blackwater fever*. The death rate due to severe malaria, even when treated in modern day intensive care units, often exceeds 30 percent, whereas in developing countries with substandard health care, persons with complicated malaria requiring blood transfusions can be at higher risk of contracting HIV and other blood-borne infections.

Of the four malaria parasites that infect humans, *Plasmodium falciparum* is the most common and the most lethal; it causes about 95 percent of deaths from malaria. More so than the other three, this species can infect a much greater proportion of red blood cells, sometimes causing death only a few hours after the rupture of red blood cells begins. In an infection with *P. falciparum*, the central nervous system can be involved, ultimately leading to confusion, seizures, and coma. For those who survive, their nervous system may be severely damaged.

Diagnosis

An active malarial infection can be diagnosed by taking a drop of the person's blood and spreading it on a microscope slide and then staining it with a special stain called Giemsa. These smears are produced as a thick and a thin smear. The microscopist then looks for the malaria parasites within the human red blood cells. Thick smears are useful in making the diagnosis; thin smears allow for species identification. Because parasites are present in the blood at intermittent cycles, smears should be evaluated every 6 to 12 hours over a period of 48 hours to improve diagnostic sensitivity. In 95 percent of cases, however, the first smear is positive for the presence of malaria parasites.

Blood testing using the polymerase chain reaction (PCR) method can also be done to detect the parasite's deoxyribonucleic acid (DNA; genetic material); however, this procedure requires a specialized laboratory, is labor intensive, and is quite expensive. Also, determination of viable versus nonviable organisms is not possible. This method may be useful to monitor the efficacy of drug treatment. A test for antibodies against the malaria parasites is available, but it can only identify prior infection.

Treatments

Various antimalarial drugs are available; however, increasing resistance by the malaria parasites has been noted, particularly to the drug chloroquine. Effective therapies include quinine sulfate, hydroxychloroquine (Plaquenil), the combination drug sulfadoxine and pyrimethamine (Fansidar), mefloquine (Lariam), the combination of atovaquone and proguanil (Malarone), and doxycycline (Doryx, Vibramycin). To improve chances for a cure, it is important to treat early using the correct drug, correct dose, and appropriate length of time. Persons infected with *P. vivax* or *P. ovale* may be treated with a second drug to prevent relapses. For drug-resistance cases, combination therapies involving the artemisinin drugs with other medicines are used, an approach referred to as artemisinin-based combination therapy (ACT).

Prevention

There is no vaccine at this time for malaria. However, because the complete genomes for *Plasmodium falciparum* and *Anopheles gambiae* have been sequenced, there is some hope that treatments such as vaccines or viruses might now be researched.

Most drugs used to treat malaria are also used to prevent it, including antibiotics such as doxycycline and tetracycline. For preventive treatment, the drug is usually started one to two weeks before travel to a malarial country, continues throughout the trip, and is also taken for four weeks after return. Even with such

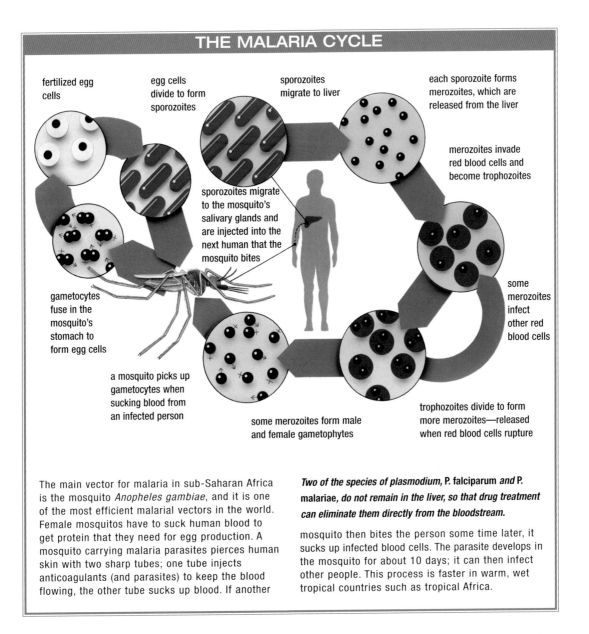

THE MALARIA CYCLE

fertilized egg cells

egg cells divide to form sporozoites

sporozoites migrate to liver

each sporozoite forms merozoites, which are released from the liver

sporozoites migrate to the mosquito's salivary glands and are injected into the next human that the mosquito bites

merozoites invade red blood cells and become trophozoites

gametocytes fuse in the mosquito's stomach to form egg cells

some merozoites infect other red blood cells

a mosquito picks up gametocytes when sucking blood from an infected person

some merozoites form male and female gametophytes

trophozoites divide to form more merozoites—released when red blood cells rupture

---

The main vector for malaria in sub-Saharan Africa is the mosquito *Anopheles gambiae*, and it is one of the most efficient malarial vectors in the world. Female mosquitos have to suck human blood to get protein that they need for egg production. A mosquito carrying malaria parasites pierces human skin with two sharp tubes; one tube injects anticoagulants (and parasites) to keep the blood flowing, the other tube sucks up blood. If another

Two of the species of plasmodium, P. falciparum and P. malariae, do not remain in the liver, so that drug treatment can eliminate them directly from the bloodstream.

mosquito then bites the person some time later, it sucks up infected blood cells. The parasite develops in the mosquito for about 10 days; it can then infect other people. This process is faster in warm, wet tropical countries such as tropical Africa.

---

preventive measures, it is still possible to acquire malaria, and preventive measures may merely delay the onset of symptoms, making diagnosis more difficult.

Attempts to minimize contact with mosquitoes can reduce the chances of contracting malaria. Insect repellent containing the chemical DEET as its active ingredient is recommended, along with wearing long sleeves and pants to decrease the chance of being bitten by mosquitoes. More recently, insecticide-treated bed nets have been shown to decrease childhood malaria and mortality from the disease.

In the 1950s, programs to eliminate malaria worldwide were implemented. These failed, however, in most malarial regions due to reasons including increased resistance of mosquitoes to insecticides, as well as increased resistance of the parasites to drugs used in treatment and political instability of some of the countries concerned. Furthermore, most people living in these countries cannot afford treatment, even though medicines to treat malaria are inexpensive by U.S. standards.

Rita Washko

See also
• Anemia • Dengue fever • Infections, parasitic • Sickle-cell anemia • Yellow fever

Male-pattern baldness

Male-pattern baldness, or androgenetic alopecia, is a common disorder that affects both men and women. It is characterized by thinning of the hair at the front of the scalp above the temples, so that the hairline recedes and reshapes. Hair loss in women is characterized by a diffusely thinned scalp, particularly from the forehead to the crown, without a receding hairline. Androgenetic alopecia is a cosmetic concern for both men and women. Treatment options have variable results.

Most cases of male-pattern baldness begin during the third or fourth decade, with progression of hair loss over time. Male-pattern baldness has many causes. People who display this condition have a genetic predisposition that is determined by many different genes. Other factors, such as poor diet and lack of exercise, also play a role. Male pattern baldness has increased greatly in Japan since the Japanese diet has become higher in fat and the lifestyle more sedentary.

Hair thins by miniaturization of the hair follicles, not just by decreased density. This process of thinning occurs over time when the combination of genetics with exposure to androgens results in the terminal (mature) hairs of the scalp slowly miniaturizing to intermediate hairs and then finally to vellus (fine) hairs. Androgens, which are the male sex hormones, include testosterone, dehydroepiandrosterone (DHEA), dihydrotestosterone (DHT), and many others. DHT is the chemical most readily linked to male-pattern baldness and is more potent than testosterone. This chemical is amplified in the scalp due to an enzyme called 5-alpha-reductase, which converts free testosterone to DHT. The overall result in those who are genetically susceptible is increased hair loss and male-pattern baldness. If a woman has baldness, she should be screened to ensure that she does not have virilism (high levels of male hormones causing masculinization). Other causes of scalp hair thinning are a thyroid disorder or anemia.

Treatments and epidemiology

Treatment of this condition is difficult, and currently there are only two medications approved by the FDA for androgenetic alopecia. Minoxidil is a topical medication that is thought to work by increasing blood flow to the follicles and increasing the time the hair is in the growth phase (anagen). The medication is best for small areas, or early stages of hair loss. It takes at least four months to start working, and it must be used indefinitely to maintain results. Finasteride is a pill that works to reduce the enzyme 5-alpha-reductase. It is not safe for use in women who can become pregnant because it causes severe birth defects. Finasteride is best used with minoxidil, and it also must be used indefinitely. It does not have any beneficial effect on hair growth in postmenopausal women.

Over the past 40 years, surgical options have become a good alternative but are limited due to high costs. Hair grafting, transfer of 2- to 4-square millimeter "plugs" to one site, is not often performed as the plugs look less natural, resembling a doll's head. In follicular unit transplantation, or micrografting, the donor pieces are individual follicular units containing one to three hairs that are then arranged as individual hair units.

Male-pattern baldness is most common in Caucasian men, then Asians and African Americans, and least often in Native Americans. It is found in more than half of all men worldwide, and up to 75 percent of postmenopausal women.

Maya Kolipakam and Richard S. Kalish

KEY FACTS

Description
Loss of head hair in men and women.

Causes
Multifactorial but mainly genetic.

Risk factors
Poor diet and lack of exercise; increasing age.

Diagnosis
Obvious from characteristic pattern of hair loss.

Treatments
The medications minoxidil and finasteride.

Pathogenesis
Progression of hair loss over time.

Prevention
No known prevention.

Epidemiology
Most common in Caucasian men, followed by Asians and African Americans.

See also
• Alopecia • Genetic disorders

Male reproductive system

The male reproductive system is comprised of the penis, testes, epididymis, vas deferens, seminal vesicles, and the prostate gland. The various disorders that affect each of these organs and structures can affect not only quality of life but also life span. In this summary of the many disorders that affect the male reproductive system, the features of the disorder will be discussed, as well as an overview of the various treatments available.

Although there are many penile disorders, the ones that are more commonly encountered include phimosis, paraphimosis, balanitis, erectile dysfunction, priapism, Peyronie's disease, condylomata acuminata, and penile cancer.

Phimosis is a disorder in which the male is unable to retract the prepuce (foreskin) behind the head of the penis. This can lead to inability to urinate as a result of blockage of the opening of the urethra. Phimosis can occur at any age. In older men who are diabetics, chronic infection may lead to phimosis and may be the initial presenting complaint. Children under 2 years of age seldom have true phimosis. Swelling, redness and tenderness of the foreskin, and the presence of purulent discharge usually cause the patient to seek medical attention. Initially, the infection can be treated with broad-spectrum antibiotics and then by gentle massaging of the foreskin over time. Ultimately, circumcision may be needed to remove the foreskin.

Paraphimosis, unlike phimosis, is the inability to replace the foreskin once retracted over the head of the penis. This is an emergency. If this condition is left uncorrected, it may cause pain and swelling and impair blood flow to the penis, resulting in necrosis and then auto-amputation of the penis. Paraphimosis can be caused by sexual activity or iatrogenically (induced inadvertently during a medical or surgical procedure), such as failing to replace the foreskin after catheter placement. Treatment of paraphimosis involves decreasing the swelling surrounding the foreskin and thus retracting the foreskin. Paraphimosis can be treated by firmly squeezing the head of the penis (glans) for five minutes to reduce the tissue swelling and decrease the size of the glans. The foreskin can then be drawn forward over the glans. Occasionally the constricting ring of foreskin requires incision under local anesthesia. Antibiotics should be given, and circumcision should be performed after the inflammation has subsided.

Balanitis is a disorder in which the skin covering the penis becomes inflamed. The disorder can manifest itself with redness, itching, pain, discharge,

RELATED ARTICLES

and encrustation. Most often, this occurs in men or boys who have not been circumcised and who have poor hygiene. Essentially, when the foreskin becomes tight, smegma, or foul-smelling substance, can be trapped underneath, ultimately leading to balanitis. Men with diabetes are at a greater risk of developing balanitis. In fact, sugar or glucose in the urine can become trapped under the foreskin and can be a breeding ground for bacteria. Other causes include allergic dermatological reactions and fungal infections. Treatment of the underlying cause forms the basis of treating balanitis. Often, if the balanitis is severe, circumcision may be the best option. Avoidance of certain soaps and products that may have been the trigger for the allergic reaction is recommended.

Erectile dysfunction is a more common disorder. This disorder is described when a man is unable to either initiate or maintain an erection. There are a multitude of reasons or causes for erectile dysfunction, including diabetes, peripheral and cardiovascular disease, alcohol abuse, smoking, and obesity. Erectile dysfunction is also associated with the treatment of prostate, bladder, and rectal cancers. Psychological causes used to be considered the most common reason for erectile dysfunction but are now thought to be the primary factors in only a few cases. There are varying treatments including medical therapy, injection therapy, vacuum erection devices, and finally, penile implants.

Priapism is a relatively uncommon disorder in which a man suffers from a painful erection that can last from several hours to several days. The erection is not usually due to sexual activity and essentially results from inability to drain a persistently engorged penis. The disorder is caused by unknown factors 60 percent of the time, whereas the remaining 40 percent can be associated with diseases such as sickle-cell anemia, leukemia, or with penile trauma, spinal cord injury, or use of medications.

The goal of treatment for priapism is to obtain detumescence, which is resolution of the erection. Acute management of priapism often involves draining the blood using a needle placed into the penis. Medications that help shrink blood vessels, which decreases blood flow to the penis, also may be used. In rare cases, surgery may be required to avoid permanent damage to the penis. Treating any

underlying medical condition or substance abuse problem is important for the prevention of priapism. Erectile dysfunction is common after prolonged priapism. Early recognition (within hours) and prompt treatment of priapism offer the best opportunity to avoid this major problem.

Peyronie's disease is a condition in which a plaque (scarlike tissue) inside the penis causes the curvature and functional shortening of the penis. This condition was first described in 1742 and is a well-recognized clinical problem affecting middle-age and older men. The plaque or scarlike tissue may be the result of trauma. Patients present with complaints of painful erection, curvature of the penis, and poor erection away from the affected area. The penile deformity may be so severe that it prevents vaginal penetration. The patient generally has no pain when the penis is not erect. Examination of the penile shaft reveals a palpable dense, fibrous plaque of varying size.

The various medical treatments for Peyronie's disease have had only limited success; these include oral vitamin E and potassium para-aminobenzoate, or intralesional injections with different medications. Surgical treatment involves either incision of the plaque followed by repair with a patch graft or plication (folding) of the tissue on the opposite side of the plaque, which cancels out the bending effect. A penile prosthesis may also be used for patients with Peyronie's disease and severe erectile dysfunction.

Condylomata acuminata is a sexually transmitted infection caused by the human papillomavirus (HPV). The effect of the virus is the development of wartlike lesions that mostly occur on the penis in males. The wartlike lesions can also be found on the scrotum and the perineum, or in the urethra, bladder, and rectum. Application of local medications or liquid nitrogen can destroy small lesions. Large lesions require laser or surgical removal. The patient's sexual partner should also be examined for the infection.

Penile cancer is an uncommon disease; in fact it comprises less than 1 percent of all male cancers in the United States. It occurs most commonly in men in their 50s, although rare cases have included children. It has been associated with chronic inflammatory disease, human papillomavirus infection, and phimosis.

MALE REPRODUCTIVE SYSTEM

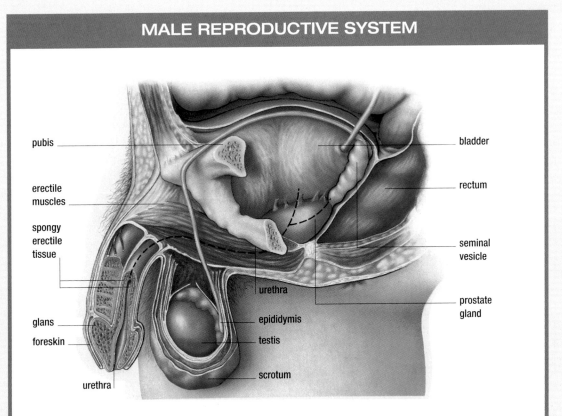

pubis

erectile muscles

spongy erectile tissue

urethra

glans

foreskin

urethra

bladder

rectum

seminal vesicle

prostate gland

epididymis

testis

scrotum

The bulbous end of the penis (glans) is protected by the foreskin (prepuce) in uncircumcised males. The penis contains three columns of spongy erectile tissue, which become engorged with blood, or erect, during sexual arousal.

The two testes hang outside the body in the scrotum. Each testis contains seminiferous tubules, which produce sperm cells, and also Leydig cells, which make the male sex hormone testosterone. The sperm mature in the coiled epididymis and travel along the vas deferens. The two vasa deferen-

The male genitals are the penis and scrotum, which holds the two testes. Internal reproductive structures are the coiled epididymis, the vas deferens, the seminal vesicle, and the prostate gland.

tia unite at the urethra, which passes through the penis and through which urine is also voided. The seminal vesicles add fluid and nutrients to the sperm to make semen, and the prostate gland also adds a milky fluid to the semen, which is discharged from the body during ejaculation.

Symptoms usually include growths and sores on the penis that may bleed or discharge. Surgery to remove the cancer is the most common treatment for penile cancer. Surgery may include wide local excision of the lesion, laser surgery, microsurgery, or penectomy (amputation of the penis). Radiation therapy or chemotherapy can also be used.

Disorders of the testes

There are many disorders that affect the testes, including trauma, torsion, varicocele, hydrocele,

hypogonadism, and cancer. The testes are in a precarious location, sitting below the protection of the muscles and bones of the pelvis. When testicular trauma does occur, it can present with severe pain, bruising, and swelling. The most serious condition occurs when a testis ruptures, causing blood to leak into the scrotum. This requires immediate surgical exploration, and the testis should be inspected to assure viability. Testicular torsion occurs when the testis twists around the spermatic cord, which results in congestion of the veins, progressive swelling, and decreased arterial supply, leading ultimately to testicular death. The symptoms are the acute onset of severe pain and swelling. The condition occurs most often when a boy is 12 to 18 years old. It can be caused by strenuous activity or trauma, or sometimes there is no apparent reason. The diagnostic test that is most useful is a color duplex ultrasound to evaluate the blood flow to the testis. If the patient is seen within a few hours of onset, manual detorsion may be attempted. However, even if this is successful, it is recommended that the patient undergo fixation of both testes. Surgical exploration is necessary in most cases to reverse the torsion or to remove the nonviable testis. After 5 to 6 hours of torsion, the testes infarct (die due to lack of blood supply).

Varicocele is a disorder in which there is an abnormal dilation of the veins in the spermatic cord, which is a connection of the testis to large blood vessels. This condition occurs more often on the left side. Varicocele can be found in about 15 percent of men. Most patients with varicocele have no symptoms. Some patients may experience dragging scrotal sensation or pain, particularly in sexually active men. The sudden development of a varicocele in an older man is sometimes a late sign of a renal tumor. On physical exam, the varicocele is often described as a "bag of worms." Varicocele is associated with male infertility. Sperm parameters may be affected in men with a varicocele. Treatment of varicocele may improve testicular function and sperm quality; however, the efficacy of the treatment should be discussed with a fertility specialist. Surgical repair of varicocele involves ligation of the veins; this can be done with open surgery, microscopic surgery, embolic therapy, laparoscopic surgery, or robotic surgery.

Hydrocele is a disorder in which fluid collects around the testis. A hydrocele may develop rapidly after local injury, radiotherapy, or infection. Chronic hydrocele is more common. Its cause is often unknown, and it usually occurs in men past the age of 40 years. Unless complications are present, active therapy is not required. The indications for treatment are a very tense hydrocele or large bulky mass that is cosmetically unpleasing and perhaps uncomfortable for the patient.

Congenital hydrocele can be seen at birth, and spontaneous resolution of the hydrocele may occur in infancy. When treatment is necessary, surgery is the definitive treatment.

Hypogonadism is a disorder in which the testes do not produce enough testosterone. Testosterone is a hormone that plays an important role in developing and maintaining physical characteristics of a man. Primary hypogonadism is a condition that occurs when there is a problem with the testes themselves. Secondary hypogonadism occurs when there is a problem with the pituitary (a gland in the brain), which sends signals to the testis to help it grow and produce testosterone. Hypogonadism can lead to decreased sex drive, decreased hair growth, decreased muscle tissue, and increased breast tissue. Treatment of hypogonadism includes testosterone replacement or, if the problem is secondary hypogonadism, replacement of pituitary hormones.

Cryptorchidism, or undescended testis, is a condition in which a testis stops its normal descent anywhere between the kidney and scrotal areas. At the time of birth, the incidence of undescended testes is 3.4 percent. The incidence of cryptorchidism in adult men is 0.7 to 0.8 percent.

Male factor infertility is a condition in which a man is unable to conceive. In fact, in nearly 40 percent of all infertility cases, the cause is attributed to a factor in the male, and in an additional 20 percent of cases the cause is attributed to both male and female factors.

Less than a decade ago, treatment for a severe male factor infertility was limited to inseminations or in vitro fertilization (IVF) using donor sperm. Today, great advances have been made to try to help infertile males. The introduction of innovative therapeutic options offer men, including those with no sperm in their ejaculate as a result of genetic conditions, a greatly improved chance to conceive their own biological offspring.

Testicular cancer occurs when abnormal cells in the testes grow uncontrollably. Testicular cancer can grow in one or both testes and can affect men at all ages. Testicular cancer usually presents with a lump or mass felt in one or both testes during a self-examination. Sometimes men present with the feeling of dull ache or heaviness on one side of the scrotum. Treatment and diagnosis of testicular cancer involves surgically removing the testis through an incision in the groin region.

Sometimes, testicular cancer spreads to nearby lymph nodes. In this case the patient may benefit from surgical removal of the affected lymph nodes. Chemotherapy or radiation therapy, or both together, can kill off cancerous cells. The cure rate for testicular cancer is extremely high (more than 90 percent). For this reason, it is very important for young men to perform self-exams so that early diagnosis can lead to early treatment.

Disorders of the epididymis

The epididymis is the coiled tube that links the testis with the vas deferens; sperm pass through this tube before they are ejaculated. The function of the epididymis is to transport, store, and mature sperm. Epididymitis is inflammation of the epididymis and can be caused by infection from the urethra or from sexually transmitted disease. Symptoms include severe pain, dysuria (pain or difficulty in passing urine), and swelling and can mimic testicular torsion in some cases. The epididymis will be markedly swollen and very tender to touch, eventually becoming a warm, red, enlarged scrotal mass indistinguishable from the testis. Fever and chills may develop, leading to bacteria in the urine or even in the bloodstream. Treatments for epididymitis include antibiotics, anti-inflammatory medications, and scrotal support. If left untreated, scar tissue can form and lead to blockage of sperm transport, which can ultimately affect fertility.

Disorders of the vas deferens and seminal vesicle

Vas deferens is a continuation of the epididymis. Vas deferens joins its corresponding seminal vesicle to form the ejaculatory duct that opens into the prostatic urethra. Sperm produced by the testes is transported through the vas deferens. The seminal vesicles are a paired, saclike, hollow organ that lie behind the prostate and bladder base. Most of the fluid part of semen is produced by seminal vesicles. Absence of vas deferens and seminal vesicle, which may be due to genetic disorders such as cystic fibrosis, or blockage of vas deferens due to infection or trauma, if occurring in both vasa deferentia, will cause male infertility.

Disorders of the prostate gland

The prostate gland is a small organ the size of a walnut that lies below the bladder and surrounds the urine channel (urethra), which carries urine. The main disorders of the prostate include prostatitis, benign prostatic hyperplasia, and prostate cancer.

Prostatitis is inflammation of the prostate gland and comprises 25 percent of men's visits to the urologist. This is the most common urological diagnosis in men under 50 years of age. Prostatitis can be classified into acute or chronic prostatitis. Prostatitis can cause symptoms of pain in the pelvic region, urgent or frequent urination, and difficult or painful urination. Sometimes it can cause patients to be unable to urinate at all (urinary retention). Acute prostatitis is usually marked by fevers and chills. Chronic prostatitis may also present without symptoms. Many patients require antibiotic treatment along with medications to improve urination.

HYDROCELE

A hydrocele is swelling that results from an excessive quantity of fluid that accumulates between the double-layered membrane that surrounds the testis. Hydroceles often develop in elderly men and infants. They can be caused by injury, infection, or inflammation, but in some cases there is no apparent cause.

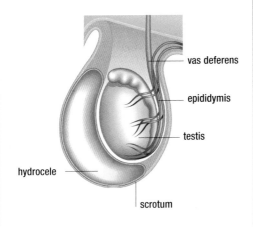

vas deferens

epididymis

testis

hydrocele

scrotum

A hydrocele causes a swelling in the scrotum, which is a type of pouch or sac in which the testes hang outside the body. The swelling may become painful, when it can be treated surgically.

Benign prostatic hyperplasia (BPH) is an enlargement of the prostate that is nonmalignant (noncancerous). Men are usually diagnosed at an older age. In fact, 50 percent of men over the age of 50 develop this disorder. Symptoms develop when the prostate enlarges and compresses the urethra. These symptoms include frequent urination, straining to urinate, and a weak stream of urine. Digital rectal examination, in which a gloved and lubricated finger is inserted in the rectum, can identify an enlarged prostate in front of the rectum. The prostate can grow large enough to block the urethra completely. In this case, a catheter may need to be inserted to allow a flow of urine. If the urine flow is blocked, kidney damage can occur. Medical treatment of BPH includes using medications to improve the urination by relaxing the muscles that surround the prostate. Some medications can shrink the prostate as well. The surgical treatment can be minimally invasive, including laser or microwave therapy, or more invasive, such as transurethral resection of the prostate, in which a specialized viewing tube—called a resectoscope — is passed along the urethra via the penis and is used to remove part of the prostate gland. Open surgery is used in very rare cases, such as when a patient has a very large (baseball-sized) prostate gland.

Prostate cancer is one of the most common cancers that develop in men. Prostate cancer occurs when there is abnormal growth of malignant cells of the prostate gland. The tumor grows slowly and is usually confined to the gland. When and if it does spread to other organs, it will usually spread to the bone, the liver, or the brain.

Symptoms are usually associated with advanced prostate cancer. The risk (predisposing) factors for prostate cancer include advancing age; this cancer usually affects elderly men. Genetic factors increase the risk; men with a family history of the disease have an increased chance of developing prostate cancer. Hormonal influences are also a risk factor, because the growth of prostate cancer is thought to be dependent on the male sex hormone testosterone. Environmental factors such as toxins, chemicals, and industrial products all increase the risk of developing the disease. The chances of developing prostate cancer increase with age. Thus, prostate cancer under age 40 is extremely rare, whereas it is common in men older

TREATMENT OPTIONS FOR PROSTATE CANCER

Retropubic radical prostatectomy. This procedure is used to remove prostatic tissue through an opening made in the abdomen. A nerve-sparing approach can be performed—if the nerves are not affected by cancer—to preserve potency. Risks include incontinence and erectile dysfunction.

External beam radiotherapy. This treatment delivers a total of 75 Gy (Gray) of radiation over 6 to 7 weeks to kill rapidly dividing cancerous cells. Long-term failure rates are higher than those seen with a prostatectomy.

Brachytherapy. Radioactive seeds are permanently implanted into the prostate gland through needles under ultrasound guidance. However, brachytherapy will not be performed if the prostate gland is very large or small or if the patient is due to have transurethral resection to remove prostate tissue.

Hormonal therapy. This therapy affects the production of the sex hormone testosterone, so that prostate tissue will atrophy. It also causes the loss of libido or erectile function.

than 80 years of age. After research, some studies have suggested that among men more than 80 years old, 50 to 80 percent of them may unknowingly have prostate cancer.

The diagnosis of prostate cancer is based on the results of a biopsy of the prostate collected via the rectum. The biopsy is usually prompted by either an abnormal digital prostate examination or an elevated prostatic specific antigen (PSA) level in the blood, a test used to screen for prostate cancer. Transrectal ultrasound is sometimes carried out at the same time. An ultrasound probe is inserted into the rectum, and scanning is carried out.

Treatment of prostate cancer includes observation, hormonal treatment, radiation treatment, including brachytherapy, chemotherapy, cryotherapy (in which tissue is destroyed by freezing), and conventional surgery. Surgery on prostate cancer can be performed by laparoscopic surgery, robotic surgery, or by an open approach.

Rowena De Souza and Run Wang

Measles

Measles is a contagious viral illness that is caused by a ribonucleic acid (RNA) virus. Although measles is a potentially dangerous disease, if children receive the MMR vaccine, the number of cases of measles decreases. Although measles mainly affects children, anybody who has not had the disease can become infected.

Measles used to be one of the most common infectious diseases of childhood before immunization became widespread. Measles virus is a member of the paramixovirus family that includes parainfluenza, mumps, and respiratory syncytial viruses. Measles has existed for many centuries, although its infectious etiology was established only in the nineteenth century. The measles virus was discovered in 1954. In the mid-twentieth century, successful immunization campaigns led to a dramatic decrease in measles cases in the developed world. In contrast, measles remains a significant cause of morbidity and mortality among children in the developing world; it caused an estimated 450,000 deaths in 2004. It is also a leading cause of blindness in African children. The Measles Initiative is a combined effort that aims to decrease morbidity and mortality from measles in the countries most heavily affected by this disease. It was launched by multiple agencies, including the Red Cross, Centers for Disease Control and Prevention, the World Health Organization, and the United Nations Children's Fund The Measles Initiative is vaccinating children at risk in many African countries and is now expanding to Asian countries as well. As a result of this campaign, measles deaths have almost halved. The campaign's goal is to reduce measles mortality by 90 percent by the year 2010. The Pan-American Health Organization has led a campaign to eliminate measles in the Western Hemisphere. The last endemic case in this part of the world was reported in 2002. The remaining reported cases of measles in countries of the Americas have been associated with importation from areas with a higher prevalence of measles.

Pathogenesis and symptoms and signs

This disease is only transmitted among humans by large air droplets. The air droplets containing the virus can survive in the environment for several hours. The person with measles remains contagious from the first day of the symptoms until approximately four to five days after the rash develops. Damage from the measles virus results in compromised function of the mucosal epithelial cells and the development of bronchitis and pneumonia.

The symptoms usually develop 10 to 14 days after exposure (incubation period), but they can start as early as 7 days or as late as 21 days after the virus enters the human body. Children less than 5 years of age or adults older than 20 years, as well as malnourished and immunocompromised individuals, are at risk for

---

KEY FACTS

Description
Measles (rubeola) is a highly contagious acute infection caused by a virus.

Causes
Measles is caused by an RNA virus that belongs to the family of paramixoviruses.

Risk factors
It is a highly contagious disease and almost everyone without previous immunity to measles is susceptible.

Symptoms
The symptoms of measles are fever, cough, coryza (runny nose), conjunctivitis, and a rash.

Diagnosis
Diagnosis is usually based on typical clinical symptoms and a history of contact if this information is available.

Treatments
Fluids and relief of fever.

Pathogenesis
The disease spreads through the air in droplets containing the virus from an infected person. The virus enters through the upper respiratory tract and invades the epithelial cells that line the respiratory tract.

Prevention
The best way to prevent measles is to maintain specific antibody protection against measles. This is commonly achieved by immunization.

Epidemiology
Measles is one of the major causes of childhood mortality in many developing countries. It is a leading cause of blindness in African children.

more severe illness and a higher chance of complications. Patients with measles develop high fevers up to 104°F–105°F (40°C–40.5°C), cough, runny nose and conjunctivitis. A typical rash helps identify measles. It develops after several days of fever and starts on the face and descends down the body and then the extremities. The rash is erythematous (red) and maculopapular; it can change its color to brown and scale before resolving. It lasts for several days and then slowly clears, starting from the face. Another very specific finding for patients with measles is Koplik's spots, white-gray patches found on the buccal mucosa of the oral cavity. They develop one to two days prior to the appearance of the rash. These are easy to miss and not always present in all the patients. Measles usually resolves on its own in an average of 14 days. The general prognosis for measles is good. Infection with measles results in lifelong immunity. Mortality from measles is associated with poor nutritional status and immunocompromised states such as HIV and cancer. Pneumonia accounts for the majority of deaths from measles.

The most common complications of measles include superinfections of the respiratory tract, such as bronchitis, pneumonia, and otitis media (ear infection). Another dangerous but rare complication of measles is encephalitis. It typically develops five to six days after the rash and results in headache, vomiting, and fever. It can also result in seizures and coma. Another illness associated with measles is subacute sclerosing panencephalitis, which is a chronic, debilitating neurological condition. It is very rare and develops years after the episode of measles.

Diagnosis and treatments

Diagnosis of measles is mostly based on the clinical presentation. In addition, a blood test called serology could be used to diagnose measles. It detects a specific immune response to the invasion of this virus: measles antibodies. Other methods, like virus isolation and detection of antigen in the mucosal cells, are also available. Another typical laboratory feature of measles is a low leukocyte count in the peripheral blood (leukopenia).

For treatment, supportive measures such as provision of fluids and relief of fever are usually necessary.

Prevention

There are two ways to prevent measles: active and passive immunization. For active immunization, a live attenuated (weakened) virus is used for vaccination in a

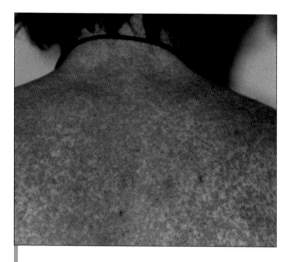

This adult male has measles and is exhibiting the typical red, blotchy rash. The symptoms are more severe in adulthood.

combined vaccine called MMR (measles-mumps-rubella). It is given twice, first at 12 to 16 months of age and later in childhood at 4 to 6 years of age. The vaccine is not given prior to 12 months of age because there are circulating maternal antibodies that are passed to the baby via the placenta. MMR vaccine is well tolerated; among the most common side effects of the vaccine are low grade fever and rash that resolve spontaneously in several days. There is no real scientific evidence to support an association of MMR with the development of autism, as some reports have suggested in the past. MMR vaccine should be given to adults born in 1957 or later if there is no evidence of specific immunity against measles. MMR vaccine should not be given if there is a history of an allergic reaction to a prior dose of MMR or allergy to the components of the vaccine (like gelatin and neomycin).

Passive immunization is achieved by the administration of specific immunoglobulin to persons exposed to measles who are not already immune. This is especially important for individuals at high risk of severe measles. Passive immunization is only indicated to prevent the disease in the event of exposure to a person with measles. In order to be effective, immunoglobulin should be given within six days of exposure to the disease.

Diana Nurutdinova

See also
• Chicken pox and shingles • Childhood disorders • Conjunctivitis • Diphtheria • Infections • Infections, viral • Mumps

Melanoma

Melanoma is the deadliest form of skin cancer. Although it accounts for only 4 percent of all skin cancers, melanoma causes more than 75 percent of all deaths from skin cancer. Melanoma cases are increasing; the rate doubles every 10 to 20 years, which is consistent with increased leisure time and the public's attraction to a tanned body. In the United States, the male death rate for melanoma has risen from 2.4 in 100,000 in 1959 to 3.8 in 100,000 in 2000.

The top layer of the skin is called the epidermis, and it is within this structure that a melanoma forms. It arises from the melanocyte, which is the pigment-containing cell responsible for skin color, located in the deepest layer of the epidermis. As in other forms of skin cancer, most melanomas are the result of the harmful effects of ultraviolet (UV) radiation, which is cumulative over a lifetime. It is the combination of the ultraviolet light injuring the deoxyribonucleic acid (DNA) in the melanocyte and the cell's inability to repair the damage that leads to uncontrolled growth.

Risk factors

Risk factors for developing melanoma include exposure to UV radiation (sun or tanning beds) and a family history of dysplastic nevus syndrome. The latter is an inherited condition in which family members develop many unusual pigmented skin lesions, which can often change and potentially progress to melanoma. Other risk factors include burning easily in the sun, a history of severe sunburns, a tendency to freckle rather than tan, and living in areas with high-intensity sunlight, such as Florida and Australia. It is also more common when an individual has irregular or unusual moles, or more than 50 moles, has xeroderma pigmentosum (a hereditary condition in which the skin cells cannot repair the DNA damage from the sun), or has an impaired immune system, from drugs or disease (HIV).

Melanoma can occur in all individuals but is more common in Caucasians, especially those with a fair complexion, light-colored eyes, and red or blond hair. When it occurs in dark-skinned individuals, it generally occurs on unexposed areas such as palms, soles,

KEY FACTS

Description

A melanoma is a dark-colored skin cancer arising from the pigmented cells of the skin (melanocytes).

Causes

Most melanomas are the result of ultraviolet radiation damage to the skin.

Risk factors

The leading risk factor is a long history of unprotected exposure to UV radiation. It is more common with advanced age, in Caucasians, and when a large number (more than 50) or unusual moles are present. Individuals with certain inherited diseases (dysplastic nevus syndrome, xeroderma pigmentosum) and immune deficiencies are also at higher risk.

Symptoms

Melanoma is heralded by the change in a preexisting mole or the development of a new dark skin growth. Worrisome signs include asymmetry of the growth, irregular borders, variation in the color, a diameter of more than 6 mm, and elevation of the lesion above the surrounding skin. The cancer can also be itchy or have a tendency to bleed or have an open sore.

Diagnosis

The diagnosis of melanoma is suspected when the above characteristics are observed and confirmed by the microscopic examination of the tissue removed.

Treatments

Surgical excision is the treatment for the primary skin lesion of melanoma. Other methods, such as chemotherapy, are used for advanced disease.

Pathogenesis

Melanoma develops from unrepaired UV radiation damage to the DNA of melanocytes. It can quickly spread to other organs through the lymph system or blood vessels.

Prevention

Limiting harmful sun exposure, protective clothing, and sunblock can prevent skin cancers. Regular skin examination and prompt treatment of suspicious lesions prevent spread and reduce the risk of death.

Epidemiology

Most commonly seen in Caucasians, especially those with fair complexions, blue eyes, and red or blond hair. It is more prevalent in areas with high-intensity sunlight. The incidence doubles every 10–20 years.

and mucous membranes. Unlike other forms of skin cancer, which occur almost exclusively in older age groups, melanoma can occur in younger people and is the most common cancer in adults under the age of 30.

Symptoms

An individual should suspect a melanoma with any changes in a preexisting dark skin lesion or development of a new mole. The "ABCs" of warning signs for melanoma are as follows: asymmetry, in which the growth is not of a uniform shape, without two similar halves; borders, in which the edges of the lesion are irregular; color (the dark color of the mole varies from one area to another); diameter, which depicts a pigmented lesion that is more than $1/4$ inch (6 mm) in diameter; and elevation, which is a growth that is higher than the surrounding skin. Other signs for concern include skin growths that are constantly itchy or bleed or darkly pigmented streaks or areas beneath a nail or on the palm or soles of the feet.

Diagnosis

A diagnosis can be made from the appearance of the melanoma, which can appear in many forms. The most common form is an enlarging, irregularly shaped black or dark brown patch (superficial spreading melanoma), usually located on the back of males and the back and lower legs of females. In the elderly, a slowly growing tan patch on sun-exposed areas may represent a lentigo maligna melanoma. It can also present as a dark raised nodule (nodular melanoma), which has the worst prognosis. There are also forms that appear on the palms or soles of the feet (acral lentiginous) and others that are not pigmented (amelanotic melanoma).

When a melanoma is suspected, it is important to remove the lesion in a timely fashion, since cure rates are very good with early detection and proper treatment. A sample or biopsy of the suspicious area is removed to be examined under a microscope. Characteristics of the appearance of the tumor, such as the location, the diameter, the presence of ulceration, and the microscopic features (tumor thickness, depth of extension, invasion of lymphatics or blood vessels) help the physician determine the best treatments and the patient's prognosis from their tumor.

Treatments and prevention

Unlike other forms of skin cancers that can be treated by a variety of methods, treatment of melanomas requires surgical excision with a margin of a normal tis-

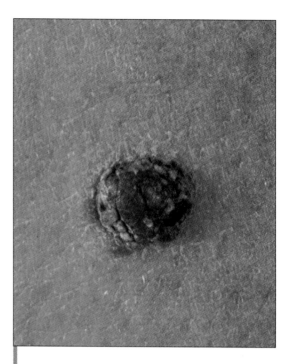

Melanomas usually grow from an existing mole, which becomes lumpy and irregular, changes shape, darkens, and sometimes bleeds or ulcerates. The mole may be itchy or tender and painful.

sue. If an enlarged lymph node is present, it may be biopsied through a needle or excised. Melanoma has a high mortality, since it can rapidly spread through the lymph system or bloodstream to other internal organs, a process called metastasizing. The addition of chemotherapy, radiation, and other modalities is used for tumors that have spread. Cure rates can approach 95 percent if detected and treated early.

Similar to other skin cancers, preventive measures include limiting the exposure to the damage inflicted by the sun's rays and tanning booths. Limiting the time of exposure (especially between the sun's peak hours of 10 AM to 4 PM), wearing protective clothing, and use of sunblocks with a sun protection factor (SPF) of 15 or greater are the standard methods. Individuals should also regularly check their skin for new moles or changes in existing ones. Those with a family history of dysplastic nevus syndrome need to have their skin examined by a dermatologist annually.

David Wainwright

See also
• Cancer • Cancer, skin • Diagnosis
• Skin disorders

Ménière's disease

Ménière's disease is a disorder of the inner ear characterized by vertigo or dizziness, tinnitus (noises in the ears), fluctuating hearing loss, and the sensation of pressure or pain in the affected ear. It is a common cause of hearing loss and typically affects only one ear.

Ménière's disease, also called idiopathicendolymphatic hydrops, is a disorder of the inner ear. It is one of the most common causes of dizziness. In most cases, only one ear is involved, but both ears may be affected in about 15 percent of patients. Ménière's disease typically starts between the ages of 20 and 50 years, with men and women being affected in equal numbers. There are about 615,000 people in the United States with Ménière's disease, with about 45,500 new diagnoses made each year.

Symptoms and causes

The symptoms of Ménière's disease occur suddenly, unpredictably, and can arise daily or as infrequently as once a year. Vertigo involves a whirling dizziness that forces the affected person to lie down and can lead to severe nausea, vomiting, and sweating. Other symptoms include tinnitus (ear noises), fluctuating hearing loss, or a full feeling or pressure in the affected ear. Typically, an attack is characterized by a combination of these symptoms, lasting several hours. A person's hearing tends to recover between attacks but over time becomes worse. The cause of Ménière's disease is unknown but is thought to occur when there is an abnormal mixing of different fluids of the inner ear.

Diagnosis and treatments

Diagnosis involves a medical history, a physical exam, hearing and balance tests, electrocochleography (ECoG), and imaging with computed tomography (CT) or magnetic resonance imaging (MRI). Electrocochleography is the recording of electrical activity of the inner ear as it responds to sound, and imaging helps confirm that symptoms are not caused by a tumor.

There is no known cure for Ménière's disease, but symptoms can be controlled by lifestyle changes, medications, and sometimes, surgery. Lifestyle changes such as a low-salt or salt-free diet, elimination of caffeine, tobacco, and alcohol, and reducing stress help keep ear fluids in balance. Furthermore, it has been found that symptoms can be alleviated by drugs that either control allergies or improve blood circulation in the inner ear.

In some cases, surgical removal of the inner-ear sense organ or severing the nerve from the affected inner ear organ can control symptoms, but there are many risks associated with these surgical procedures. Recently, the administration of the antibiotic gentamycin directly into the middle-ear space has been used to control vertigo. Thus, until a cure is found, treatment of symptoms appears to be the best way to cope with Ménière's disease.

Rashmi Nemade

KEY FACTS

Description
A disorder of the inner ear that gets worse over time.

Causes
Abnormality in the volume of fluid in the inner ear.

Symptoms
Fluctuating vertigo, in which there are attacks of a spinning sensation, hearing loss, tinnitus (a roaring, buzzing, or ringing sound in the ear), and a sensation of fullness in the affected ear.

Diagnosis
Tests for hearing, balance, electrocochleography (ECoG), computed tomography (CT), or magnetic resonance imaging (MRI).

Treatments
Antivertigo and antinausea drugs; lifestyle changes such as cutting out alcohol, caffeine, and cigarette smoking, avoiding stress, and a regular schedule of eating and sleeping; in some cases, surgery may be recommended.

Pathogenesis
Abnormal mixing of inner-ear fluids that affects hearing and balance.

Prevention
There is no known way of preventing the development of Ménière's disease.

Epidemiology
It is estimated that there are about 615,000 people with Ménière's disease in the United States and 45,500 newly diagnosed cases each year.

See also
• Ear disorders

Meningitis

Meningitis is an inflammation of the meninges, the thin membranes that surround the brain and spinal cord. Between the meninges is the subarachnoid space, which contains cerebrospinal fluid (CSF). Meningitis develops when the subarachnoid space becomes infected, usually from outside organisms carried in the bloodstream. This infection typically involves the entire surface of the meninges.

Inflammation of the meninges—meningitis—can be caused by various infectious agents, most commonly viruses and bacteria. It may occur as a complication of another infectious illness such as syphilis, Lyme disease, or tuberculosis. Other microorganisms such as protozoa and fungi may also cause meningitis. In addition, certain medications, cancers, and other diseases can inflame the meninges—but these are very rare occurrences.

Pathogenesis

Many of the bacteria or viruses that can cause meningitis are fairly common and more likely associated with other everyday illnesses. At other times they spread to the meninges from an infection elsewhere in the body, such as the heart and lungs. The infection can start in the skin, gastrointestinal tract, or urinary tract. From there, the microorganism enters the blood and travels through the body and enters the central nervous system. Bacteria can also spread directly to the meninges from a nearby severe infection such as a serious ear infection (otitis media) or nasal sinus infection (sinusitis). Bacteria can also enter the central nervous system (CNS) from head surgery or after blunt head trauma, such as skull fracture.

In otherwise healthy individuals, the subarachnoid space is relatively resistant to microorganisms even during persistent bacteremia (presence of viable bacteria in the bloodstream). Cell-mediated immunity and antibody-mediated destruction of bacteria are the predominant defense mechanisms in the central nervous system. Once infection in the subarachnoid space is established, the invading microorganism can rapidly multiply to high levels, resulting in severe inflammation of the meninges.

Viral meningitis is relatively more common and far less serious than bacterial meningitis. It often remains undiagnosed because the symptoms are similar to those of the viral infection influenza. Most cases of viral meningitis are caused by a group of viruses called enteroviruses, which are viruses that can affect the stomach. These viruses account for 80 to 92 percent of

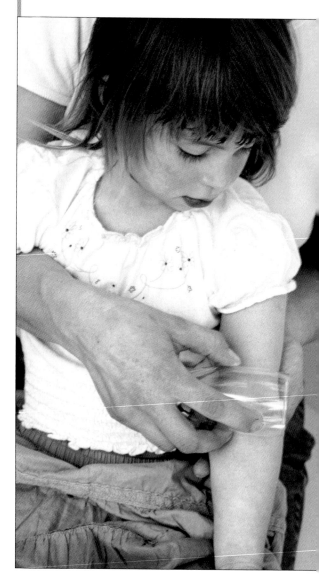

A mother is testing her young daughter for meningitis. Because a meningitis rash is blotchy and does not fade under pressure, a simple test is to press a glass against the skin. If the rash does not fade, medical help must be called at once.

all cases of viral meningitis. Anyone can get viral meningitis; however, it occurs most often in children during the summer and fall months and resolves spontaneously after 7 to 10 days. Many other types of viruses, such as herpes viruses, lymphocytic choriomeningitis virus, Epstein-Barr virus (which causes mononucleosis), varicella zoster virus (which causes chicken pox and shingles), and paramyxovirus (which causes mumps), can also cause meningitis.

Bacterial meningitis is less common than viral meningitis, but it is much more serious and can be life threatening if not treated promptly. Many types of bacteria, such as streptococcus, E. coli, and *Listeria monocytogenes*, are common causes of meningitis in newborns. *Streptococcus pneumoniae* and *Neisseria meningitidis* are more frequent in children older than two months of age. *Hemophilus influenzae* type B (Hib) was the leading cause of meningitis in children in the United States, but the widespread use of Hib vaccine as a routine standard immunization has dramatically reduced the frequency of this type of meningitis since the 1990s. In developing countries, *Mycobactrium tuberculosis* is a common cause of bacterial meningitis. Bacterial meningitis can occur in adults or children, but is more common in the very young (infants and young children) and elderly people (those more than 60). College students and teenagers are at a relatively higher risk for the disease due to time spent in close contact in dormitories with their peers.

Symptoms

Symptoms of meningitis vary but often include the classic triad of headache, fever, and stiff neck. Other symptoms include sensitivity to light (photophobia), nausea, vomiting, drowsiness, body aches, and confusion. Weakness, loss of appetite, shaking chills, profuse sweats, cranial nerve palsies (weakness of 3rd, 4th, 6th, and 7th cranial nerves) occur in between 10 and 20 percent of patients with meningitis. Generalized seizures occur in up to 40 percent of patients. Kernig's sign, in which extension of the knee with hips flexed is met with strong passive resistance, and Brudzinski's sign, in which passive flexion of the neck causes flexion of the leg, are observed in up to 50 percent of patients and are suggestive of meningitis. The presence or absence of the signs, however, does not make a definitive diagnosis of meningitis.

Symptoms in very young children may be particularly difficult because they often lack the classic signs mentioned earlier. Babies with meningitis may be irritable, less active, vomit, and refuse to eat. Normally, infants who are not feeling well are comforted when their mother picks them up. However, a baby with meningitis may show increased irritability when picked up and gently rocked when an attempt is made

---

KEY FACTS

Definition

Meningitis is an inflammation of the meninges, the thin membranes that surround the brain and spinal cord.

Causes

Meningitis is triggered by microorganisms that cause inflammation of the meninges.

Risk factors

Extremes of age, alcoholism, severe liver disease, renal disease, HIV and AIDS, malignancy, non-functional spleen due to sickle-cell disease, and diabetes. Living in close quarters, prolonged or close contact with a patient with meningitis, and direct contact with a patient's oral secretions (kissing or coughing) are considered increased risks for acquiring the infection.

Symptoms

Classic triad of headache, fever, and stiff neck in adults. In children, symptoms may include irritability, decreased activity, vomiting, refusal to eat, fever, jaundice, rashes, weak sucking, and bulging fontanelles (soft spots on an infant's skull).

Diagnosis

Analysis of cerebrospinal fluid (CSF) for signs of infection; clinical presentation suggestive of meningeal inflammation.

Treatment

For viral meningitis, treatment is relief of symptoms, bed rest, and analgesics. For bacterial meningitis, there must be prompt early diagnosis, broad-spectrum antibiotics given early, and treatment of complications, such as shock and abnormal electrolyte levels in the blood.

Pathogenesis

Microorganisms enter the blood and travel through the body and enter the central nervous system or spread directly to the meninges from a nearby severe infection.

Prevention

Routine immunization of young children and adolescents with vaccine against *Pneumococcus*, *Hemophilus*, and *Neisseria* (Hib, Menactra T, and pneumococcal vaccine).

Epidemiology

20,000 to 25,000 cases of bacterial meningitis in United States yearly; about 2,000 Americans die of meningitis each year; greatest group at risk for meningitis are children between 1 and 24 months.

to comfort him or her (paradoxical irritability). Other symptoms of meningitis in infants can include jaundice (a yellow tint to the skin), stiffness of the body and neck (neck rigidity), a lower than normal temperature, poor feeding, a weak suck, and a high pitched cry, and bulging fontanelles (membranous junction between two surfaces of the skull bones).

Meningitis can also lead to skin rashes (50 percent of meningococcal meningitis), seizures, and loss of consciousness in the latter stages of the disease. Viral meningitis has similar symptoms to bacterial meningitis, such as fever, headache, nausea, vomiting, and body aches. These signs and symptoms are preceded by several days of a nonspecific, acute febrile (feverish) illness with malaise and loss of appetite.

Diagnosis

The most important diagnostic test for meningitis is to examine a sample of cerebrospinal fluid. The fluid is removed from the spinal canal with a needle in a procedure called a lumbar puncture. The classic symptoms and a lumbar puncture analysis that shows purulent spinal fluid (sign of inflammation) are usually all that is required for diagnosis.

Cerebrospinal fluid is examined for numbers and types of blood cells (complete blood count), for levels of substances such as glucose and protein, and for presence of microorganisms, which may be cultured, or propagated, for identification. In meningitis, the white blood cell count is elevated with a predominance of immature forms. Conversely, severe infection can be associated with a low white blood cell count. The results of glucose and protein analyses will depend on the severity of the disease.

Treatments

Treatment for meningitis depends on the cause of the infection. Viral meningitis comprises the majority of cases, with most people getting better in about two weeks. Mild cases of viral meningitis may only need home treatment, including fluids to prevent dehydration and control of pain and fever.

Bacterial meningitis will require hospital admission and a course of intravenous antibiotics. The disease is regarded as a medical emergency because death can occur within hours if bacterial meningitis is not treated promptly. Broad-spectrum antibiotics should be started before test results become available, on the presumption that all cases are bacterial in nature until proven otherwise. Appropriate antibiotic treatment can reduce the mortality rate of meningitis to below 15

percent. Corticosteriod drugs can reduce or prevent complications, such as hearing loss, that are associated with *Hemophilus influenzae* meningitis.

Prevention

Routine immunization of young adolescents will help prevent this rare but serious infection. Vaccines against the most common causes of bacterial meningitis (*Streptococcus pneumoniae* and *Neisseria meningitidis*) are recommended for people at high risk of infection. These include older adults and children, those with a weakened immune system, and those with a nonworking spleen. People traveling to areas, such as sub-Saharan Africa, where meningitis is prevalent should receive the *Neisseria meningitidis* vaccine.

The Centers for Disease Control and Prevention (CDC) now recommends the new vaccine Menactra T for protection against certain strains of *Neisseria meningitidis* for children age 11 and 12 years, teens entering high school, and college freshmen living in dormitories. Children between 2 months and 5 years should be vaccinated against *Hemophilus influenzae* type B bacteria. Pneumococcal conjugate vaccine (pneumovac) is part of the regular immunization for all children younger than 2 years in the United States. CDC recommends pneumovac for children 2 to 5 years with chronic heart disease, lung disease, or cancer. It is also recommended for adults older than 65, as well as those with chronic heart disease, diabetes, or sickle-cell anemia.

Epidemiology

There are 20,000 to 25,000 cases of bacterial meningitis in United States each year, and 2,000 people die of meningitis each year. There is an incidence of 4 to 10 cases per 100,000 people in the United States. The people at greatest risk for acute bacterial meningitis include children who are between 1 and 24 months of age. Adults older than 60 years account for 1,000 to 3,000 cases of acute bacterial meningitis each year in the United States and for more than 50 percent of all deaths related to meningitis. Worldwide, bacterial meningitis accounts for about 1.2 million cases annually.

Isaac Grate

See also
- Brain disorders • Childhood disorders
- Infections, bacterial • Infections, fungal
- Infections, parasitic • Infections, viral
- Lyme disease • Syphilis • Tuberculosis

Menopausal disorders

A set of symptoms and disorders commonly associated with menopause, a natural event that occurs in a woman's life as part of the aging process. Menopause is defined as 12 consecutive months without menstrual periods that is not due to an unrelated disease or other condition.

Menopause is either natural, with the gradual cessation of menstrual periods, or it can be induced or surgical, which is the cessation of ovarian function due to the surgical removal of the ovaries or as a result of chemotherapy or radiation therapy. There are more than 40 million menopausal or post-menopausal women in the United States, of whom almost half are over 65 years old. As life expectancy increases, most women will spend one-third of their life postmenopausal. Many women experience a relatively trouble-free menopause with just mild symptoms, but some women are seriously affected with symptoms and disorders that impact severely on their lifestyle.

Causes and risk factors

In the ovaries about 600,000 eggs are present at birth, 300,000 at the onset of menstruation, and fewer than 10,000 at the time of menopause. This normal decline is caused by the genetically programmed death of the eggs. Follicle-stimulating hormone (FSH) is one of the hormones the brain sends to the ovaries to develop the eggs. When a healthy egg is stimulated, it grows and produces estrogen. As the number of viable eggs declines, the level of FSH rises. When there are no viable eggs left, no more estrogen is produced by the ovaries, and FSH levels become even higher in an effort to stimulate the ovaries.

These hormonal changes and the irregular menstrual cycles that are associated with menopause typically start at about age 47, with menopause being completed by about age 52. This time period between the beginning and completion of menopause is called the climacteric.

About 1 percent of women are affected by premature menopause, which is the spontaneous cessation of menstrual periods before the age of 40 years. Factors associated with earlier menopause include a woman's mother's age when she experienced menopause,

KEY FACTS

Description
A set of symptoms associated with menopause, which is the cessation of menstrual periods due either to the natural loss of ovarian activity between the ages of 45 and 55, the surgical removal of the ovaries, chemotherapy, or radiation therapy, or the spontaneous cessation of periods prior to the age of 40, called premature menopause.

Causes and risk factors
Early menopause is linked to a woman's mother's age at menopause, nulliparity (never having delivered a baby), current cigarette smoking, genetic abnormalities, early onset of puberty, living at high altitudes, left-handedness, lower education and socioeconomic status, type 1 diabetes, and blindness. Late menopause is associated with having delivered many babies, obesity, prior use of oral contraceptives, and higher socioeconomic status.

Symptoms
Hot flashes, night sweats, sleep disturbances, vaginal dryness, pain and problems with intercourse, urinary incontinence (leaking urine unintentionally), mood changes, or problems with memory or concentration.

Diagnosis
There is no single perfect test for menopause. The diagnosis is confirmed by an elevated level of the hormone FSH (the signal the brain sends to the ovaries to tell them to make eggs), which rises dramatically when the ovaries do not respond because there are no longer any viable eggs. Menopause may also be suspected from the associated symptoms.

Treatments
Treatments are geared toward the specific medical issue or symptom.

Pathogenesis
The genetically programmed normal loss of ovarian function results in an estrogen-deficient state that affects many different systems or body parts, including bones, brain, breasts, skin, colon, urogenital (urinary and genital tract), and cardiovascular systems.

Prevention
There is no accepted way to delay or prevent menopause, although there are interventions and drugs that can help treat symptoms.

Epidemiology
There are more than 40 million menopausal and postmenopausal women in the United States.

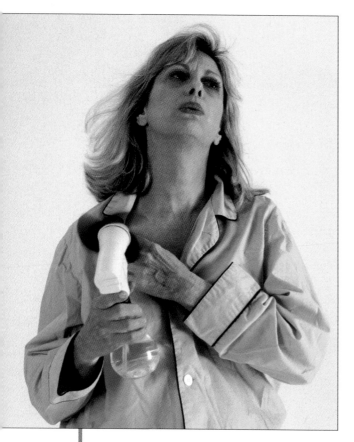

The most common complaints of menopause are vasomotor symptoms. These include hot flashes and night sweats—temporary reddening of the upper body with a sensation of heat, followed by sweating.

nulliparity (having no children), current smoking, genetic abnormalities (which may limit ovarian function), abnormally early puberty, living at high altitudes, left-handedness, lower education and socioeconomic status, type 1 diabetes, and blindness. Late menopause is associated with having given birth to several children, obesity, prior use of oral contraceptives, and higher socioeconomic status.

Symptoms and diagnosis

Vasomotor symptoms, which include hot flashes and night sweats, remain the most common and bothersome complaints faced by menopausal women, with up to 85 percent of menopausal women affected. Other associated symptoms include sleep disturbances, vaginal dryness, pain and problems with sexual intercourse, urinary incontinence (leaking urine unintentionally), mood changes, and problems with memory or concentration.

Although there is no perfect way to diagnose menopause, measuring the FSH level in the blood is the best single test. Menopause may also be suspected from the associated symptoms.

Pathogenesis

As the ovaries produce fewer hormones, including estrogen, many organ systems may be affected, including the cardiovascular and vasomotor systems, which are concerned with the constriction and dilation of blood vessels, the brain, breasts, urogenital tract (bladder and vagina), bones, colon, and skin.

Treatments and prevention

Treatments exist for each system affected by menopause. Cardiovascular disease, which includes heart attacks and stroke, is the leading cause of death in postmenopausal women, killing more women than all cancers combined. Treatment is geared toward lifestyle measures such as stopping cigarette smoking, managing weight and fat distribution, ensuring good nutrition, checking blood pressure, increasing physical activity, and lowering cholesterol.

Hot flashes usually go away (regardless of treatment) within five years in most women. About one-quarter of menopausal women will have flashes for up to ten years, and an unfortunate 10 percent of women can experience hot flashes for even longer. Treatment includes lifestyle modification such as dressing in layers of clothing, which can be sequentially removed when a flash comes on, and avoiding triggers such as spicy food. Various drugs or herbal preparations may help; hormone replacement therapy, which boosts the estrogen levels in the body, is the most effective medical treatment, and black cohosh the best herbal preparation. Estrogen creams may also be used to treat other menopausal symptoms such as vaginal dryness.

Osteoporosis, which is the loss of bone (and bone density) from the skeleton, is one of the biggest health problems in older women following menopause; it commonly leads to brittle bones and fractures of the hip, spinal column, or other bones. Exercise, calcium supplementation, and drugs are the mainstay to minimize this age-related disease.

Roxanne Vrees and Gary Frishman

See also

- Blindness • Diabetes • Female reproductive system • Fractures
- Menstrual disorders • Obesity
- Osteoporosis • Smoking-related disorders

Menstrual disorders

Menstrual disorders include any interference with the normal menstrual cycle, menstrual pain, unusually heavy or light bleeding, and delayed or missed menstrual periods. A regular menstrual cycle occurs between 21 to 35 days, with 3 to 10 days of bleeding. Interruptions in this cycle can result in amenorrhea (cessation of menstruation), oligomenorrhea (infrequent menstrual cycles) menorrhagia (heavy bleeding), menometrorrhagia (irregular heavy bleeding) and dysmenorrhea (severe menstrual cramps).

Most women experience a form of menstrual disorder at some time. A regular menstrual cycle begins between the ages of 12 and 13 years. Most cycles occur between 21 and 35 days, with 3 to 10 days of bleeding and 1 to 1½ fluid ounces (30 to 40 ml) of blood loss. A typical menstrual cycle occurs about every 28 days, unless a woman is pregnant or moving into menopause. When the menstrual cycle is abnormally disrupted, a menstrual disorder may be occurring.

Menstrual disorders include amenorrhea (the cessation of menstruation), oligomenorrhea (infrequent menstruation), menorrhagia (heavy bleeding), menometrorrhagia (irregular heavy bleeding), dysmenorrhea (severe menstrual cramps), and premenstrual syndrome (PMS); emotional symptoms a week preceding menses. The physical and emotional symptoms accompanying these irregularities in the menstrual cycle may cause serious anxiety and distress for patients and their families and diminish the quality of life.

Symptoms and signs

Symptoms of menstrual disorders vary depending on the cause. Most menstrual disorders are caused by a hormonal imbalance or a dysfunction that is related directly to the female reproductive organs. A common cause of menstrual irregularity is polycystic ovary syndrome (POS), in which there is anovulation (lack of ovulation), which can result in oligomenorrhea or menometrorrhagia. The lack of progesterone associated with anovulation in POS can predispose a woman to endometrial cancer. In primary amenorrhea, the only symptom is delayed menstruation; in secondary amenorrhea, menstruation stops for at least three months.

Heavy bleeding and fatigue due to the loss of iron-rich blood are the symptoms of menorrhagia. In this type of menstrual disorder, blood flow soaks through a tampon or pad every hour for several hours, or a period lasts more than seven days. Symptoms of primary dysmenorrhea include severe cramping, pelvic pain, nausea, and vomiting and diarrhea. The symptoms may be stronger on one side of the body than the other. In secondary dysmenorrhea, the pain might feel like regular menstrual cramps but lasts longer than normal and occurs throughout the month. Another

---

KEY FACTS

Description
Painful menstruation; too light or too heavy bleeding during menstruation; frequent or infrequent menstruation; premenstrual syndrome.

Causes
Hormonal imbalance; the most common is polycystic ovary syndrome.

Risk factors
Excessive exercise, eating disorders, stress, and medical conditions such as fibroids, bleeding disorders, or diabetes.

Symptoms
Too much or too little blood flow or lower abdominal and pelvic pain radiating to the thighs and back during menstruation; debilitating emotional symptoms the week before menses.

Diagnosis
Laboratory tests for hormone levels, MRI or ultrasound imaging.

Treatments
Hormone replacement therapy or treatment of pain.

Pathogenesis
Fluctuation of ovarian hormones leading to irregular or ceased menstrual cycles.

Prevention
Healthy exercise and nutritional program, as well as dietary supplements and vitamins.

Epidemiology
Amenorrhea affects 2–5 percent of childbearing women; menstrual cramps or painful periods affects up to 90 percent of all women; heavy bleeding occurs in about 9–14 percent of all women. About 13–18 percent of women have symptoms severe enough to interfere with work and daily activities.

menstrual disorder is PMS, which is used to describe emotional symptoms like mood swings in the week preceding menses. If PMS is severe and debilitating, it is also known as premenstrual dysphoric disorder (PMDD).

Causes and risks

Since *menstrual disorders* is a general term to describe pathological variations in the menstrual cycle, the causes of each component are different. Lifestyle choices such as excessive exercise or low body weight can lead to primary amenorrhea. Medical conditions causing amenorrhea include Turner's syndrome, a birth defect related to the reproductive system, or ovarian problems. Secondary amenorrhea can be caused by pregnancy, breast-feeding, sudden weight loss or gain, intense exercise, stress, endocrine disorders affecting the thyroid, pituitary, or adrenal glands, and surgical procedures affecting the ovaries, including removal of the ovaries, cysts, or ovarian tumors. Amenorrhea is common in athletes or dancers and is frequently associated with two other disorders—reduced bone mass and eating disorders. This combination is sometimes called the female athlete triad.

Heavy or irregular bleeding during menstruation is a symptom of an underlying condition rather than a disease itself. It is usually related to a hormonal imbalance but can be caused by fibroids, cervical or endometrial polyps, the autoimmune disease lupus, pelvic inflammatory disease (PID), blood platelet disorder, a hereditary blood factor deficiency, or possibly, some reproductive cancers. Having these other conditions may increase the risk of menstrual disorders in a particular individual.

Dysmenorrhea is usually related to the production of prostaglandins, naturally occurring chemicals that cause an inflammatory reaction. Women with severe menstrual pain have higher levels of prostaglandin in their menstrual blood than women without such pain. In some women, prostaglandins can cause some of the smooth muscles in the gastrointestinal tract to contract, resulting in the nausea, vomiting, and diarrhea that some women experience. Other causes of dysmenorrhea include fibroids, PID, an intrauterine device, uterine, ovarian, bowel, or bladder tumor, uterine polyps, inflammatory bowel disease, scarring or adhesions from surgery, and endometriosis or adenomyosis, conditions in which the endometrial lining grows in other areas of the pelvic cavity. As in menorrhagia, having any of these conditions increases the risk for menstrual disorders. The likely causes of PMS or PMDD are hormonal imbalances.

Diagnosis and treatments

Menstrual disorders are diagnosed by considering family and medical history, eating and exercise habits, lifestyle, stress levels, changes in body weight, and a pelvic exam. Routine blood tests are done to measure hormone levels and to check for pregnancy. A diagnosis may include an endometrial biopsy in which a small amount of tissue is scraped from the lining of the uterus for examination. An ultrasound of the pelvic area typically allows visualization of any internal structural anomalies. Similarly, surgical procedures may include laparoscopy, in which a thin tube with a camera attached is inserted through a small incision below or through the navel, or a hysteroscopy, in which a thin tube with a camera attached is inserted into the vagina and up through the cervix; these allow internal views of the abdominal cavity and uterus, respectively.

Treatments for menstrual disorders depend on which type of disorder is diagnosed. In the case of amenorrhea, simple changes in lifestyle such as reducing the intensity of exercise, maintaining an appropriate weight, and reducing stress levels may solve the problem. Surgery is recommended only in rare cases in which amenorrhea is linked to ovarian cysts, vaginal blockage, or uterine anatomical abnormalities. It is essential to determine the cause before treating menorrhagia. Medical therapies may help, but occasionally surgery is indicated. In most cases, surgery involves removing the lining of the uterus temporarily or permanently. There are a number of procedures that can achieve this goal, such as a dilation and curettage, endometrial biopsy, endometrial resection, and endometrial ablation. Primary dysmenorrhea is handled with drugs and nonmedical treatments. Drugs include either over-the-counter nonsteroidal anti-inflammatory drugs (NSAIDS) or prescription medications such as oral contraceptives that provide cycle control and reduce menstrual blood flow.

Nonmedical treatments include using a heating pad on the abdomen or taking warm baths to reduce discomfort. Taking B vitamins, magnesium, and omega-3 fatty acid supplements may also help. Menstrual disorders are diverse and complicated and require medical consultation.

Rashmi Nemade

See also
• Anemia • Cancer, ovarian • Cancer, uterine • Endometriosis • Female reproductive system • Fibroids • Menopausal disorders

Mental disorders

Mental disorders is a broad generic term to describe affective or emotional instability, behavioral dysregulation, and cognitive impairment. Specific illnesses known as mental disorders include major depression, anxiety disorder, schizophrenia, bipolar disorder, and attention-deficit hyperactivity disorder. Mental illnesses can be of biological or psychological origin and can impact everyday functioning.

A mental disorder can have an effect on every aspect of a person's life, including thinking, feeling, mood, and outlook, as well as areas of external activity, such as family and marital life, sexual activity, work, recreation, and management of material affairs. In addition, because mental illnesses are disabling and last for many years, they take a tremendous toll on the emotional and socioeconomic capabilities of relatives who care for the patient, especially when the health care system is unable to offer treatment and support at an early stage. Sufferers typically seek treatment only when psychiatric symptoms make it very difficult to function, but early treatment, when symptoms are mild or moderate, will generally lead to a better long-

term outcome. As with many physical diseases, the diagnostic process is complex. Diagnosis remains subjective, although it is becoming increasingly evidence-based and scientific, which includes careful and detailed assessment of patient histories and current and past symptoms.

Mental disorders vary from one person to another and may be mild, severe, or anything between. Even in one person, symptoms can vary over time from their most severe to complete remission. These disorders are episodic, and occasional bouts may be triggered by stress or other life factors. Appropriate treatment of the disease can help stabilize the course of the illness and reduce or eliminate waxing and waning symptoms.

Some mental conditions can be cured in the sense that the symptoms go away or the patient no longer suffers significantly, but the underlying vulnerability remains. Psychiatry and related disciplines embrace a wide spectrum of techniques and approaches for treating mental illnesses. These include the use of psychoactive drugs to correct biochemical imbalances in the brain or to relieve depression, anxiety, and other painful emotional states. Medicine has been unable to completely cure mental disorders. However, many

RELATED ARTICLES

conditions, such as schizophrenia, bipolar disorder, and depression, can be treated with medication.

Psychotherapies seek to treat mental disorders by psychological means and involve communication between the patient and a trained person in the context of a therapeutic interpersonal relationship between them. The function of the psychiatrist is to provide support, therapy, and, if necessary, medications to address the symptoms. Behavioral therapy concentrates on changing or modifying observable pathological behaviors by the use of conditioning and other experimentally derived principles of learning. Each disorder is likely to have its own cause. It has generally been settled that both "nature" and "nurture" contribute to major psychiatric disorders. All of the major disorders show strong signs of heritability, with bipolar disorders showing the highest incidence of inheritance.

At the start of the twentieth century, there were only a dozen recognized mental disorders. By 1952 there were 192, and by the early twenty-first century there were approximately 375. This increase could be a result of more effective diagnosis and better characterization of mental disorders, an increase in incidence of mental disorders, or an increase in familiarity with diagnostic methods, described in the *Diagnostic and Statistical Manual of Mental Disorders*, fourth edition (DSM-IV).

Causes

Mental disorders may be caused by a number of factors, or the confluence of several factors. Different schools of thought, including the biological, psychological, and social, offer different explanations, although most current theories hold that a combination of all three factors can contribute to the development of an individual's illness.

Many mental disorders have a biological component; that is, a person with a mental disorder may have a difference in brain structure or function, through either genetic or environmental vulnerabilities (such as exposure to alcohol in utero). Additionally, some argue that neurotransmitter imbalance may cause mental disorders. Even when biochemical abnormalities have been found in mental patients, it is difficult to know whether they are the cause or the result of the illness, or of its treatment, or of other consequences. Despite

these problems, progress has been made in unraveling the biochemistry of affective disorders, schizophrenia, and some of the dementias. Neurotransmitters play a key role in transmitting nerve impulses across the microscopic gap (synaptic cleft) that exists between neurons. The release of such neurotransmitters is stimulated by the electrical activity of the cell. Among the main neurotransmitters are norepinephrine, dopamine, and serotonin. Some neurotransmitters excite or activate neurons, while others act as inhibiting substances. Abnormally low or high concentrations of neurotransmitters at sites in the brain are thought to change the synaptic activities of neurons, thus ultimately leading to the disturbances of mood, emotion, or thought found in various mental disorders.

Many genetic studies have shown that mental disorders, such as bipolar disorder or schizophrenia, can be inherited. When one parent is found to have the disorder, the probability that his or her children will develop schizophrenia is at least 10 times higher (about 12 percent risk) than it is for children in the general population (about 1 percent risk). If both parents are schizophrenic, their children stand anywhere from a 35 to 65 percent probability of becoming schizophrenic. If one member of a pair of fraternal twins develops schizophrenia, there is about a 10 percent chance that the other twin will also develop the disorder. If one member of a pair of identical twins has schizophrenia, the other identical twin has at least a 40 to 50 percent chance of developing the disease. Genetic factors seem to play a less significant role in the causation of other psychotic disorders and in personality disorders, and they seem to be even less of a factor in the causation of neuroses.

Psychological explanations have also been offered for the causes of mental disorders. Individual conflict, stress, or trauma may lead to the development of mental disorders. Social explanations suggest that mental disorders may be caused by significant events in the environment. For example, people living in poor communities or households tend to have a higher incidence of mental disorders. Freudian and other psychodynamic theories view neurotic symptoms as arising from internal conflict, that is, as being caused by conflicting motives, drives, impulses, and feelings held within various components of the mind. Behavioral theories for the causation of mental disorders rest largely upon the assumption that the symptoms or symptomatic behavior found in persons with various neuroses (particularly phobias and other anxiety disorders) can be regarded as learned behaviors that have built up to conditioned responses.

Prevalence

According to recent reports, the presence of a major mental disorder, including depression, bipolar disorder, and schizophrenia, is the most common cause of disability in the United States. Approximately 23 percent of North American adults will suffer from a clinically diagnosable mental disorder in a given year, but less than half of them will suffer from symptoms that severely impact their daily lives. Approximately 9 to 13 percent of children under the age of 18 experience problems with mental disorders that significantly affect their daily performance. It is suggested that many young people diagnosed with mental disorders early in life will recover with appropriate treatment and may be only mildly affected later in their lives.

Worldwide prevalence varies widely, from about 4 to 25 percent, with an average ranging between 9 and 17 percent. Anxiety disorders are the most common disorders, with mood disorders following. Substance discords and impulse-control disorders are consistently less prevalent.

Diagnosis

Diagnosis is the process of identifying an illness by studying its signs and symptoms and by considering the patient's history. The diagnosis of mental disorders is usually done by a licensed mental health professional or a medical doctor. Diagnosis usually involves a number of sources and instruments, including a personal history, a physical exam, an evaluation of behavior, a symptom inventory, a condition-specific instrument (such as the Beck depression inventory), and other information suggested by the history. Information obtained from the interview, along with observations of the patient, will form the basis of a preliminary diagnosis.

One method for diagnosing different mental disorders is to classify individuals according to the same or related clinical symptoms. Therefore, based

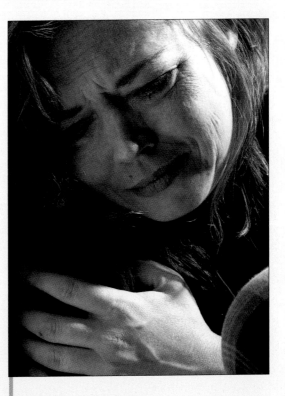

Symptoms of mental disorders can vary from very mild to severe. The symptoms tend to be episodic and can be triggered by stress and other life factors.

on the classification of a depressive illness, it may be appropriate to consider prescribing antidepressant drugs when preparing treatment plans.

The two most frequently used systems of psychiatric classification are the International Classification of Diseases, produced by the World Health Organization, and the DSM-IV, produced by the American Psychiatric Association. The DSM-IV differs from the International Classification in its introduction of precisely described criteria for each diagnostic category; its categorizations are usually based upon the detailed description of symptoms.

Categorization

Mental disorders have been categorized into groups relating to their common symptoms according to the DSM-IV, compiled by the American Psychiatric Association. There are many different categories; some contain many illnesses and others only a few.

There are many disorders that are usually first diagnosed in infancy, childhood, or adolescence.

Children are usually referred to a psychiatrist or therapist because of complaints or concern over the child's behavior or development by a parent or some other adult. Family problems, particularly difficulties in the parent-child relationship, are often an important causative factor in the symptomatic behavior of the child. For the practice of child psychiatry, the observation of behavior is especially important, as the child may not be able to express his or her feelings in words. Examples include attention disorders in which children show a degree of inattention and impulsiveness that is markedly inappropriate for their stage of development. Gross overactivity in children has many causes, including anxiety, or the effects of living in institutions.

Also included are conduct disorders, the most common psychiatric disorders in older children and adolescents, accounting for nearly two-thirds of disorders in those aged 10 and 11 years. In conduct disorders, abnormal conduct more serious than ordinary childlike mischief persistently occurs. Lying, disobedience, and aggression may be shown at home, and truancy, delinquency, and deterioration of work may occur at school. Important causative factors are the family background, such as broken homes, unstable and rejecting families, institutional care in childhood, and a poor social environment.

Infantile autism begins in the first two years of life. The child shows an inability to make warm emotional relationships, has a severe speech and language disorder, and exhibits a desire for sameness in which he shows distress if thwarted from his stereotyped behavior. There is some evidence to support genetic and organic factors in causation. Treatment involves management of the abnormal behavior, training in life skills and occupational activities, and counseling for the family.

Delirium, dementia, amnesia, and other cognitive disorders are another group of mental disorders. There are several types of psychiatric syndromes that arise from organic brain disease; the most prominent are dementia and delirium. Dementia is the loss of

MENTAL DISORDERS

DISORDERS	SYMPTOMS	TREATMENT
Schizophrenia	Delusions, hallucinations, and withdrawal from reality	Drugs, psychotherapy, and supportive therapy
Bipolar disorder	Depression and mania	Antidepressant drugs, cognitive psychotherapy, ECT
Anxiety disorders	Palpitations, sweating, dizziness, trembling, dry mouth	Psychotherapy, antidepressant drugs, short-term anti-anxiety drugs, and cognitive behavioral therapy
Somatoform disorders	Symptoms of physical illness but no organic disorder is found; these disorders are called hypochondriasis and hysteria	Psychotherapy and psychiatry
Dissociative disorders	Alteration in someone's motor behavior and sense of identity	Psychotherapy
Eating disorders	Lowered food intake or overeating binges	Psychotherapy and diet counseling; hospitalization

such intellectual abilities as memory, thinking, remembering, paying attention, judging, and perceiving, without an accompanying disturbance of consciousness. The syndrome may also be marked by the onset of personality changes. Dementia is usually a chronic condition and frequently worsens over the long term. Delirium is a diffuse or generalized intellectual impairment marked by a clouded or confused state of consciousness, an inability to attend to one's surroundings, difficulty in thinking coherently, a tendency to perceptual disturbances such as hallucinations, and difficulty in sleeping.

Delirium is generally an acute condition and does not last long. Other specific psychological impairments associated with organic brain disease are amnesia (a gross loss or disorder of recent memory and time sense without other intellectual impairment), recurring or persistent hallucinations or delusions, or marked personality changes.

In old age the most common causes of dementia are Alzheimer's disease and cerebral arteriosclerosis. There is no specific treatment for the symptoms of dementia; the underlying physical cause needs to be identified and treated when possible. The aims in the care of the demented patient are to relieve distress, prevent behavior that might result in accident, and optimize remaining physical and psychological faculties.

Mental disorders due to a general medical condition are diagnosed when there is evidence from the patient's history, physical exam, or other laboratory results that show that the symptoms are a direct physiological consequence of a general medical condition. The symptoms can include any of the various categories of symptoms in the DSM-IV. These can include, but are not limited to, delirium and dementia, psychosis, depression, anxiety, and personality changes. Many different types of medical conditions can lead to the development of mental disorders, such as AIDS, diabetes, multiple sclerosis, asthma, rheumatoid arthritis, Parkinson's disease, or cardiovascular disease. To treat these mental disorders, it is necessary to treat the underlying medical disorder.

Substance-related disorders

This category refers to maladaptive behavior associated with the regular nonmedical use of substances that affect the central nervous system. Substance abuse implies a sustained pattern of pathological use resulting in impairment of the drug abuser's social or occupational functioning. Substance dependence implies tolerance, in which markedly increased amounts of the drug must be administered to achieve the same effect, and withdrawal, in which symptoms follow the cessation of drug use or decreases in the dose of the substance.

Schizophrenia and other psychotic disorders

Schizophrenia is the single largest cause of admission to a mental hospital, and it accounts for an even larger proportion of the permanent populations of such institutions. It is a severe and frequently chronic illness that typically first manifests itself during the teen years or during early adult life. More severe levels of impairment and personality disorganization are reached in schizophrenia than in almost any other mental disorder. The principal clinical signs of schizophrenia are delusions, hallucinations, a loosening or incoherence of a person's thought processes and train of associations, deficiencies in feeling appropriate to normal emotions, and a withdrawal from reality.

A delusion is a false belief that is firmly held despite obvious or objective evidence to the contrary. The delusions of schizophrenics may be persecutory, grandiose, religious, sexual, or hypochondriacal in nature, or they may be concerned with other topics. Hallucinations are false sensory perceptions that are experienced without an external stimulus but that nevertheless seem real to the subject. The thought disorders may consist of a loosening of associations, so that the speaker jumps from one idea or topic to another unrelated one in an illogical, inappropriate, or disorganized way. Among the so-called negative symptoms of schizophrenia are a blunting or flattening of the person's ability to experience (or at least to express) emotion, indicated by speaking in a monotone and by a peculiar lack of facial expressions.

It can be estimated that approximately one-third of schizophrenic patients make a complete recovery and have no further recurrence, one-third have recurrent episodes of the illness, and one-third deteriorate into chronic schizophrenia with severe disability. Family, twin, and adoption studies provide strong evidence to support an important genetic contribution, but the mode of inheritance is not known. Stressful life events are known to trigger or quicken the onset of schizophrenia or to cause relapse. Some abnormal neurological signs have been found in schizophrenics, and it is possible that brain damage, perhaps occurring at birth, may be a cause in some cases. Various biochemical abnormalities have been reported in schizophrenics, but the evidence for the causal relevance of these abnormalities is incomplete. The most successful treatment approaches combine the use of drugs, psychotherapy, and supportive therapy. Psychotherapy serves to relieve the patient's feelings of helplessness and isolation, buttress his or her healthy or positive tendencies, and help him or her to distinguish between psychotic perceptions and reality and to deal with any underlying emotional conflicts that might be exacerbating the condition.

Mood disorders

These disorders are usually restricted to two abnormalities of mood: depression and mania.

Depression is characterized by a sad or hopeless mood, pessimistic thinking, a loss of enjoyment and interest in one's usual activities and pastimes, reduced energy and vitality, increased fatigue, slowness of thought and action, loss of appetite, and disturbed sleep or insomnia.

Mania is characterized by an elated or euphoric mood, quickened thought and accelerated, loud or voluble speech, overoptimism and heightened enthusiasm and confidence, inflated self-esteem, heightened motor activity, irritability, excitement, and a decreased need for sleep.

The DSM-IV defines two major disorders involving depression and mania: bipolar disorder and major depression. A person with bipolar disorder typically experiences discrete episodes of depression and then of mania, lasting for a few weeks or months, with intervening periods of complete normality.

Severe and long-lasting depression without the presence of mania is classified by the DSM-IV as major depression. Depression is a much more common illness than mania, and there are indeed many sufferers from depression who have never experienced mania. Major depression may occur as a single episode, or it may be recurrent. It may also exist with or without melancholia and with or without psychotic features. It seems that both psychosocial and biochemical mechanisms are important in causing depression. Of the latter factor, the best-supported hypotheses suggest that the faulty regulation of the release of one or more naturally occurring amines at sites in the brain where the transmission of nerve impulses takes place may be one cause, with a deficiency of the amines resulting in depression, and an excess causing mania. The treatment of major depressive episodes usually requires antidepressant drugs; electroconvulsive therapy may also be helpful, as may cognitive psychotherapy.

Anxiety disorders

Anxiety has been defined as a feeling of fear, dread, or apprehension that arises without a clear or appropriate real-life justification. Anxiety may arise in response to apparently innocuous situations or may be out of proportion to the actual degree of the external stress. Anxiety also frequently arises as a result of subjective emotional conflicts of which the person may be unaware. The symptoms of anxiety are physical, psychological, and behavioral. Anxiety, especially during panic attacks, can manifest itself in a distinctive set of physical signs that arise from overactivity of the sympathetic nervous system or from tension in skeletal muscles. The sufferer experiences palpitations, dry mouth, dilation of the pupils, shortness of breath, sweating, abdominal symptoms, tightness in the throat, trembling, and dizziness. Aside from the actual feelings of dread and apprehension, the psychological symptoms include irritability, difficulty with concentration, and restlessness. Anxiety may also be manifested in avoidance behavior, for example, running away from the feared object or situation.

Anxiety disorders include phobias, panic disorders, generalized anxiety disorders, obsessive-compulsive disorders, and post-traumatic stress disorders. Phobias are neurotic states accompanied by intense dread of certain objects or situations that would not normally have such an effect. Anxiety disorders in which the anxiety is not aroused by any specific object or situation can basically be subsumed under the headings of panic disorder and generalized anxiety disorder. In obsessive-compulsive disorder, an traumatic stress disorder, symptoms develop in an individual after he or she has experienced a psychologically traumatic event. The traumatic events can include serious automobile accidents, rape or assault, military combat, torture, incarceration in a concentration camp or death camp, and such natural disasters as floods, fires, or earthquakes. A feature of this condition is the person's reexperiencing the traumatic event in nightmares and in intrusive daytime fantasies.

Somatoform disorders

In these conditions, the physical symptoms of the person suggest the presence of organic disease but no such organic disorder can be found upon physical examination and investigation. Instead, there is positive evidence that the symptoms are caused by psychological factors. The production of these symptoms is not under voluntary control.

The sufferer of somatization disorder demands medical attention, but no organic cause is found. The terms *hypochondriasis* and *hysteria* that traditionally designated these disorders are still widely used by psychiatrists.

Factitious disorders

These are characterized by physical or psychological symptoms that are voluntarily self-induced; they are distinguished from hysteria, in which the physical symptoms are produced unconsciously. In factitious disorders, although the person's attempts to create or exacerbate the symptoms of an illness are voluntary, such behavior is neurotic in that the individual is unable to refrain from it; that is, his or her goals, whatever they may be, are involuntarily adopted.

In malingering, by contrast, the person simulates or exaggerates an illness or disability to obtain some kind of discernible personal gain or to avoid an unpleasant situation; for example, a prison inmate may simulate madness to obtain more comfortable living conditions.

It is important to recognize factitious disorders as evidence of psychological disturbance. Treatment is of the underlying conflicts

Dissociative disorders

Dissociation is a syndrome in which one or a group of mental processes are split off, or dissociated, from the

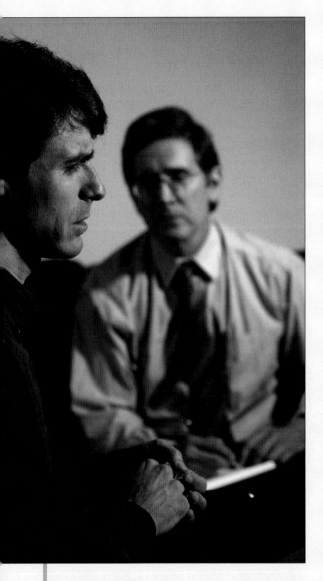

A psychiatrist works with a patient during a therapy session. For less severe forms of mental illness, psychotherapy and behavioral therapy are the treatments that are generally preferred.

individual experiences obsessions or compulsions, or both. Obsessions are recurring words, thoughts, ideas, or images that, rather than being experienced as voluntarily produced, seem to invade a person's consciousness despite his or her attempts to ignore, control, or suppress them.

Compulsions are urges or impulses to perform repetitive acts that are apparently meaningless, unnecessary, stereotyped, or ritualistic. In post-rest of the psychic apparatus so that their function is lost, altered, or impaired. In dissociative disorders there is a sudden, temporary alteration in the person's consciousness, sense of identity, or motor behavior. There may be an apparent loss of memory of previous activities or important personal events, with amnesia for the episode itself after recovery. These are rare conditions, and it is important to exclude organic causes.

Multiple personality is a rare dissociative disorder in which two or more distinct, independent personalities develop in an individual. Each of these personalities inhabits the person's conscious awareness to the exclusion of the others at particular times.

This disorder frequently arises as a result of traumas that were suffered during childhood and is best treated by psychotherapy, which seeks to reunite the various personalities into a single, integrated one.

The causes of depersonalization are obscure, and there is no specific treatment for it. When the symptom arises in the context of another psychiatric condition, treatment is aimed at that illness.

Sexual and gender identity disorders

Sexual and gender identity disorders are related to issues of gender identity. The person has preferences for unusual or bizarre sexual practices or objects.

In transsexualism the person feels a discrepancy between anatomical sex and the gender the person ascribes to himself or herself. The sufferer claims to be a member of the other sex, for example "a female spirit trapped in a male body." He or she may assume the dress and behavior and participate in activities commonly associated with the other sex and may even use hormones and surgery to achieve the physical characteristics of the other sex. The cause of the condition is unknown. Psychiatric treatment is generally supportive in type.

Paraphilias, or sexual deviations, may be classified into disorders of sexual object (for example, fetishes, transvestism, zoophilia, and pedophilia) and of the sexual act (such as exhibitionism, voyeurism, sexual masochism, and sexual sadism). The causes of these conditions are generally not known.

Behavioral, psychodynamic, and pharmacological methods have been used with varying efficacy to treat these disorders.

Eating disorders

Anorexia nervosa is characterized by a body weight more than 25 percent below standard, amenorrhea, a fear of loss of control of eating, and an intense desire to be thin. Though grossly thin, patients nevertheless believe themselves to be fat. They go to enormous lengths to resist eating food and to lose weight, including food avoidance, purging, self-induced vomiting, and vigorous exercise. The condition appears to start with the patient's voluntary control of food intake in response to social pressures such as peer conformity. The disorder is exacerbated by troubled relations within the family. Bulimia nervosa refers to episodic grossly excessive overeating binges. These may alternate with episodes of self-induced vomiting.

Sleep disorders

A sleep disorder is any difficulty with sleep, including difficulty falling asleep or staying asleep, difficulty staying awake during the daytime (excessive sleepiness), too much sleep, difficulty sleeping during normal hours at nighttime, abnormal behaviors during sleep that disrupt sleep, or unrefreshing sleep. Sleep deprivation is a symptom of a sleep disorder. The most common types of sleep disorders include insomnia (a significant lack of high-quality sleep), sleep apnea (an interruption of breathing during sleep), restless leg syndrome (a neurological disorder characterized by uncomfortable, tingly, or creeping sensations in the legs, which creates an uncontrollable urge to keep them moving), periodic limb movement disorder (that is, episodes of rhythmic jerking of the feet or legs during sleep, to the point of disrupting sleep), and narcolepsy (a condition in which someone falls deeply asleep at any time through the day, sometimes with loss of muscle power and hallucinations).

Treatment for the various sleep disorders can include medication, various behavioral therapies, and lifestyle changes.

Impulse-control disorders

These conditions are usually associated with a disorder of personality. There is a failure to resist desires, impulses, or temptations to perform an act that is harmful to the individual or to others.

The individual experiences a feeling of tension before committing the act and a feeling of release or gratification upon completing it. The behaviors involved include pathological gambling, setting fires (pyromania), and impulsive stealing (kleptomania).

Adjustment disorders

These are neurotic conditions in which there is an inappropriate reaction to an external stress occurring within three months of the stress. The symptoms may be out of proportion to the degree of stress, or they may be maladaptive in the sense that they prevent the individual from coping adequately in his social or occupational setting. These disorders are often associated with other neurotic conditions such as anxiety neurosis or minor depression.

Personality disorders

A personality disorder is a deeply ingrained, long-enduring, maladaptive, and inflexible pattern of thinking, feeling, and behaving that either significantly impairs an individual's social or occupational functioning or causes him or her subjective distress. Personality disorders are not illnesses but rather are pronounced accentuations or variations of personality in one or more of its traits. The causes of personality disorders are obscure. There is undoubtedly a constitutional and therefore hereditary element in determining personality type. Psychological and environmental factors are also important in causation; for instance, the association of antisocial personality disorders with other features of social deviance is found in some families and in members of lower socioeconomic groups.

There are numerous different types of personality disorders. Some of them include paranoid personality disorder, in which there is a pervasive and unjustified suspiciousness and mistrust of others, whose words and actions are misinterpreted as having special significance for, and as being directed against, the individual. In affective personality disorder, the trait of anxiety may be persistent and highly developed; a chronic depressive may be persistently gloomy and pessimistic, or may show excessive swings of mood. Someone with explosive personality disorder has a tendency to sudden emotional rages or tantrums that result in physical assault on others. An individual with histrionic personality disorder will be overly dramatic and have intensely expressed behavior, a tendency to call attention to oneself, a craving for novelty and excitement, and tendencies toward dependency. In dependent personality disorder, the person lacks the mental energy and ability to act on his or her own initiative and therefore passively allows others to assume responsibility for major aspects of his or her life. Antisocial personality disorder is marked by a personal history of chronic and continuous antisocial behavior, in which the rights of others are violated, and by poor or nonexistent job performance. It is manifested in persistent criminality, sexual promiscuity or aggressive sexual behavior, and drug use. People with this disorder are impulsive, mendacious, irresponsible, and callous; they feel no guilt over their antisocial acts and fail to learn from their mistakes. In the narcissistic personality disorder, there is a grandiose sense of self-importance and a preoccupation with fantasies of success, power, and achievement. Avoidant personalities are excessively sensitive to social rejection, humiliation, and shame, have low self-esteem, and are deeply upset by the slightest disapproval of others; they are consequently unwilling to enter into relationships but crave affection and acceptance. *Passive-aggressive personality disorder* is the term applied to people who respond aggressively and negatively to demands made upon them by using such passive means as procrastination, dawdling, intentional inefficiency, or deliberate forgetfulness.

Treatments

Psychiatry and related disciplines embrace a wide spectrum of techniques and approaches for treating mental illnesses. These include various types of medications and therapies, either alone or in combination. Certain drugs have been demonstrated to have beneficial effects upon mental illnesses. Antidepressant, antipsychotic, and anti-anxiety drugs are thought to achieve their therapeutic results by the selective inhibition or enhancement of the quantities, action, or breakdown of neurotransmitters in the brain.

Antipsychotic drugs have a calming effect that is valuable in the relief of agitation, excitement, and violent behavior in psychotic patients. The drugs are quite successful in reducing the symptoms of schizophrenia, mania, and delirium, and they are used in combination with antidepressants to treat psychotic depression. The drugs suppress hallucinations and delusions, alleviate disordered or disorganized thinking, improve the patient's lucidity, and generally make him or her more receptive to psychotherapy.

Anti-anxiety medications most commonly used in the treatment of anxiety are the benzodiazepines, or minor tranquilizers, which have replaced barbiturates because of their vastly greater safety. The advantage of benzodiazepines is that they calm the patient without the marked sleep-inducing effects of barbiturates, so that a degree of wakeful alertness is maintained and the individual can carry on his or her daily activities. Smaller doses have a calming effect and alleviate both the physical and psychological symptoms of anxiety. Larger doses induce sleep, and some benzodiazepines are marketed as hypnotics. The benzodiazepines are among the most widely prescribed drugs in the developed world, and controversy has arisen over their excessive use by the public.

Antidepressant medications are prescribed for many patients suffering from depressive illness who gain symptomatic relief from treatment with these drugs. Successful treatment with such drugs relieves all the symptoms of depressive illness, including disturbances of sleep and appetite, loss of sexual desire, and decreased energy, interest, and concentration. Once a good response has been achieved, the drug should be continued in reduced dosage for a further six months. Research has shown that such maintenance treatment greatly reduces the risk of relapse during that time.

Mood-stabilizing medications, such as lithium, are effective in the treatment of an episode of mania. Lithium can drastically reduce the elation, overexcitement, grandiosity, paranoia, irritability, and flights of ideas that are typical of people in the manic state. The most important use of lithium is in the maintenance treatment of patients with bipolar affective disorder (manic-depressive illness) or with recurrent depression. When given while the patient is well, lithium may prevent further mood swings, or it may reduce either their frequency or their severity. Its mode of action is unknown.

Valproate and carbamazepine, anticonvulsant drugs, have been shown to be effective in the treatment of mania and in the maintenance treatment of bipolar affective disorder. It may be combined with lithium in bipolar affective patients who fail to respond to either drug alone. Electroconvulsive treatment (ECT) induces a convulsion in a person by passing an electric current through the brain. The duration of the convulsive activity in the brain appears to determine its therapeutic effects, while the intensity of the electrical stimulus plays a role in determining its unwanted side effects, particularly the short-term memory impairment in the patient immediately after treatment.

Several controlled trials have shown that ECT is effective in treating melancholia in patients suffering from a depressive illness. Whenever rapid improvement is important, ECT is preferred to the treatment of depression with drugs. This is so in cases of severe depression when the patient's life is endangered because of refusal of food and fluids or because of serious risk of suicide, as well as in cases of depression with psychosis after childbirth, when it is desirable to reunite the mother and baby as soon as possible.

Psychotherapy is the treatment of mental discomfort, dysfunction, or disease by psychological means by a trained therapist who adheres to a particular theory of both symptom causation and symptom relief. It is usual to contrast two main forms of psychotherapy: dynamic and behavioral. They are conceptually different; behavioral therapy concentrates on alleviating a patient's overt symptoms, which are attributed to faulty learning, while dynamic therapy concentrates on understanding the meaning of symptoms and understanding the emotional conflicts within the patient that may be causing those symptoms. In their pure forms the two approaches are very different, but in practice many therapists use elements of both.

The repertoire of drugs used in the treatment of mental illness has continued to grow as new drugs are developed or new applications of existing ones are discovered, and research on the biochemical and genetic causes of mental disease continues to make gradual headway in explicating the causes of various disorders. The triad of psychotherapy, drugs, and behavioral therapy afford an unprecedented array of approaches, techniques, and procedures for alleviating symptoms or curing people altogether of mental disorders.

Lori M. Lieving and Oleg V. Tcheremissine

Mental retardation

Mental retardation produces a below-average level of intellectual functioning that leads to limitations in daily living skills. Children with mental retardation learn and develop more slowly than others, and their disability continues in adulthood. The condition, which varies in severity, becomes apparent before children reach the age of 18. Supervision and training can enhance an affected person's quality of life and increase independence.

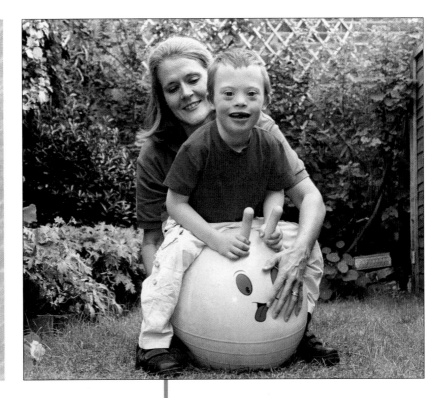

A child with Down syndrome plays in the garden. Down syndrome is a chromosomal abnormality, in which there are three copies of chromosome number 21 instead of two. The condition is thus also called trisomy 21. Children with this condition usually have below-average intellectual function, which causes learning problems.

Mental retardation (MR) demonstrates a pattern of slow learning of basic skills in language and movement (motor skills) that becomes apparent before the age of 18 and often persists throughout adulthood.

People with mental retardation have low intelligence-quotient (IQ) scores, and their adaptive skills are affected because of their intellectual limitations. Examples of adaptive skills are those skills that allow them to function in everyday life. They can include communication, home or living skills, self-care and social skills, academic skills, or job-related skills. Children who have mental retardation typically reach each developmental milestone much later than other children of the same age group.

There are four different degrees of mental retardation, as outlined in the *Diagnostic and Statistical Manual of Mental Disorders*, fourth edition (DSM-IV). People with mild mental retardation have IQ scores between 50 and 70 and can achieve academic skills up to about sixth-grade level. These individuals are able to live independently, with additional support. People with moderate mental retardation have IQ scores between 35 and 55. They can complete daily living tasks with moderate supervision and can func-

tion successfully, usually living in supervised environments such as group homes. Severe mental retardation is defined as an individual with an IQ between 20 and 40. These individuals can master basic self-care skills and some communication, but usually live in a group home. Finally, profound mental retardation is indicated by IQ scores of less than 20 or 25, and people affected to this degree require a high level of supervision to carry out most day-to-day activities.

The American Association on Mental Retardation (AAMR) has also developed a widely accepted diagnostic classification system, which assumes a positive viewpoint and focuses on the capabilities of the individual rather than on his or her limitations. The categories describe the level of appropriate support required, including intermittent, limited, extensive, and pervasive support.

Causes

The causes of mental retardation can arise either during pregnancy or after birth. Prenatal causes of mental retardation can include genetic factors, as well as illnesses or physical or social problems in the mother. About 30 percent of cases of mental retardation are the result of genetic abnormalities. Two of the most common inherited genetic disorders are Down syndrome and fragile X syndrome, which are both characterized by mental and physical disabilities. Single-gene defects such as phenylketonuria (PKU), which disrupts the body's metabolic processes, can also lead to brain damage and mental retardation. In most people with mild mental retardation, no cause is identified.

Risk factors and symptoms

Some of the risk factors are incidents during pregnancy that prevent the infant's head, brain, or central nervous system from developing properly in the uterus and may lead to learning impairments. Factors may include excessive alcohol consumption by the mother; maternal glandular disorders and infections such as toxoplasmosis; and physical problems (for example, high blood pressure) in the mother.

After birth, childhood illnesses, including chicken pox or hyperthyroidism (an excess production of thyroid hormones) can cause mental retardation if not treated appropriately. Childhood injuries, such as a blow to the head or violent shaking, can also cause sufficient brain damage to lead to mental retardation. Infants with insufficient levels of mental and physical stimulation because of malnutrition, abuse, or inadequate health care can also incur permanent learning impairments.

The symptoms of mental retardation are a low IQ score and impaired functioning in the skills needed to live independently. Children with mental retardation may reach developmental milestones, such as crawling, walking, and learning to talk, later than other children. They may also have trouble speaking clearly, remembering information, solving problems, and thinking logically, and their social skills may be limited.

The severity of symptoms varies and is related to the timing and duration of the factors that caused the disability. If retardation is caused by damage to the developing infant during pregnancy, then the symptoms are often apparent from birth or early infancy, especially in severe cases. If the causes of mental retardation occurred after birth, then motor and other skills that were learned during infancy or childhood may suddenly become difficult to complete.

Diagnosis

If mental retardation is suspected, diagnostic investigations begin with the compilation of a full medical, family, and educational history. This is followed by a number of intellectual tests. For a diagnosis of retardation, three criteria must be present. First, a person must have an IQ below 70. Individuals undertake standard intelligence tests to assess their intellectual functioning and learning capabilities. Standardized

KEY FACTS

Description

Significantly below-average intellectual functioning and significant impairment of daily living skills.

Causes and risk factors

Inherited genetic abnormalities are a common cause and account for around 30 percent of mental retardation. Illnesses or other conditions affecting a woman during pregnancy can prevent proper development of the infant in the uterus, leading to mental retardation. Events occurring after birth, including childhood illnesses or injuries and inadequate physical or emotional care, can also cause learning difficulties.

Symptoms

Low IQ scores and limited ability in the skills needed to live independently. Affected children usually reach developmental milestones later than others.

Diagnosis

An IQ of less than 70 and significant limitations in two or more areas of adaptive behavior diagnosed before the age of 18.

Treatments

Special education, training, and supervision. Medication can reduce the symptoms of associated disorders that may interfere with the quality of life and learning.

Pathogenesis

Symptoms become apparent slightly before or at the beginning of the school years. More severe forms of retardation are recognized earlier than milder forms.

Prevention

Genetic counseling and proper prenatal care can help reduce the chances of retardation developing.

Epidemiology

An estimated 2 to 3 percent of the population, about 7 to 8 million people, of the United States have some degree of mental retardation. This varies from mild to severe. It is thought that about 800,000 children are affected by some form of mental retardation in the United States.

tests may include the Stanford-Binet Intelligence Scale, the Weschler Intelligence Scales, or the Kaufman Assessment Battery for Children. Such tests allow a complete assessment of motor, language, learning, and problem-solving skills and provide a specific assessment of IQ.

Second, the individual must experience significant limitations in two or more areas of adaptive behavior (the ability to perform daily activities required for personal and social sufficiency). To determine whether limitations are present, a person's functioning is compared to that of other individuals within the same age range. Specific skills that are considered adaptive include living skills (getting dressed, attending to personal hygiene), communication skills (participating in conversations and following instructions), and social skills with peers and family.

To fulfill the third criterion, signs of intellectual and adaptive impairment must be present before the age of 18. The onset and duration of symptoms is determined from interviews with parents, teachers, or caregivers.

Treatments

Although there is no cure for established MR, support and teaching can be provided to enable most people to develop their potential. The foundation of treatment for MR is to develop a comprehensive management plan for the condition. This plan should include special education, behavioral and occupational therapy, and community services that provide social support and respite care for families affected by mental retardation. Mainstreaming in education (mixed-ability classes) aims to raise the standard of students with MR and encourage higher-level students to take leadership roles.

Federal legislation allows mentally retarded children to be tested and provided with free appropriate training within the school system between the ages of 3 and 21. Early intervention programs help train children with mental retardation in basic skills such as daily hygiene and feeding. In early adulthood, individuals receive training in living and job skills to enable them to live as independently as possible.

There is no specific medication for mental retardation, but individuals may be prescribed several drugs to treat the problems that are sometimes associated with retardation, including aggression, depression, hyperactivity, and self-injury. Although these medications do not treat the specific symptoms of mental impairment, they may prevent problems that could interfere with basic-skills training. For example, drug therapy may help reduce aggression directed toward a caregiver or teacher.

Pathogenesis

Mild MR is likely to be diagnosed after children reach school age. Although social skills may be sufficient in a preschool child, academic and intellectual deficiencies usually become apparent when the child begins elementary school. Individuals with moderate MR are usually diagnosed earlier than those with mild retardation because basic communication deficiencies will appear before a child reaches school age. With a relatively high level of supervision, these individuals usually become competent at occupational tasks. Severe MR is usually apparent at a young age because speech is minimal and motor coordination is poor. Such children typically require extensive supervision, although behavioral approaches can be useful in training them to communicate nonverbally and learn self-care. Individuals with profound MR are severely limited in communication and motor skills and, even as adults, need constant supervision and care.

Prevention and epidemiology

In a family with a history of genetic disorders associated with mental retardation, genetic counseling prior to pregnancy or birth can help reduce the incidence of retardation. In addition, ensuring proper prenatal and postnatal care can help minimize complications that may lead to mental retardation.

The prevalence of mental retardation is approximately 2 to 3 percent of the general population. The highest incidence is in school-age children, peaking between the ages of 10 and 14. Mental retardation is typically more common among men than women. Usually, higher-than-average mortality rates are found among individuals with severe or profound mental retardation, most likely because of complications arising from associated physical disorders. This is particularly so in people with Down syndrome if they have severe mental retardation.

Oleg Tcheremissine and Lori Lieving

See also
• Asperger's syndrome • Attention-deficit hyperactivity disorder • Birth defects
• Blood poisoning • Disabilities • Down syndrome • Fetal alcohol syndrome • Fragile X syndrome • Genetic disorders • Language and speech disorders • Learning disorders
• Mental disorders • Phenylketonuria
• Rubella • Toxoplasmosis

Metabolic disorders

The metabolism involves all the physical and chemical processes that take place in a human body. Disorders of metabolism caused by gene defects can disrupt the way that enzymes work. If an enzyme concerned with important body processes is defective, organs can be damaged or the production of vital hormones can be affected. Disorders also occur when the body lacks an enzyme needed for breaking down food elements; for example, phenylalanine, a constituent of protein, can cause a toxic buildup that may damage a developing

Genes pass on hereditary characteristics, and there are thousands of genes on each chromosome. Genes are made up of lengths of deoxyribonucleic acid (DNA) that contain a long code specifying which of the 20 amino acids found in the blood and in the cells are selected, and in what precise order, to form proteins. Each gene is a sequence of DNA, and each gene codes for a protein. Most of the proteins are enzymes, and there are thousands of different enzymes; specific enzymes are chemical activators that are responsible for construction and normal functioning of the body. Without enzymes, these reactions would be absent or fatally slow. Metabolism is conducted largely under the influence of enzymes, resulting in growth or repair.

Mutations are small errors in the genetic code of genes that can result in incorrect production of enzymes, lack of enzyme production, malfunctioning enzymes, or nonfunctioning enzymes. The defective enzymes resulting from these mutations cause metabolic disorders.

Some hereditary disorders can be diagnosed in the fetus using amniocentesis, chorionic villus sampling, or blood or urine sampling. The physician may recommend dietary changes to compensate for the deficiencies. Metabolic disturbances are classified as follows: those that affect the breakdown of amino acids; those that relate to carbohydrate or sugar metabolism; those related to fat or lipid metabolism; and those that relate to minerals in the blood.

Amino-acid metabolism

Amino acids are the building blocks of proteins. There are about 20 amino acids essential for human metabolism, including phenylalanine, tyrosine, and leucine. Hereditary amino-acid anomalies are mainly concerned with the way that they are broken down. Disorders of amino acid metabolism are phenylketonuria, homocystinuria, tyrosinemia, maple syrup urine disease, and about 35 other rare genetic disorders. The inborn error of metabolism phenylketonuria (PKU) is characterized by a defective enzyme, which normally would break down the amino acid phenylalanine into tyrosine. If phenylalanine is not excluded from the diet, it builds up in the blood and causes problems in the nervous system, including epilepsy and learning difficulties. The amino acid is found in most protein foods, so a modified diet is needed.

RELATED ARTICLES

Children with homocystinuria have an inherited condition in which they are unable to metabolize the amino acid homocystine because they lack an enzyme called cystathionine beta-synthase, which breaks down homocystine. As a result, there is a buildup of toxic by-products, which causes a variety of symptoms. Homocystinuria is rare; it affects about 1 in 200,000 to 335,000 people worldwide.

Homocystinuria is inherited in an autosomal recessive pattern, which means that the child gets the defective gene from both parents (see GENETIC DISORDERS). The gene *CBS* makes the enzyme cystathionine beta-synthase, which processes the amino acid methionine and is involved in the chemical pathway of homocystine. Mutations in the gene disrupt the function of the enzyme, resulting in the buildup of homocystine and other toxic substances in the blood.

Homocystinuria has several features of Marfan's syndrome, including a tall, thin build with long limbs, spidery fingers, high arches, knock-knees, spinal curvature, and osteoporosis. Behavioral and psychiatric conditions, as well as mental retardation, are common. Children are screened for homocystinuria at birth with a blood test, and it is then confirmed by a test measuring enzyme function in the liver or in skin cells. Genetic testing also can reveal the mutation in the cystathionine beta-synthase gene.

Children with tyrosinemia cannot metabolize the amino acid tyrosine. The condition is inherited through an autosomal recessive trait, which means that both parents must carry the gene. Mutations in the *FAH*, *HPD*, and *TAT* genes cause a shortage of one of the enzymes that breaks down tyrosine in a complex five-step process, causing damage to the liver, kidneys, nervous system, and other tissues. There are three types of tyrosinemia, each with distinctive symptoms caused by a deficiency of a different enzyme.

Type I, the most serious, appears in the first few months of life when the child does not gain weight. Other symptoms include vomiting, diarrhea, yellowing of the skin and whites of eyes, a cabbage-like odor, and a tendency to nose bleeds. Liver and kidney failure, problems affecting the nervous system, and an increased risk of cancer can occur. Worldwide, type I tyrosinemia affects about 1 in 100,000 individuals and is common in children of French-Canadian or Scandinavian descent.

INBORN ERRORS OF METABOLISM

The dark urine of one of his pregnant patients puzzled Alexander Garrod (1857–1936), a London physician. He was reminded of a group of physicians in the Middle Ages, who believed they could determine what was wrong with the body by studying urine. From his studies, he realized his patient had a condition now called alkaptonuria. When she gave birth to a child that had blackened urine, Garrod postulated that this condition was caused by some inborn error of metabolism that the mother had passed to the child. Garrod's work received little attention until the 1940s when geneticists, working with fruit flies, first realized that certain inherited conditions were caused by inborn errors of metabolism.

Since genetics has become better understood and the human genome decoded, knowledge about many genetic disorders has grown, and metabolic enzymes are the subjects of continued investigations.

Type II affects the eyes, the skin, and mental development. Symptoms begin early in life and include excessive tearing of the eyes, abnormal sensitivity to light, eye pain and redness, painful skin sores on the palms and soles, and mental retardation. Occurrence is less than 1 in 250,000 people.

Type III, which is rare, has only a few cases in the medical literature. Characteristic features include mental retardation, seizures, and loss of balance and coordination.

The three types of tyrosinemia are caused by deficiencies in different enzymes that affect tyrosine. An experimental drug, which blocks the production of the toxic substances, may help children with type I, and often these children require a liver transplant. Restriction of tyrosine in the diet may help children with type II but not type I.

Children with maple sugar urine disease (MSUD) have obvious symptoms in the first few days of life. First, the urine has the odor of burned maple sugar, and the child refuses to eat, is lethargic, and has convulsions in the first few days of life. Amino acids accumulate in the blood, causing toxic effects.

Both parents must carry the gene for MSUD. First described in 1954, MSUD affects about 1 in 120,000 live births and is common among Mennonites, affecting about 1 in 760 births in this group. Several states require testing at birth for this condition. Treatment for MSUD is a lifelong restriction of foods that contain the three amino acids. Adhering closely to the restricted diet may enable people with MSUD to live long and relatively healthy lives.

Carbohydrate metabolism

Complex carbohydrates (polysaccharides) are starches, cellulose (fiber), and gums. Humans do not have enzymes to break down cellulose but do have enzymes to break down starches. Cellulose is valuable as dietary fiber. Simple carbohydrates (sugars; monosaccharides or disaccharides) result from the breakdown of polysaccharides. The final product is the monosaccharide glucose, which is the principal fuel of the body. Bread, pasta, rice, and other carbohydrate-containing foods have long chains of complex carbohydrates. Enzymes must break down the chains before the body can use glucose for energy. If a required enzyme is missing, carbohydrates can accumulate in the bloodstream and cause problems.

METABOLIC SYNDROME OR SYNDROME X

People with metabolic syndrome, also called syndrome X, have a cluster of major risk factors for cardiovascular disease. Affected people have very high blood levels of glucose, often due to insulin resistance, and high blood levels of triglycerides and cholesterol. They may also have high blood pressure, kidney disorders, and blood-clotting disorders. People with metabolic syndrome tend to have a sedentary lifestyle, be overweight, and have a high intake of carbohydrates, often in the form of alcohol. Their fat is usually concentrated in the abdominal cavity (an "apple-shaped" body). Some researchers believe there is a genetic basis for the syndrome, involving neurotransmitters in the brain. Genetics appears to load the gun, but behavior and lifestyle pull the trigger, resulting in life-threatening heart and cardiovascular disease.

Disorders related to carbohydrate metabolism are glycogen storage diseases, diabetes, hereditary fructose intolerance, and gout.

Glucose and glycogen storage diseases

Diabetes occurs in two ways. The most serious form, type 1, is caused by the failure of the pancreas to produce insulin. Type 2 diabetes has a variety of causes, including insulin resistance. It is also known as maturity-onset diabetes and is caused by a relative insufficiency of insulin as a result of impaired sensitivity of cells to the actions of the hormone. Other important factors are obesity, which requires larger amounts of insulin; abnormal beta cell function; and excessively raised intracellular triglycerides. The rise in obesity has been accompanied by a rise in the prevalence of type 2 diabetes, which has the same serious complications as type 1 diabetes.

The opposite is true with hypoglycemia. When too little glucose circulates in the blood, body cells cannot produce energy. The condition can occur if the dose of insulin that a diabetic person takes is too large, if they miss a meal, or they take excessive physical activity. Common symptoms are weakness, trembling, dizziness, rapid heart rate, and cold perspiration. Headache or confusion may follow. In most cases, treatment is to take a simple carbohydrate or sugar that will raise the blood glucose level in 10 to 15 minutes.

Many glucose, or simple sugar molecules, linked together form glycogen. The body uses glucose as the main source of energy, but glucose not immediately used is stored in the liver, muscles, and kidneys in the form of glycogen. When one of the enzymes essential to the process of forming or breaking down of glycogen is missing, the person may have a glycogen storage disease. About one in 20,000 infants inherit some form of glycogen storage disease. Inheritance is autosomal recessive.

Some of the storage disorders have few symptoms. Others are fatal. The symptoms vary considerably among the types. The following disorders are types of glycogen storage diseases.

Type 0 causes an enlarged liver with an accumulation of fat inside the liver cells. It also affects the muscles.

Type IA, or von Gierke's disease, causes an

enlarged liver and kidney, slowed growth, and very low blood sugar levels. There may also be abnormally high levels of acid, fats, and uric acid in the blood.

Type IB affects the liver and kidneys and causes a low white blood count. Recurring infections in the mouth and intestines may lead to Crohn's disease, an inflammatory disease that affects the intestines.

Type II, or Pompe's disease, affects all organs.

Type III, or Forbe's disease, causes an enlarged liver or cirrhosis, low blood sugar levels, muscle and heart damage.

Type IV, or Andersen's disease, causes cirrhosis in juveniles, muscle damage, and heart failure in adults.

Type V, or McArdie's disease, causes muscle cramps during physical activity.

Type VI, or Her's disease, enlarges the liver with episodes of low blood sugar when fasting, but often there are no symptoms.

Type VII, or Tarui's disease, affects skeletal muscles and red blood cells.

Diagnosis of glycogen storage disorder is made by chemical examination of a sample of muscle or liver to determine which enzyme is missing. Treatment depends on the type of disease. For most people, eating several small high-carbohydrate meals daily prevents blood sugar levels from dropping. The inability to metabolize galactose, one of the sugars found in milk, causes the disorder galactosemia. The enzyme deficiency affects about one in 40,000 to 50,000 people and if left untreated can cause brain damage, cataracts in the eyes, and kidney and liver problems. A routine blood test to detect the disorder is required of newborns in almost all states. Eliminating milk and other fruits and vegetables that might contain galactose is essential. People with the disorder must restrict galactose throughout their lives.

A metabolic inability to utilize fructose causes a by-product of fructose to accumulate in the body, blocking the formation of glycogen and its conversion to energy. In people with this condition, very small amounts of fructose or sucrose cause low blood sugar levels with symptoms of sweating, confusion, and occasionally seizures and coma. Chemical examination of the liver determines if the enzyme is missing.

Treatment involves excluding fructose found in fruits, sucrose, and sorbitol from the diet. Sometimes

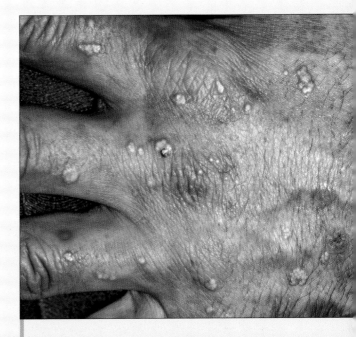

Cysts and scars on this hand are a result of **Porphyria cuatanea tarda,** *a type of porphyria that results from a defective enzyme in the liver. The enzyme normally breaks down substances called porphyrins, but in its absence, porphyrins build up in the skin, which then becomes sensitive to light. Any exposure of the skin causes blistering and scarring.*

people will excrete fructose in urine, a hereditary condition called fructosuria. This condition is harmless and needs no treatment but can lead to an incorrect diagnosis of diabetes.

Lipid metabolism

Specific enzymes called lipases break down fats or lipids or fats in the body. However, if the enzyme is not present, specific fatty substances can accumulate over time and damage tissues and organs. These abnormalities are called lipidoses, or fatty acid oxidation disorders. Most of these conditions are rare and found in certain ethnic groups. The following disorders are related to fat metabolism.

Gaucher's disease is the most common form of lipidosis, causing toxic products to accumulate in tissues. The disease, which is common in Ashkenazi Jews of eastern European descent, leads to an enlarged liver and brownish pigmentation of the skin. Many people with Gaucher's disease can be treated with enzyme replacement therapy.

WAS KING GEORGE III MAD OR MISUNDERSTOOD?

King George III of England, who reigned during the American Revolution, was known for his bizarre behavior, which often resulted in him being constrained in a straitjacket or chained to a chair. In the 1970s medical investigators revisited the king's medical records and found a symptom of porphyria: dark red urine. Researchers have found that one trigger of porphyria in adults is exposure to arsenic. They knew that the king had used a skin cream with arsenic and that the powder of his wig contained the chemical. Later it was found that the king had been given a compound of antimony with traces of arsenic for his mental illness. Mary Queen of Scots may also have suffered from porphyria.

Niemann-Pick disease also affects Jewish people. The effect of the disease is an accumulation of sphingomyelin, a product of fat metabolism, and cholesterol buildup. None of the three types of this disease can be cured, and children tend to die of infection or central nervous system disorders. It is similar to Tay-Sachs disease, another genetic disorder, which causes a fatal buildup of substances called sphyngolipids in the brain.

Fabry's disease causes glycolipid, a product of fat metabolism, to accumulate in tissue. This disorder is due to a defective gene carried on the X chromosome and is only seen in males. Affected men can live into adulthood but develop kidney failure and heart disease.

Tangier disease is a rare genetic disorder characterized by an enlarged liver and spleen in later life. The person may also have reoccurring neuropathy, which is disease of the nerves.

Porphyrias and metal accumulations

Deficiencies involved in the production of heme, the chemical compound that gives blood its red color, causes a group of disorders called porphyrias. Two groups of porphyrias occur, according to where the dysfunction occurs. They are hepatic porphyrias, which involve the liver, and erythropoitic porphyrias, which are related to the formation of the red blood cells in the bone marrow.

Three major findings characterize porphyrias: sensitivity to light and a tendency to develop rashes; neuropsychiatric disorders such as delusions; and severe abdominal pains or cramping followed by vomiting or constipation. Other signs and symptoms may include numbness and tingling that can result in weakness and paralysis, and sensitivity to light, causing the skin to redden, become painful, feel hot, or puffy. The urine of affected people is often dark red, purplish, or brown.

Porphyrias can be autosomal dominant or autosomal recessive, depending on the type. In autosomal dominant disorders, the gene that is defective is dominant compared to the normal gene, so that only one copy of the dominant gene is needed to cause a disorder. In autosomal recessive disorder, the faulty gene is recessive compared to the normal gene, so that two copies of the faulty gene (one copy from each parent) are needed to produce the disorder.

Some types of porphyria begin in early childhood, some at puberty, and others begin during adulthood. Diagnosis involves blood or urine tests that measure chemicals involved in heme production. Treatments include maintenance of electrolyte balance and an increase of carbohydrate intake. The porphyrias are lifelong conditions, but with good long-term management, the person can expect extended periods without significant problems.

Hemochromatosis is a condition caused by increased iron absorption that leads to an accumulation of iron in tissue. Symptoms include fatigue, pain, impotence, absence of menstrual period, and palpitations. The disease may be fatal if untreated.

Wilson's disease is a rare autosomal recessive inherited disease that is primarily caused by an accumulation of copper in tissues all over the body, especially the liver, brain, kidneys, and cornea. Due to an unknown metabolic abnormality, the liver does not excrete copper in the bile. Symptoms include tremors, spasticity, and rigidity. Diagnosis is based on finding increased amounts of liver and urinary copper. Treatment involves taking the drug penicillamine for life.

Evelyn Kelly

Migraine

Migraine is characterized by intense pulsing or throbbing pain in one area of the head, accompanied by extreme sensitivity to light and sound, nausea, and vomiting. Some people can predict the onset of a migraine because it is preceded by an "aura," a type of visual disturbance that appears as flashing lights, zigzag lines, or a temporary loss of vision. Migraine is three times more common in women than in men.

Migraine headaches are a legitimate biological disease consisting of severe, painful headaches and extreme sensitivity to light and sound. Migraines can often be recurring and disabling. These types of headaches are also associated with nausea and vomiting. Some migraine sufferers also experience an aura, a warning in which visual disturbances appear as flashing lights, zigzag lines, or even a temporary loss of vision that forecast an oncoming migraine.

Typically, people with migraine tend to have recurring attacks triggered by eating certain foods, a lack of food or sleep, exposure to light, or hormonal irregularities (only in women). Anxiety, stress, or relaxation after stress can also be triggers.

About 13 percent of the U.S. population—28 million Americans—suffer from migraines. Migraine is more common than asthma, diabetes, and coronary artery disease combined. It afflicts both women and men, but three times more women experience migraine. The first attack usually occurs before the age of 30, but even children as young as 2 years can be affected by migraine. Migraine is a chronic, recurrent disease. Although some people have attacks several times a month, sufferers typically experience an average of two attacks per month, which can last any duration between 4 and 72 hours.

Causes

Although the cause of migraines is unknown, there are many theories put forward by the medical and research communities. For many years, it was believed that migraines were linked to the dilation and constriction of blood vessels of the dura mater (the outer covering of the brain). However, recent evidence has led investigators to believe that migraine is caused by inherited abnormalities in genes that control the activities of certain cell populations in the brain. A predominant theory is that migraines are caused by functional changes in the trigeminal nerve system, a major pain pathway in the nervous system, and by imbalances in brain chemicals such as serotonin, which regulates pain messages passing through this pathway. During a migraine, serotonin levels drop. Researchers believe this causes the trigeminal nerve to release substances called neuropeptides, which travel to the dura mater. There, they cause blood vessels to become dilated and inflamed. The result is a headache. Because levels of magnesium, a mineral involved in the functioning of neurons, also drop right before or during a migraine, it is possible that low amounts of magnesium may cause nerve cells in the brain to misfire.

KEY FACTS

Description

A headache of intense pulsing or throbbing pain in one area of the head.

Causes

Unknown but there are many theories.

Risk factors

Family history and being young and female, along with a number of triggers including hormonal changes, certain foods, stress, sensory stimuli, changes in the environment or schedule, and certain drugs.

Symptoms

Recurring attacks of severe pain on one or both sides of the head, nausea, vomiting, and sensitivity to light and sound.

Diagnosis

Medical history; physical exam; CT or MRI scan.

Treatments

Drugs for pain relief and prevention.

Pathogenesis

Drop in serotonin thought to cause the trigeminal nerve to release neuropeptides, causing inflammation of the brain's outer covering (dura mater).

Prevention

Avoiding migraine triggers.

Epidemiology

More than 28 million Americans—three times more women than men—suffer from migraine headaches.

Risk factors

Whatever the exact mechanism of migraine headaches, a number of factors may trigger them. Common migraine headache triggers include hormonal changes, sensory stimuli, foods, stress, changes in the environment or schedule, and certain drugs. Although the exact relationship between hormones and headaches is not clear, fluctuations in the hormones estrogen and progesterone seem to trigger migraine headaches in many women. Women with a history of migraines often have reported headaches immediately before or during their menstrual periods. Others report more migraines during pregnancy or menopause. Hormonal drugs, such as contraceptives and hormone replacement therapy, also may worsen migraines. Sensory stimuli such as bright lights and sun glare can produce headaches, as can pleasant scents, such as perfume and flowers, and unpleasant odors, such as paint thinner and secondhand smoke. Certain foods appear to trigger headaches in some people. Common offenders include alcohol, especially beer and red wine; aged cheeses; chocolate; fermented, pickled or marinated foods; aspartame; caffeine; monosodium glutamate, which is a key ingredient in some Asian foods; certain seasonings; and many canned and processed foods. However, skipping meals or fasting also can trigger migraines. Behavioral aspects such as stress, intense physical exertion, including sexual activity, changes in sleep patterns (too much or too little sleep), or changes in the weather, season, altitude, barometric pressure, or time zone may provoke migraines as well. Also, certain drugs can aggravate migraines. Thus, there are many aspects to migraine triggers. Triggers are not the same for everyone; what causes a migraine in one person may relieve it in another.

The definite risk factors for developing migraines are family history and being young and female. Migraine is often hereditary. In fact, a child has a 50 percent chance of becoming a sufferer if one parent suffers and a 75 percent chance if both parents suffer. The fact that young women are more likely to suffer from migraines possibly reflects the puzzling relationship between migraines and hormones. Many people find that their attacks of migraine lessen and are not as severe as they get older.

Signs and symptoms

Migraine headaches are characterized by throbbing head pain, usually located on one side of the head and often accompanied by nausea and sensitivity to light or sound or both. The combination of disabling pain and associated symptoms often prevents sufferers from performing daily activities. Symptoms, incidence, and severity vary by individual. Less than a third of sufferers experience what is called an aura. They may see flashes of light, blind spots, zigzag lines, and shimmering lights and may experience vision loss and numbness prior to the head pain and other symptoms.

Diagnosis

Typically, diagnosis of migraine is simple, involving only a medical history and physical examination. Occasionally, CT (computed tomography) or MRI (magnetic resonance imaging) scans and lumbar puncture are conducted to rule out underlying causes.

Treatments

Drugs are the primary treatment for migraine. Drugs for migraines fall into two classes: pain-relieving drugs that stop pain once it has started, and preventive drugs that reduce or prevent a future migraine headache. Pain-relief drugs such as nonsteroidal anti-inflammatory drugs (NSAIDs) can treat the inflammation in the dura mater, whereas drugs called triptans and ergots can treat the blood-vessel dilation in the brain and dura mater, and others still can treat nausea and vomiting. Preventive drugs can reduce the frequency, severity, and length of migraines and may increase the effectiveness of pain-relieving drugs used during migraine attacks. Preventive drugs include cardiovascular drugs, antidepressants, NSAIDs, antiseizure drugs, and cyproheptadine, an antihistamine. Overall, there are many treatment options for people who suffer from migraine headaches.

Epidemiology

Sources from the American Medical Association report that approximately 6 percent of men and 18 percent of women suffer from migraine in the United States. The age range of those people most likely to report migraine is 24 to 44 years. People who suffer from migraine typically have 24 to 35 attacks each year.

Rashmi Nemade

See also
• Alcohol-related disorders • Allergy and sensitivity • Anxiety disorders • Childhood disorders • Diagnosis • Environmental disorders • Genetic disorders • Hormonal disorders • Nervous system disorders • Nutritional disorders • Treatment

Miscarriage

A miscarriage, also known as a spontaneous abortion, is a pregnancy that spontaneously ends before the fetus is able to live outside the uterus. *Therapeutic abortion* is the equivalent term for an elective termination of pregnancy, which lay people often refer to as an abortion. About 15 to 20 percent of women who know they are pregnant will spontaneously miscarry. However, many pregnancies end before women even realize they are pregnant. Miscarriages generally occur before 20 to 22 weeks of pregnancy and most take place in the first trimester (first three months of pregnancy). Miscarriage is the most common problem in early pregnancy.

Genetic abnormalities, such as too few or too many chromosomes, are the most common reason for miscarriages. This is especially true during the early part of a pregnancy. Less commonly, a medical problem with the mother can lead to a miscarriage. These problems include uncontrolled diabetes mellitus or the uterus being abnormally structured, which prevents the normal growth and development of a pregnancy.

The single biggest risk factor for miscarriage is the increasing age of the mother. This probably relates to a higher risk of chromosomal abnormalities, and a woman more than 40 has a risk of miscarriage of 40 percent or more. Smoking more than 10 cigarettes each day or consuming more than 30 ounces (880 ml) of alcohol per month also increase the chance of a miscarriage. Taking in 500 milligrams or more of caffeine per day has been linked to an increased rate of miscarriage. One cup of coffee contains 0.003 to 0.005 ounces (100 to 135 mg) of caffeine. Infections, such as herpes, may be linked to miscarriage. Contrary to popular belief, abdominal injuries in early pregnancy, such as falling down stairs or having a motor vehicle accident, are unlikely to result in miscarriage.

If a woman has had one previous miscarriage, the probability of miscarriage during her next pregnancy is not significantly elevated and remains at about 20 percent. After two miscarriages, the probability of miscarriage is 28 percent, but it rises to 43 percent after three previous miscarriages. However, the majority of pregnancies still result in the delivery of a baby, even in women who have had three miscarriages.

Symptoms

The most common symptoms of miscarriages are vaginal bleeding or abdominal cramping, or both, similar to a very heavy period. The vaginal bleeding can vary from light spotting to (rarely) hemorrhaging requiring a blood transfusion. There are different types of miscarriages. Passing all the pregnancy tissue is known as a complete miscarriage. If some of the pregnancy tissue is not passed and remains in the uterus, this is known as an incomplete miscarriage. A threatened miscarriage is when a woman has bleeding but the pregnancy is ongoing. Threatened miscarriages occur in up to 50 percent of pregnancies, but only half of these will miscarry. An inevitable miscarriage is one

KEY FACTS

Description
Spontaneous ending of a pregnancy before the fetus is able to survive outside the womb (uterus).

Causes
Usually genetic (chromosomal) abnormalities of the fetus. Less commonly, medical problems with the mother such as uncontrolled diabetes or structural abnormalities.

Risk factors
Advancing age, previous miscarriages, smoking, alcohol or drug use, high caffeine intake.

Symptoms
Vaginal bleeding or abdominal pain, or both.

Diagnosis
Pelvic examination; blood tests; ultrasound.

Treatments
Surgical procedure (dilatation and curettage); drugs that cause the uterus to pass any remaining tissue; observation.

Prevention
Treat any correctable causes, such as malformation of the uterus; avoidance of tobacco and drugs.

Epidemiology
15 to 20 percent of women who know they are pregnant have a miscarriage. Many miscarriages occur before women know they are pregnant.

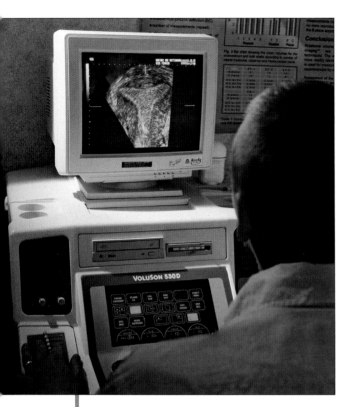

A gynecologist performs an ultrasound scan on a woman's uterus. The uterus shows a congenital deformation called uterus arcuatus; it has a Y shape instead of a rounded top. This malformation may result in infertility or miscarriage.

in which the cervix (the lower opening of the uterus) is open. Although the pregnancy is still inside the uterus, a miscarriage cannot be avoided.

Septic miscarriages are uncommon, accounting for less than 2 percent of all miscarriages. Septic miscarriages result from an infection in the uterus, often due to a foreign object being placed in the uterus, such as during an illegal abortion. In addition to bleeding and pain, symptoms of septic miscarriage include fever, chills, and possibly a thick, yellow-green, foul-smelling vaginal discharge. A septic miscarriage can be very dangerous if not treated in a timely manner.

Diagnosis

The most helpful blood test in early pregnancy is the beta human chorionic gonadotropin (B-hCG) test. This test confirms the presence of a pregnancy, and serial measurements can help determine whether it is healthy. An ultrasound uses sound waves without radiation to examine pregnancies for their location and health and is very useful in diagnosing miscarriages. A

pregnancy cannot usually be seen with an ultrasound until about five weeks of age. If the pregnancy is more than six weeks old, a fetal heartbeat may be seen. Obversation of a fetal heartbeat on ultrasound is a reassuring sign that the pregnancy is likely to continue.

Treatments

Treatments for miscarriages include surgery, drug treatment, or observation. Surgical treatment consists of a dilatation and curettage (D and C) or, later in pregnancy, a dilatation and evacuation (D and E). Both of these involve gently dilating the cervix and removing the pregnancy contents inside the uterus. Surgery is the fastest way to treat a miscarriage and is the preferred choice for women who are bleeding heavily or have a septic miscarriage. Although very safe, the risks of this surgery include damaging the uterus or causing an infection. These complications may diminish future fertility. Management with drugs is an option for women whose pregnancy is less than 12 weeks and who wish to avoid surgery. Currently, misoprostol is the drug most commonly used to treat miscarriage in the United States. The most common side effects from misoprostol are nausea, vomiting, and severe cramping. This treatment results in successful expulsion of the pregnancy 70 to 90 percent of the time. A dilatation and curettage may need to be done if the treatment with misoprostol is unsuccessful. Observation, or expectant management, is the third option for women without significant bleeding, cramping, or signs of infection. Most miscarriages will be naturally expelled within the first two weeks after diagnosis. If this does not happen, the woman can then undergo surgery or treatment with drugs.

Emotional impact of miscarriage

Grieving and a profound sense of loss often accompany a miscarriage, with the intensity of these symptoms varying among patients. Frequently, women blame themselves for their loss. It is often helpful to explain to patients that most miscarriages are due to genetic abnormalities and reassure them that they did not cause the miscarriage. Also, it is important to explain that one miscarriage does not lessen a woman's chance of having a successful pregnancy in the future.

Emily White and Gary Frishman

See also
- Birth defects • Diabetes • Ectopic pregnancy
- Genetic disorders • Pregnancy and childbirth
- Smoking-related disorders

Mononucleosis

Also called the "kissing disease," mono, and Pfeiffer's disease in North America and glandular fever in other countries, mononucleosis is characterized by sore throat, fever, and enlarged lymph nodes, particularly those in the neck. The disease most commonly affects people between the ages of 12 and 20 years.

Mononucleosis was first described in Germany in 1889 as *drusenfieber*, meaning "glandular fever." In 1920, the term *infectious mononucleosis* was applied to six college students who developed an illness that was characterized by fever and an increased count of white blood cells called lymphocytes. Since then, research has shown that 90 percent of mononucleosis syndromes are a result of infection with the Epstein-Barr virus (EBV). Other infections that have symptoms that may resemble mononucleosis include acute toxoplasmosis, a protozoan infection obtained from cats or from eating raw meats; acute cytomegalovirus (CMV) infection, a viral infection of white blood cells; hepatitis B, a viral infection that can cause liver inflammation; and infection with human immunodeficiency virus (HIV), which in its early stages has symptoms similar to those of mononucleosis.

Herpes family of viruses

EBV is a virus in the herpes family that has a predilection for infecting B lymphocytes. Once inside these cells, the virus can become a persistent, lifelong (but generally silent) infection, reactivating when the immune defenses weaken. EBV is nearly ubiquitous in humans, with 90 to 95 percent of adults harboring evidence of past infection. The virus is transmitted by intimate contact, often through saliva, hence the nickname "kissing disease." Asymptomatic carriers can shed the virus in their saliva for over a year and sometimes intermittently throughout their life.

Symptoms and signs

Mononucleosis occurs in a wide range of ages from childhood to adulthood, but in developed countries the disease most commonly affects preadolescents and adolescents. Young children often do not have symptoms. Classically, adolescents with mononucleosis have the triad of moderate to high fever, sore throat, and enlarged lymph nodes. These symptoms occur after a four- to seven-week incubation, during which people may have milder symptoms, such as headache, fatigue, and a slightly raised temperature. Other symptoms that may occur include rash, enlargement of the spleen, swelling around the eye, yellowing of the white of the eyes (jaundice), anemia, and neurological syndromes. There is an interesting phenomenon in which patients who are treated with the antibiotic amoxicillin for the possibility of a streptococcal throat infection, but who actually have Epstein-Barr infection, develop a rash.

KEY FACTS

Description

A syndrome characterized by fever and enlarged lymph nodes caused by a number of different pathogens.

Causes

Predominantly caused by the Epstein-Barr virus, but also by HIV, *Toxoplasma* protozoa, hepatitis B virus, and the cytomegalovirus. Transmitted by intimate physical contact, including via passage of saliva during kissing.

Risk factors

Close contact with someone suffering from mononucleosis.

Symptoms and signs

Fever, sore throat, enlarged lymph nodes, fatigue, malaise, enlarged spleen, rash. Complications include splenic rupture, tonsil enlargement, persisting fatigue, and neurological syndromes.

Diagnosis

Blood tests, including a complete blood count and finding a heterophile antibody. Serology may be done to help confirm the diagnosis.

Treatments

Supportive care.

Pathogenesis

May result in chronic fatigue syndrome.

Prevention

Physical activity limited to prevent splenic rupture and to allow the body to recover from fatigue.

Epidemiology

Nearly all humans infected by adulthood. Once infected, the virus can persist in an individual in a silent state, reactivating when the immune system weakens.

Diagnosis

Mononucleosis should be suspected in patients who display the classic triad of symptoms. The addition of blood tests help confirm the diagnosis. A complete blood count and a smear of blood may show an elevated lymphocyte count and a small percentage of atypical lymphocytes. These abnormal lymphocytes are large, with generous cytoplasm, and often are seen to be sticking to nearby cells. Liver enzymes may also be elevated on blood tests. Serology studies, the measurement of a person's immune response against an antigen, can be helpful in diagnosing the specific cause of mononucleosis.

In about 90 percent of patients with a mononucleosis syndrome due to EBV, the diagnosis can be made by finding a heterophile antibody. This is an antibody found in infected people that has the ability to clump sheep red blood cells. In the same blood sample, specific antibodies against EBV can also be screened for.

If evidence of EBV cannot be confirmed, further serological tests can be carried out to look for the other potential causes of mononucleosis, including tests for HIV, CMV, *Toxoplasma*, and hepatitis viruses.

Treatments

Therapy for mononucleosis is mainly supportive. Providing adequate rest, fluids, and nutrition, along with pain control with acetaminophen or nonsteroidal anti-inflammatory drugs such as ibuprofen, are usually all that is needed.

Complications

A rare, but potentially life-threatening complication of mononucleosis due to Epstein-Barr infection involves the spleen. About 50 percent of people with mononucleosis due to EBV will have splenic enlargement. Very rarely, this enlargement can lead to rupture and disastrous internal bleeding. Although half of these cases are spontaneous, it is important that infected individuals, especially those with an enlarged spleen, limit participation in contact sports.

Recovering from the tiredness brought on by mononucleosis may take several weeks or even months. Experts recommend limiting activity for at least three weeks after the start of the illness for noncontact sports, and a minimum of four weeks for contact sports such as football. However, if the spleen is still enlarged after four weeks, it is prudent to continue to limit activity. Athletes should return to activity gradually, as the fatigue from the illness may prevent them from reaching preinfection activity levels until several months later.

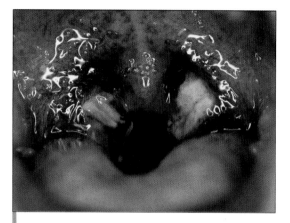

This inflamed throat, with the tonsils covered in a thick white coating, is a typical symptom of mononucleosis. This infection is usually caused by the Epstein–Barr virus, which belongs to the herpes virus family.

Another potentially dangerous complication of mononucleosis is the extreme enlargement of the tonsils, lymphoid tissue located on both sides of the back of the throat. These can grow and touch one another—a condition that is often called "kissing tonsils"—which can lead to airway obstruction that requires placement of a mechanical airway.

A more common complication often seen by physicians is fatigue and sleepiness that persists for months after the acute illness. Usually these individuals improve, and their symptoms will resolve in less than six months, but some continue to have fatigue for over a year. It is thought that EBV triggers chronic fatigue syndrome in these people.

Other rare complications of mononucleosis due to Epstein-Barr infection include encephalitis (infection and inflammation of the brain) and a rare syndrome known as Guillain-Barré syndrome. In this syndrome the coating of the nerve axons is destroyed, starting from the toes, and gradually progresses up the body, resulting in an ascending paralysis. However, most people do make a complete recovery from the syndrome, although some suffer repeated attacks and have a residual weakness.

Edward Cachay and Sanjay Mehta

See also
- Epstein-Barr infection • Guillain-Barré syndrome • Hepatitis infections • Herpes infections • Infections, viral • Liver and spleen disorders • Paralysis • Prevention • Throat infections

Mood disorders

Mood disorders, also known as affective disorders, are a group of disorders that display an abnormal range of moods that fluctuate between extremes of lows and highs and result in impairment in social and occupational functioning. They are one of the most ancient and common mental disorders affecting the general population.

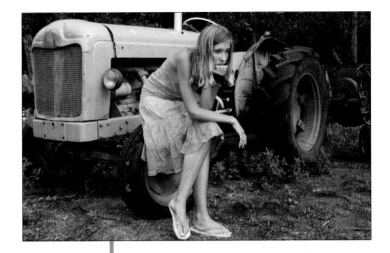

M ood disorders are defined by their patterns of mood episodes. Depressive disorders include major depression and dysthymic disorder. Bipolar disorders consist of bipolar I, bipolar II, and cyclothymic disorder.

People who have affective disorders, such as bipolar disorders, may feel elated and depressed at the same time. Two chemicals in the brain, serotonin and norepinephrine, are imbalanced and are believed to influence mood swings.

Causes of mood disorders

The exact causes are unknown, but genetic, biochemical, psychosocial, and environmental factors each may contribute. The genetic factor for depressive disorder suggests that first-degree relatives are 2 to 3 times more likely to have a major depressive disorder. Twin studies reported 50 percent of identical twins and 10 to 25 percent of fraternal twins are affected with depressive disorders.

First-degree relatives of patients with bipolar disorder are 8 to 18 times more likely to develop the illness. Twin studies reported 75 percent of identical and 5 to 25 percent of fraternal twins are affected with bipolar disorders.

Biochemical causes of mood disorders include a decrease in certain neurotransmitters (brain chemicals) such as serotonin, norepinephrine, and dopamine. Individuals with bipolar disorder may have increased norepinephrine, serotonin, and dopamine in the central nervous system (CNS).

Stressful life events more often cause a first episode of mood disorders (major depressive disorders and bipolar I disorders). The loss of one parent before age 11 most often causes depression at a later age. Environmental stressors, for example, the death of a relative or of a spouse, are most often associated with the onset of depression.

Risk factors

In addition to the above factors, certain medical conditions, including thyroid diseases, adrenal diseases, and hormonal imbalance are risk factors for developing a mood disorder. Other known risk factors are certain medications, such as antihypertensive medications, bronchodilators, and levodopa. The abuse of central nervous system (CNS) depressants such as alcohol and sedative-hypnotics or CNS stimulants such as amphetamines and cocaine, viral infections such as mononucleosis, and HIV infection can all increase the chance of developing a depressive disorder.

Major depression

The symptoms of major depression include feelings of intense sadness that cause daily life to become very difficult. A person with major depression tends to be in a depressed mood most of the day, loses interest in pleasurable activities, has changes in appetite or body weight (increased or decreased), has feelings of worthlessness or excessive guilt, insomnia or hypersomnia, decreased concentration, restlessness or slowness, fatigue or loss of energy, recurrent thoughts of death, and suicidal ideations or attempts.

The criteria for diagnosis of major depression are that a person must have at least two weeks of either a depressed mood or the loss of interest or pleasure in nearly all activities. The individual must have at least five of the symptoms. These symptoms cannot be due to substance abuse or medical conditions, and they must cause social or occupational impairment.

Hospitalization is indicated if the patient is at risk of suicide or unable to care for him- or herself. Selective serotonin reuptake inhibitors (SSRIs), tricyclic antidepressants, and atypical antidepressants are types of antidepressant medications. Electric shock treatment is recommended for a person with a severe form of depression that is not responsive to medications. Psychotherapy (counseling) for major depression includes supportive, cognitive, and behavioral therapy. The natural course of depressive episodes is from 6 months to 13 months, and if left untreated, depressive episodes are self-limiting.

There is a 50 percent risk of having a subsequent major depressive episode within the first two years after the first episode. About 15 percent of patients will eventually commit suicide.

Antidepressant medications significantly reduce the length and severity of symptoms. To reduce the risk of subsequent episodes, antidepressants could be used prophylactically between major depressive episodes. Approximately 75 percent of patients are treated successfully with medications.

The average age of the onset of major depression is 40. Women are twice as likely to be affected with this disorder as men. Lifetime prevalence is 15 percent; in the elderly the prevalence is from 25 to 50 percent. There are no ethnic or socioeconomic differences associated with this disorder.

KEY FACTS: DEPRESSIVE DISORDERS

Description
Depressive disorders are mood disorders with both severe and mild forms of depression.

Causes
Unknown, but genetic and bio-psychosocial factors may each contribute.

Risk factors
Genetic factors, medical conditions, stressful life events, and a decrease in brain chemicals, such as serotonin and dopamine.

Symptoms
Depressed mood, decreased interest, change in appetite, sleep disturbances, poor concentration, worthlessness or guilt, and suicidal ideation.

Diagnosis
Evaluation by a psychiatrist.

Treatments
Antidepressants and psychotherapy are usually recommended.

Pathogenesis
Affects people of all ages and is recurrent. The usual duration of major depression if untreated lasts for 6–13 months. Suicide rate is about 15 percent with major depression.

Prevention
Antidepressant medications, which can also be given prophylactically between episodes of illness, reduce the length and severity of symptoms.

Epidemiology
Around 15 million people in the U.S. suffer from depression in a given year, which is about 7 percent of the population. Women are twice more likely to have depression than men.

Dysthymic disorder

Symptoms consist of someone having a depressed mood for the majority of the time on most days, poor concentration, difficulty making decisions, change in appetite (loss of appetite or overeating) and sleep (insomnia or excessive sleep), low energy or fatigue, low self-esteem, and feelings of hopelessness.

For a diagnosis of dysthymic disorder to be confirmed, the person must have at least two of the above symptoms for two years or more, and must never have been without the symptoms for more than two months at a time. There is no major depressive episode.

Cognitive therapy and insight-oriented psychotherapy are most effective. Antidepressant medications are given that are similar to those prescribed for major depression, except that the treatment is of shorter duration for dysthymic disorder. These treatments are useful when they are used concurrently.

Twenty percent of patients will develop major depression, 20 percent will develop bipolar disorder, and 25 percent will have lifelong symptoms.

Medications and psychotherapy similar to those used for major depression are commonly used. Daily exercise and stress management could be helpful.

Lifetime prevalence is 6 percent. It is 2 to 3 times more common in women. The onset of this disorder is before age 25 in 50 percent of patients. It is a chronic and less severe form of major depression.

Bipolar I disorder

Also known as manic depression, a person with bipolar disorder tends to alternate between periods of high activity or mania and low energy levels with abnormal depression. Manic symptoms also include inflated self-esteem or grandiosity; increase in goal-directed activity (occupational or social or both); easy distractibility; decreased need for sleep; racing thoughts or ideas; hypertalkative or pressured speech (rapid and uninterruptible); excessive involvement in pleasurable activities that have a high risk of negative consequences, for example spending sprees, hypersexuality, and driving while under the influence of drugs and alcohol.

To be sure of a definitive diagnosis for bipolar I disorder, the patient must show a period of abnormally and persistently elevated, expansive, or irritable mood, which lasts at least one week and which includes at least three of the symptoms above. These symptoms should not be a result of general medical conditions or substance abuse, and they must cause impairment in social and occupational functioning.

Medications (mood stabilizers) such as lithium, carbamazepine, or valproic acid can help. Supportive psychotherapy, group therapy, and family therapies are used when the patient is well controlled with medication. Electroconvulsive therapy (ECT) is usually used only for patients who do not improve with medications.

Untreated manic episodes generally last about three months. The course is usually chronic with relapses. More frequent relapses are associated with a longer history of manic symptoms. Bipolar I disorder has a worse prognosis than major depressive disorder. Lithium prophylaxis between episodes helps to decrease the risk of relapse of bipolar I disorder.

Onset is usually before age 30. Women and men are equally affected with this disorder. Lifetime prevalence is 1 percent. There are no ethnic differences associated with bipolar I disorder.

Bipolar II disorder

Hypomanic (an abnormality of mood resembling mania) symptoms include elevated mood, inflated self-esteem, decreased need for sleep, hypertalkative, racing thoughts or ideas, distractibility, and hyperactivity with high potential for painful consequences. The depressive symptoms exhibited are similar to those of major depression.

The criteria for a definitive diagnosis of bipolar II disorder are that the person is required to have a history of one or more major depressive episodes—and at least one hypomanic episode of abnormal mood that lasts for 4 days. During these episodes, the person has no impairment in either social or occupational functioning.

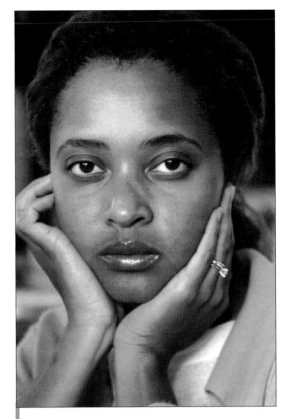

Many mood disorders are more common in women and they often begin at a crucial period in someone's life. However, they do vary in severity. Mood stabilizers and psychotherapy can help many people.

Medications and psychotherapy are the treatment of choice and are similar to the treatment of bipolar I disorder. Caution must be taken for patients on antidepressants, because there is a possibility of a switch to mania with tricyclic antidepressants and some SSRIs.

Bipolar II disorders tend to be recurrent and chronic, requiring long-term treatment. Mood stabilizers such as lithium and psychotherapy are helpful in preventing bipolar II disorders.

Lifetime prevalence for bipolar II disorders is 0.5 percent. The disorder is slightly more common in women. The onset of this disorder is usually before age 30. There are no ethnic differences associated with this disorder.

Cyclothymic disorder

This is a milder form of bipolar disorder consisting of recurrent mood symptoms associated with hypomania (like mania but of lesser intensity) and dysthymic mood. There are numerous periods of hypomanic symptoms and periods of dysthymic disorder symptoms for two years. However, the symptoms are less severe than bipolar I, bipolar II, and major depression. Cyclothymic disorder is not diagnosed if a person has had a manic episode or a major depressive episode. Mood stabilizers such as lithium, valproic acid, and carbamazapine are usually helpful.

This disorder has a chronic course. About one-

KEY FACTS: BIPOLAR DISORDERS

Description
Bipolar disorders are mood disorders with episodes of mania and major depression, hypomania, and mild to moderate depression with low grade mania.

Causes
Both genetic and environmental factors appear to play a role.

Risk factors
Decrease in brain chemical such as dopamine and serotonin; stressful life events; genetic factors, and certain medical conditions.

Symptoms
Elevated mood; decreased need for sleep; inflated self-esteem; racing thoughts or ideas; distractibility; hyperactivity; hypertalkative; risk-taking behavior; may or may not have an episode of major depressive symptoms. Hypomanic symptoms with bipolar II; mild manic and depressive symptoms with cyclothymic disorder.

Diagnosis
Evaluation by a psychiatrist.

Treatments
Medications (mood stabilizers and antidepressants) and psychotherapy.

Pathogenesis
Untreated manic episodes usually last for 3 months with bipolar I disorder. The course is usually chronic with relapses for all types of bipolar disorders.

Prevention
Mood stabilizers such as lithium and valproate. Psychotherapy may help prevent bipolar II disorders. For bipolar I disorders, lithium as a prophylactic between episodes helps decrease risk of relapse.

Epidemiology
Bipolar disorder affects about 6 million people in the United States, that is, about 2.5 percent of the U.S. population who are 18 years or more in a given year.

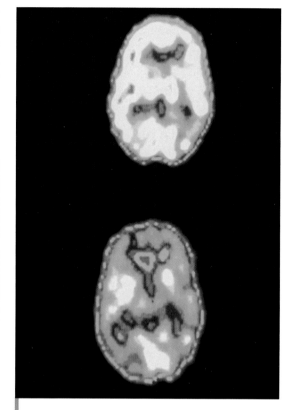

These axial PET scans are of a normal brain (top) and the other from a patient with a depressive illness. The brain of the person suffering from depression shows a markedly lower brain activity than that of the normal brain. The activity in the brain is processed to produce color coded images; areas of activity in these scans are yellow.

third of cyclothymic patients are eventually diagnosed with bipolar disorder (I and II). A person with cyclothymia may seldom feel the need to seek medical attention for their mood symptoms.

The lifetime prevalence of this disorder is less than 1 percent. The onset is usually between the ages of 15 to 25. Cyclothymic disorder occurs equally in men and women.

Nurun Shah

See also
- Adrenal disorders • Bipolar disorder
- Brain disorders • Depressive disorders
- Diagnosis • Environmental disorders
- Genetic disorders • Hormonal disorders
- Prevention • Psychotic disorders
- Schizophrenia • Sleep disorders
- Thyroid disorders • Treatment

Motion sickness

Motion sickness, seasickness, and airsickness are all essentially the same condition: unease followed by nausea and vomiting during motion or travel. For reasons that are unclear, some people are more prone to motion sickness than others.

For a person to be able to balance, the brain must receive sensory input from three very different sources. Input from the eyes tells the person where the horizon is and the position of the head and the body in space. Input also comes from the muscles, tendons, and joints of the lower extremities (the so-called proprioceptive system) and from motion sensors in both inner ears. The inner ear comprises the organ of hearing, or the cochlea, and the organ of balance, which includes structures called the utricle, saccule, and semicircular canals. Electrical impulses from these three distinct inputs are processed in the part of the brain called the cerebellum, and the patterns of these impulses are integrated in the brain. This information tells a person exactly his or her position in space. In simple terms, the brain can be compared to a computer receiving simultaneous information from three different sources and matching them for symmetry. Should there be a mismatch between these inputs, conflicting information reaches the brain. The confusion results in dizziness, or giddiness, or even vertigo. This sensory conflict is thought to be the cause of motion sickness.

For example, a person sitting at the back of a bus reading a book does not see any movement, and his or her eyes send information to the brain that his or her head is stationary. However, as the bus moves, the inner ears are unconsciously informing the brain that the head and body are in motion. As a result, the brain becomes confused, and this confusion is thought to be the underlying cause of motion sickness.

Symptoms and signs and prevention

Motion sickness is often characterized by a feeling of dizziness and fatigue, which may progress to headache, nausea, and vomiting. Stopping the motion stops the symptoms of motion sickness.

Prevention is best performed by sitting in an area of a vehicle that pitches and rolls the least, such as over the wings in an airplane. On boats or ships, staying above deck in midship and facing forward, in the direction of travel, appears to be efficacious for seasickness. To prevent motion sickness in an automobile, sitting in the front with eyes open is preferable to sitting at the back in a car with eyes closed. When these strategies do not work, medications may be required.

Over-the-counter (OTC) medicines such as promethazine, dimenhydrinate, and meclazine are all effective when taken an hour before a short trip. For longer trips, scopolamine patches may be worn behind the ear for three days at a stretch. There is some evidence that ginger root may be as effective as some of the OTC medications. Acupressure may be helpful, but its true effectiveness has yet to be studied in a systematic fashion.

Arun Gadre

KEY FACTS

Description
Nausea and other symptoms induced by motion.

Causes
Conflicting sensory information from the eyes, inner ears, and proprioceptive system.

Risk factors
Road, sea, and air travel.

Symptoms
Dizziness (or giddiness); vertigo; fatigue; nausea and vomiting; headache.

Diagnosis
From symptoms.

Treatments
Stopping the motion; OTC preparations such as promethazine, dimenhydrinate, and meclazine (for short trips), and scopolamine patches (for long trips); ginger root; possibly acupressure bands.

Pathogenesis
Conflicting sensory information in the brain results in nausea and other symptoms.

Prevention
Sitting in the least rocky part of a moving vehicle and facing forward with eyes open.

Epidemiology
Very common, affecting millions of people in the United States.

See also
• Ear disorders

Motor neuron disease

A group of debilitating disorders that involve progressive degeneration of the nerves (motor neurons) that control muscle movement, motor neuron disease (MND) causes loss of voluntary muscle control, stiffness, paralysis, and muscle wasting. The disorder sometimes runs in families. Some forms of motor neuron disease are linked to gene mutations, but in the majority of cases the cause is unknown. There is no cure for motor neuron disease, but medications can help relieve symptoms.

Motor neuron disease (MND) was first recognized in 1869 by a French neurologist, Jean-Martin Charcot, who described a group of disorders that involved loss of motor neurons, the nerve cells that exert functional control over muscles. Some of these nerve cells are called lower motor neurons; they directly activate muscles and are primarily located in the spinal cord. The lower motor neurons that control facial expression, speech, and swallowing are found in the brain stem. When these cells degenerate, the muscles associated with them lose the ability to function; they become weak and eventually paralyzed. Muscle activity is also indirectly regulated by the upper motor neurons, which are located in the front part of the brain and which influence the activity of the motor neurons in the brain stem and spinal cord. When upper motor neurons die, the muscles that they regulate become slower and weaker; movements lose their smoothness and fine control, becoming clumsy, exaggerated, or "spastic."

Motor neuron disease is prevalent worldwide and affects an average of 6 people in every 100,000 of the total population. Men are more frequently affected, accounting for 60 percent of all cases.

Four types of MND are recognized, depending on which motor neurons are involved in the degeneration process. Lou Gehrig's disease, also called amyotrophic lateral sclerosis (ALS), is the most common form and involves loss of both upper and lower motor neurons. The limb muscles are usually affected first, followed by the facial, swallowing, and speech muscles.

Another form of MND that may involve both types of motor neurons is progressive bulbar palsy, which commonly strikes older women. In this disease, the motor neurons in the brain stem are most vulnerable, but in some cases only upper motor neurons are affected. The first noticeable symptom of progressive bulbar palsy is weakness in the muscles of swallowing or speech.

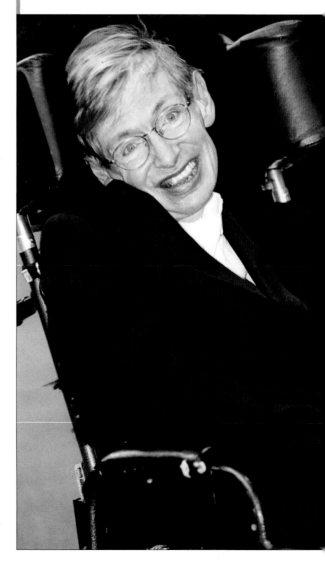

Stephen Hawking has suffered from motor neuron disease for more than 40 years, yet he is renowned in the world of physics. He writes scientific papers and gives lectures using his computerized voice synthesizer.

Progressive muscular atrophy (PMA) is an uncommon form of MND and involves only lower motor neurons. Primary lateral sclerosis (PLS) is rare, progresses slowly, and involves only upper motor neurons.

Causes

Although the causes of MND remain unknown, much has been learned about factors that might trigger the disease. Motor neurons are large cells, and their high energy requirements and specific protein composition may make them particularly vulnerable to damage.

A breakthrough in research came in the early 1990s when scientists learned that levels of glutamate (a chemical messenger in the nervous system) are very high in patients with Lou Gehrig's disease (ALS) and concluded that glutamate toxicity may be the cause of the illness.

A subsequent research study revealed that 5 percent of patients with the type of ALS that runs in families have a mutation in the gene for superoxide dismutase, an enzyme that mops up harmful waste products called free radicals. This enzyme is normally protective of motor neurons, which produce high levels of free radicals, but it is toxic in its mutated form.

Other gene variations have also recently been discovered in ALS. Some of these genetic alterations do not cause ALS but predispose a person to get the disease. The genes involved include those that make the proteins for building the internal scaffold of neurons, the formation of blood vessels, the detoxification of chemicals like pesticides, and the movement of molecules and small specialized structures within cells. Scientists believe that these gene variations will collectively reveal a common pathway leading to the development of all forms of MND.

The role of viruses as a trigger factor for MND has long been suspected, although as yet the role that viruses play in this disease is not scientifically proven.

Environmental toxins, such as pesticides and heavy metals (lead, arsenic, and mercury) are being investigated, especially with regard to geographical disease clusters. Dietary toxins have also been given serious consideration. The high incidence of ALS on the Pacific island of Guam prior to 1960 was linked to the local practice of consuming bats that feed on toxic cycad seeds. As the practice declined, so did the prevalence of the disease. However, a direct link between diet and MND has been difficult to establish. Individuals are also reported to have developed MND following electrical injuries from lightning strikes or high voltage shocks.

KEY FACTS

Description

There are four types of the disease, involving progressive degeneration of motor neurons, muscle stiffness and wasting, and paralysis.

Causes

Not known in 90 percent of cases; in 10 percent of cases the disease is a form that runs in families and may be linked to mutated genes.

Risk factors

The disease is most likely to affect people of Caucasian origin (93 percent of cases) and to occur between the ages of 50 and 70 years. Men are at slightly higher risk than women.

Symptoms

Fatigue, weakness, muscle stiffness, overactive reflexes, slurred speech, difficulty with swallowing, uncontrollable laughing, crying. Although mental faculties are rarely affected, dementia may occur in some cases.

Diagnosis

No definitive test; other diseases are ruled out by electromyography, blood and urine tests, brain and spinal cord MRIs, nerve conduction measures, spinal tap, muscle and nerve biopsies.

Treatments

No known cure. Drug treatment with Riluzole slows progression. Medication and therapy provide symptomatic relief.

Pathogenesis

MND starts in midlife and has a rapid progression; symptoms spread and occasionally reach a plateau. Average survival is 2–5 years from diagnosis; 10 percent of affected people survive 5–10 years.

Prevention

Genetic counseling is offered when the disease runs in families.

Epidemiology

Worldwide the disease affects 6 people per 100,000 of total population; 5,600 new cases are diagnosed annually in the United States. High prevalence in Pacific islands before 1960.

Symptoms

MND usually strikes in midlife between the ages of 50 and 70, although a juvenile form develops in a minority of cases. Among individuals there is considerable variation in the symptoms. Initially symptoms are limited to fatigue, weakened grip, twitching, clumsiness, and cramping in limb muscles. Deterioration is rapid as the disease spreads and affects the individual's capacity to walk, swallow, speak, and carry out everyday activities.

The senses and sexual function remain unaltered by MND. Bowel and bladder functions are not directly affected but are influenced by prolonged immobility and swallowing and eating difficulties. If there are swallowing problems, small pieces of food can enter the lungs and cause infections, such as pneumonia. Mental faculties are, for the most part, unimpaired; however, dementia is associated with a rare, rapidly deteriorating form of Lou Gehrig's disease. Uncontrollable laughing or crying may be related to the degeneration of motor neurons that regulate these functions. Quality of life declines precipitously as the motor neurons that control respiratory muscles deteriorate and mechanical assistance is needed with breathing. Death is commonly due to respiratory failure or pneumonia.

Although the progression of the disease may slow down, or reach a plateau, symptoms remain irreversible. Rare individuals, like physicist Stephen Hawking, live with MND for more than four decades and continue to be intellectually very productive.

Diagnosis

There is no single diagnostic test for MND. Diagnosis rests on examinations by a neurologist and tests that rule out other diseases, including tumors, metabolic disorders, multiple sclerosis, and myasthenia gravis. Recordings of muscle activity (electromyograms), measures of the speed at which electrical signals are conducted along nerves, muscle biopsies, and MRI (magnetic resonance imaging) of the brain and spinal cord may also be necessary. A decrease in muscle electrical activity is linked with MND. Much research is targeted on discovering a biomarker (a specific chemical substance) that is shared by all MND patients and that can be used for a definitive diagnosis.

Treatments

For many years, little could be done to help people with MND, and there is still no cure. The only FDA-approved medication for treating MND is the anti-glutamate drug Riluzole, which slows the progression of the disease. However, there are medications that provide relief of symptoms like spasticity, excess salivation, anxiety, stress, depression, and pain. Relaxation exercises, pain management, and various therapies (physical, occupational, and speech) make life more comfortable. Special devices are available that promote mobility and aid in tasks such as turning keys, holding utensils, opening doorknobs, and pulling up zippers. If a person cannot swallow easily, sometimes a surgical

gastronomy procedure will be carried out. This creates an opening in the stomach or small intestine in which a permanent feeding tube is inserted, through which nutrition can be given.

Home services, medical devices, and help with planning for the inevitable march of the disease allow a person with MND to live more independently and achieve a better quality of life. The roles of advocacy groups and volunteer organizations, in addition to support from family and friends, are very important for improving patient well-being.

A number of methodologies and drug therapies that are currently undergoing studies and clinical trials show promise for the future treatment of MND. These include dietary supplements of the compounds creatine and oxandrolone (an anabolic steroid), which are aimed at maintaining or building up muscle mass. Antioxidants like vitamin E, coenzyme Q10, and porphyrins are being tested in cocktails with other drugs, including Riluzole, in an attempt to arrest motor neuron degeneration. Growth factors (proteins that nourish nerve cells) are also targeted at preventing loss of motor neurons.

Other proteins, like sodium valproate, which protect motor neurons, are also being evaluated. The drug thalidomide, which has anti-inflammatory action, is being assessed for its ability to stop motor neuron degeneration. Antibiotics are being tested for their influence on delaying the onset of disease and prolonging survival. In addition, various techniques involving gene therapy are being evaluated, and methods that can induce stem cells to develop into motor neurons are being used to grow motor neurons from MND patients so that disease mechanisms can be studied.

Pathogenesis

The progression of MND is relentless. Average survival is 2 to 5 years from the time of diagnosis, although about 10 percent of patients live for 5 to 10 years. Deterioration is slower if only lower motor neurons are affected, although the outlook is grave if these include motor neurons in the brain stem.

Sonal Jhaveri

See also
- Alzheimer's disease • Genetic disorders
- Huntington's disease • Language and speech disorders • Leukodystrophy
- Lou Gehrig's disease • Mental disorders
- Nervous system disorders • Spinal disorders • Substance abuse and addiction

Multiple sclerosis

Multiple sclerosis (MS) is a progressive disease of the central nervous system (CNS). The CNS is composed of the brain and spinal cord, and within are numerous nerves. Each nerve is composed of a nerve cell body and its processes, called axons. Nerves are like electrical wiring that transmits electrical impulses by which the brain and spinal cord control the function of many body parts. Myelin is a fatty substance that acts as insulation for many of the axons of the CNS. The myelin sheath helps speed the pace of electronic impulses in the CNS so that signals are sent rapidly over relatively long distances.

In MS, there is a selective destruction of the myelin sheath, a process called demyelination, resulting in significant impairment of transmission of electrical impulses. Demyelination probably results from inflammation, a process caused by the accumulation of immune cells like T- and B- lymphocytes and macrophages. These cells can directly injure myelin, the cell that produces it in the CNS (called the oligodendrocyte or the underlying axon), or may indirectly cause similar injury via the secretion of inflammatory substances.

Clinical symptoms of MS depend upon which area of the CNS is affected. For example, if the optic nerve, which supplies the eye, is affected, there can be loss of vision. If the connections for movement of the eyes are affected in the brainstem, then there can be double vision. If damage occurs in the spinal cord, there can be paralysis and numbness of the legs.

A definite cause for MS is not known, but there are a few hypotheses. Infection is a possible cause. For decades, viruses and bacteria have been implicated in MS. Viruses like human herpes virus-6, Epstein-Barr virus, retroviruses, and bacteria such as *Chlamydia pneumoniae* have been implicated but never clearly shown to be the cause.

Autoimmunity is another likely possibility. There are several such diseases of the body, affecting many different organ systems. It is believed that some factor turns the immune system against the body; possibly triggered by one of the infectious agents above.

MS has been shown to be hereditary, but many genes may be involved, so the risk of vertical transmission is still quite low, in the order of 3 to 5 percent.

Risk factors

The mean age of onset of MS is 30 years. The onset is usually between 18 to 60 years, but there are many instances in which MS has occurred in children, adolescents, and the elderly.

Gender is a factor. Women tend to be affected slightly more frequently than men, with a female-to-male ratio of 1.77 to 1 (an oddity peculiar to most autoimmune diseases).

Geographical and racial distribution are relevant factors. MS is common in Europe, Canada, northern United States, New Zealand, and southern Australia. However, race is a major determinant of MS risk. Caucasians have the highest risk. Persons of African, Asian, and Native American origin have the lowest risk. However, persons migrating from a place of higher risk to a place of lower risk carry their risk with them, especially if they migrate before the age of 15 years. The same applies to persons of lower risk migrating to high-risk areas.

There is a genetic influence. The risk of MS is highest for siblings (2 to 5 percent) and decreases for children, aunts, uncles, and cousins. Among siblings, the risk is the highest for identical twins (monozygotic): up to 20 to 25 percent.

Environmental factors such as climate, diet, and toxins have been implicated as risk factors. According to a few studies, persons residing in areas with low exposure to the sun, resulting in vitamin D deficiency, may be at higher risk of MS.

Symptoms

Clinical symptoms reflect the areas of CNS that are damaged. Typically, patients will experience loss or blurring of vision, double vision, facial pain like an electric shock (called trigeminal neuralgia), slurring of speech, loss of sensation, tingling sensations, discomfort like an electric shock on bending the neck forward, paralysis, stiffness of the limbs, loss of balance, tremulousness, loss of coordination, bladder or bowel disturbances, impotence, change of personality, and poor mental functioning, such as memory disturbances. A common unexplained symptom is severe fatigue, which may be out of proportion to other clinical symptoms or signs. Depression is also quite common.

There are two typically common phenomena associated with MS. The first is Uhtoff's phenomenon, in which symptoms worsen with an increase in body temperature or exposure to heat and improve with reduction of the temperature. The second is l'Hermitte's sign, in which the patient experiences a shocklike sensation, usually running from the head down the back of the spine, upon bending the neck forward.

There are four types of multiple sclerosis, depending on symptoms and the course it follows.

KEY FACTS

Description
Autoimmune inflammatory demyelinating disease of the CNS.

Causes
Unknown, but genetic loading, environmental triggering, and autoimmunity all play a role.

Risk factors
None proven, but being a white female in the 20 to 30 age range, growing up and living in high-risk areas are clear risk factors. There are no clear dietary or other risk factors.

Symptoms
Most typical symptoms are episodic loss of neurological function with recovery, such as: unilateral loss of vision, numbness or tingling, paralysis, bladder or bowel disturbances, and lack of coordination or loss of balance.

Diagnosis
Primarily a clinical diagnosis involving the demonstration of clearly separate areas of the CNS being affected at different times. Diagnosis supported by MRI findings of white matter lesions and cerebrospinal fluid findings of increased immunoglobulin-G with the presence of oligoclonal bands.

Pathogenesis
An autoimmune inflammatory disease that attacks multiple ares of the CNS, causing the degradation of myelin, followed by loss of axons.

Treatments
Symptomatic therapy to improve quality of life and disease-modifying drugs to alter the natural disease course leading to slowed progression.

Prevention
Nothing proven.

Epidemiology
Most common in Caucasians and in high risk areas like Europe, northern United States, Canada, New Zealand, and southeastern Australia.

Relapsing remitting MS. The patients experience attacks of neurological symptoms, usually with new signs, that last for at least 24 to 48 hours before subsiding. Typically, an MS attack evolves over hours to days and can build over several days, lasting several weeks. Recovery from attacks is variable, in some cases complete, but in others there is residual deficit. Steroid treatments help to reduce the duration of attacks, but seem to have no influence on the outcome.

Primary progressive MS. From the onset, there is gradual worsening of the neurological symptoms and signs over months to years. There is generally no improvement, but at times the course might waver. Patients do not experience any attacks. Though progression is generally unstoppable, the rate of deterioration is quite variable, and very slow protracted courses are not atypical.

Secondary progressive MS. Evolving from the relapsing-remitting course, attacks start to diminish, residual deficits build, but between any perceived attacks or in the complete absence of relapses, there is steady progression, not unlike that which is seen with primary progressive disease.

Progressive relapsing MS. A rarer condition, but usually patients appear to be primary progressive disease, then they begin having attacks. The course seems to follow that of primary progressive disease.

Pathologically, there have also been four subtypes of MS described, but there does not seem to be a particular association with any clinical subtype.

It is important to know the particular type of MS since the management differs for each group. Patients with relapsing remitting MS tend to have more inflammation and therefore do better than the other types with regard to treatments.

There are some variants of MS, which are conditions somewhat similar to MS and often grouped with MS.

Optic neuritis. This is a condition involving the optic nerve, resulting in loss of vision and pain on moving the eyes. One or both eyes may be affected. Patients may have only recurring episodes of optic neuritis, while others clearly evolve into typical MS.

Neuromyelitis optica. Also called NMO (Devic's disease), this condition often involves devastating bilateral optic neuritis and large demyelinating destructive spinal cord lesions. Although originally described as a monophasic illness, more typically it is a relapsing condition that can be quite disabling, with each attack building on the other. Patients most often have a measurable specific antibody in their blood that characterizes the condition. Patients often have loss of vision in one or both eyes in a progressive pattern, usually with paralysis of or loss of sensation in the limbs, and bladder disturbances. A form of MS in Japan called optico-spinal MS is most commonly NMO.

Slow progressive myelopathy. There is demyelination of the spinal cord and it progresses slowly. Patients may present with stiffness and weakness of the lower limbs and bladder disturbances. There are still such cases that evolve with or without a history of transverse myelitis; they lack all the features of primary progressive MS.

Acute tumorlike (tumorigenic) MS. The patients present with confusion or paralysis similar to that seen with brain tumors. The cause, however, is large-scale demyelination of areas of the brain that have the appearance and presentation of a brain tumor. Despite the presentation, these lesions tend to recover well, and the course is no different from typical MS.

Marburg variant of MS. A severe progressive widespread demyelinating condition often leading to death. This condition is still quite rare, but many individual cases have been reported.

Diagnosis

The diagnosis of MS must be established prior to considering any therapy. Diagnosis is based primarily on clinical presentations and is supported by laboratory findings. An international committee have recently published revised criteria focused on making an accurate diagnosis. They are based on the ability to demonstrate a condition that affects at least two separate areas of the CNS on at least two separate occasions (dissemination in place and time). Patients should have suffered at least two attacks of neurological symptoms lasting at least 24 to 48 hours in the absence of flu or fever (see Uhtoff's phenomenon, above). These attacks should be verified by a physician to ensure that separate areas of the CNS have been affected. For example, one attack could be the loss of vision and another numbness of the legs, indicating that as a minimum there are lesions both in the optic nerve and spinal cord. The symptoms should be accompanied by findings on clinical examination involving two separate parts of the nervous system. The current appearance of clear new lesions on magnetic resonance imaging (MRI) remote from a first episode (see below) would qualify for evidence of new activity over time.

If there is only one attack or clinical finding of involvement of only one part of the nervous system, additional tests of cerebrospinal fluid (CSF) and radiological investigations like MRI are advised in

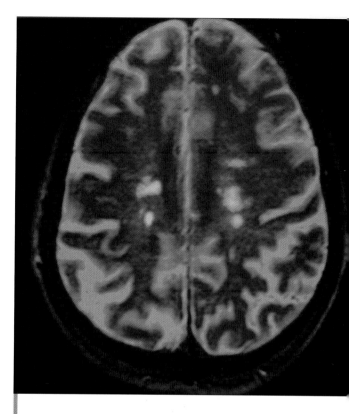

An MRI scan of a brain of someone suspected of having multiple sclerosis shows some damaged areas (pink). These are the result of plaques or damaged patches in the myelin sheath that surrounds nerve fibers.

order to ascertain the risk of the attack evolving to MS. Patients who have "silent" lesions on their MRI after only one attack (areas of involvement that do not correspond to symptoms or signs) are termed *clinically isolated syndrome*; this is most likely an early form of MS.

In patients with MS, typically there is an increase in immunoglobulin G in the spinal fluid that resolves as bands on protein separating gels (electrophoresis). These bands have been termed *oligoclonal* (*oligo* is a Greek word meaning "few"; *clonal* pertains to a clone, that is, one or a few genetically identical cells). They are not specific for MS, but in the absence of CNS infections, they are supportive of an MS diagnosis. There is still no specific test for MS, but many potential leads in serum and spinal fluid are being examined.

MRI is used increasingly in the diagnosis of MS. Some believe a normal MRI virtually rules out MS, even if the MRI is done early. During an MRI, the brain and spinal cord are subjected to a magnetic field that stimulates water molecules to become excited. When the magnetic field is removed, the water molecules relax and the energy they emit is measured. The computer converts this energy to an image. Areas containing more water will give off more energy. Typically, areas of inflammation contain more water, and this is the case with most MS plaques of demyelination. Demyelinated areas of the brain and spinal cord have a characteristic appearance on MRI that differentiate them from other conditions. They appear predominantly in the CNS white matter, and their number, distribution, and evolution over time are characteristic of MS. There are specific areas in the brain that typically harbor MS plaques. These are the periventricular region (area surrounding the CSF spaces in the brain), corpus callosum (white matter connecting the left and right hemispheres of the brain), and the centrum semiovale (white matter above the ventricles of the brain). In computed tomography, a dye called gadolinium can be used to enhance newer lesions.

Pathogenesis

The cause of MS is unknown, but the main evidence that MS is an autoimmune disease comes from pathological studies showing the presence of T cells and macrophages within MS lesions. These cells are vital to protect the body from infections. What causes immune cells to attack CNS myelin is unknown, but a popular theory suggests this could be due to molecular mimicry. This refers to the introduction to the body of a foreign protein (usually from an infectious agent such as a virus) that is similar in structure to a protein in myelin. The immune system becomes primed to locate the foreign protein, but instead launches an attack against CNS myelin, leading to chronic demyelination (MS). Removing the myelin exposes the underlying axons to inflammatory substances. It is this progressive loss of axons that probably represents the progression seen in all forms of MS. Destruction of myelin may or may not be followed by some regeneration or repair.

Treatments

There are now several proven effective treatments for some forms of MS.

Acute attacks. Typically a short course (3 to 5 days) of high dose steroids (oral or intravenous) can shorten the duration of an attack, but does not seem to impact on the final disability. For more severe attacks, plasma exchange has been shown to be effective.

Relapsing remitting MS. There are now five approved and proven effective immunomodulatory treatments that reduce the number of attacks and also slow MRI activity. Some, but not others, have been shown to slow disease progression. First line agents are the interferons and glatiramer acetate; second line agents (because of potentially more toxic side effects) are mitoxantrone and natalizumab. Interferon beta-1a and beta-1b have both been shown to reduce attacks and MRI activity and to slow disease progression. Glatiramer acetate reduces attacks and MRI activity. Mitoxantrone reduces attacks and MRI activity and slows progression, but it is a chemotherapeutic drug with potential toxic effects that can cause irreversible heart damage and increase the risk for leukemia. Natalizumab, a newly approved humanized mouse monoclonal antibody, reduces attacks, slows MRI activity, and slows progression, but it is also associated with a rare irreversible brain disease called PML, caused by a virus.

Secondary progressive MS. There are no approved or proven treatments for this form of MS, though for years immunosuppressive agents have been used with varying and limited success. It seems that timing is key; if these agents are used when there is still evidence of ongoing inflammation, they will be more effective. Once a slow progressive course ensues, they seem to be of limited benefit. Agents such as cyclophosphamide, azathioprine, methotrexate, and others have all been tested.

Primary progressive MS. No effective therapy has been shown to alter the course of this form of MS.

Prevention and epidemiology

There is no way of preventing MS, although studies have been initiated that focus on correcting activated Vitamin D levels.

The highest prevalence of MS is 30 to 60 in 100,000 or more in Europe, northern United States, Canada, New Zealand, and southeastern Australia. In the United States the prevalence is 0.1 percent, or a total of 250,000 to 400,000 persons. A lower prevalence is seen in the southern United States, northern Australia, the Mediterranean basin, South America, and the white population of South Africa. The lowest prevalence is seen in Asia, Africa, and parts of South America and Mexico. Race is an important predictor of susceptibility to MS and may be reflective of genetic differences. MS is most prevalent in Caucasians and affects Africans, Asians, and to a lesser degree, Amerindians.

Monica Badve and Mark Freedman

See also
- Environmental disorders • Genetic disorders • Immune system disorders
- Nervous system disorders

Mumps

Mumps is a viral infection that usually occurs in children, resulting in swelling of the cheek area. However, a vaccine has been in use since the 1960s, so actual cases are fairly rare. If an adult becomes sick, mumps may cause mild cases of meningitis, encephalitis, or orchitis.

The term *mumps* is an old English word for either "bumps", "grimace," or "mumble." It always involves swelling of the cheeks. Mumps was also commonly referred to as epidemic parotitis before the vaccine was introduced and the prevalence of the virus was significantly reduced.

Causes and risk factors

Mumps is an acute systemic viral infection, which occurs mainly in children. The virus is a member of the paramyxovirus family, which includes parainfluenza and the measles viruses in humans as well as animal pathogens such as the Newcastle disease virus and simian viruses. The virus is passed through contact with droplets from sneezing, coughing, or any personal contact with infected saliva. Although contagious, it is not as easily spread as chickenpox or measles. Most children are vaccinated against the disease, but children in school or day care settings are most likely to come in contact with the virus.

Symptoms, signs, and diagnosis

The virus usually incubates for 14 to 24 days. Symptoms include a loss of energy and little appetite, chills, headaches, and a fever as high as 104°F (40°C). Once symptoms appear, within 12 to 24 hours the patient will probably have painful swelling of the parotid area (saliva glands in the cheeks just in front of the ears). The skin over the gland will usually be hot and flushed, but there will not be a rash. Sometimes only one side will be swollen, and as it shrinks, the other side will swell, or both sides may swell at once. The parotitis usually lasts three to four days.

An infected person is infectious from three days before the symptoms start until nine days after the symptoms appear.

It is estimated that 30 percent of patients have subclinical symptoms needing no treatment. In adult cases of mumps, complications are more common. One complication is a mild case of meningitis, an inflammation of the brain and spinal covering causing a stiff neck, headache, vomiting, and lack of energy. It usually resolves within seven days. Mumps meningitis only occurs in about one in 20 cases of mumps.

Another complication is encephalitis, an inflammation of the brain that can cause seizures, a high fever, or even an inability to feel pain. Encephalitis may cause permanent brain damage. In normal cases, encephalitis is usually resolved within one or two weeks,

KEY FACTS

Description

A short-term viral infection best known for causing parotitis.

Causes

A paramyxovirus transmitted through contaminated saliva.

Risk factors

Close proximity to unvaccinated children such as at schools or day care centers.

Symptoms

Parotitis, chills, headache, loss of appetite, loss of energy, fever, and complications in adults may cause meningitis, encephalitis, or orchitis.

Diagnosis

Examination by experienced medical personnel; lab tests of saliva.

Treatments

If uncomplicated, the infection is self-limiting and will be allowed to run its course. Antibiotics may be prescribed for complications.

Pathogenesis

The virus causes an infection of the upper respiratory tract that spreads to the lymph nodes. Infection of the lymphocytes causes a blockage of the ducts in the salivary glands.

Prevention

Childhood immunization from 12 to 15 months along with the measles and rubella vaccine.

Epidemiology

Before the vaccine was licensed in 1967, there were approximately 200,000 cases each year in the United States. Currently there are less than 1,000 cases reported each year in the United States.

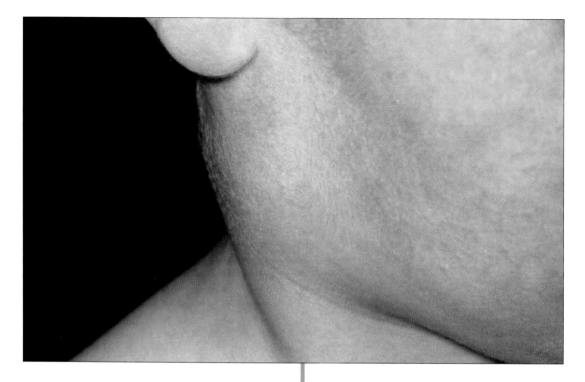

A young child with mumps (infectious parotitis) has an in-flamed parotid gland. The swelling can cause difficulty chewing, and swallowing may be painful. Sometimes a child will have fever and headache, but many children will merely feel slightly unwell.

and it only occurs in one or two cases out of 10,000. Finally, orchitis, which is relatively common in post-pubertal males, is a swelling of the scrotum that causes severe pain, fever, and nausea. One out of four men with mumps will have orchitis, but it does not cause any sterility and will usually subside after five to seven days. Most cases of mumps can be diagnosed by a trained medical professional on physical examination, but confirmation of the presence of the mumps virus may require additional lab tests of saliva, urine, or cerebrospinal fluid.

Treatments and prevention

There is no treatment for mumps. However, a vaccine for mumps has been licensed and administered to the public since 1967. The vaccine contains live, attenuated mumps virus and is administered usually when children are 12 to 15 months of age in combination with the measles and rubella vaccines (MMR vaccine).

The World Health Organization, the British Medical Association, and the American Academy of Pediatrics all endorse the vaccine and its safety. However, some parents choose not to have their children vaccinated because of personal beliefs or fear of a connection between the immunization and autism.

Pregnant women should avoid getting vaccinated until after they give birth because of the risk of birth defects or miscarriage.

Before the vaccine was licensed, 200,000 cases of mumps were reported every year in the United States. The virus usually peaked between January and May, with epidemics occurring at two- to five-year intervals. Since the advent of the vaccine, the occurrence of mumps has decreased substantially.

In the event that the vaccine does not build up a sufficient quantity of mumps antibodies, most children will recover from the illness in several days and be immune to further illness after having it once. The most important thing in normal cases of mumps is to keep the patient fed and hydrated since swallowing and chewing will be painful. Citric beverages should be avoided because they will sting the swollen cheeks. Blended foods can help keep the patient nourished. Painkillers may help reduce the pain of the swollen parotid glands.

Graeme Stemp Morlock

See also
• Immune system disorders • Infections, viral • Meningitis

Muscle system disorders

The basic functional unit of the muscular system is the muscle fiber. Muscle fibers, or cells, are made of filaments that move against each other to produce contractions, or shortening of the fibers, when stimulated by electrical signals generated by nerves or by adjacent muscle fibers.

The filaments in muscle fibers are typically arranged into units called sarcomeres, bounded on either end by Z discs. Between the Z discs is a structure called the M line. Two types of filaments produce muscle contractions. Thin filaments, made of the protein actin, are anchored to the Z discs. Thick filaments, made of the protein myosin, are anchored to the M line.

Where the two types of filaments overlap, thick filaments attach to the thin filaments on either side of them. When stimulated, the thick filaments pull the thin filaments toward the M line, thus shortening the overall length of the muscle fibers, ultimately shortening the length of the muscle itself.

There are three types of muscle tissue: skeletal, smooth, and cardiac. Skeletal muscle produces the voluntary movements of the body, such as walking, writing, or throwing a ball. The muscles that give shape to the body, such as the curves of the shoulder, the arms, or the legs, are skeletal muscles. Because of the sarcomere structure, skeletal muscle has a striated, or banded appearance (it is also referred to as striated muscle).

Skeletal muscles produce movement by antagonistic movement; one muscle pulls on a joint in one direction, while another muscle pulls on the joint in an opposing direction. Flexor muscles cause a limb to curl or bend, such as in the bending of the arm at the elbow. Extensor muscles do the opposite, such as making the arm straighten out at the elbow. Abduction is movement of a limb away from the midline of the body, such as when someone reaches out to the side and up in one sweeping gesture. Its opposite, adduction, is movement of a limb toward the midline, such as when the arms fall back down to the sides. Rotation is turning of a bone around its longitudinal axis. Opposing muscles rotate the head to the right and to the left when one shakes one's head.

Cardiac muscle produces involuntary movement in the contractions of the heart. Cardiac muscle fibers are similar in structure to those of skeletal muscle; thus they have a striated appearance, but they also feature intercalated discs, structures that connect the ends of adjacent cardiac muscle fibers to each other.

Smooth muscle is responsible for most involuntary movements within the body. Peristalsis, the rhythmic contractions that move food and waste products through the digestive tract, is driven by smooth muscle. The size of the pupil, which controls the amount of light that enters the eye, is regulated by smooth muscle. Contractions of the urinary bladder and contractions of the uterus are produced by smooth

RELATED ARTICLES

muscle. Passage of blood into capillary beds likewise is controlled by smooth muscle.

Smooth muscle is so named because, while its fibers contain thick and thin filaments that interact to produce muscle contractions, they are not arranged in the regular pattern of sarcomeres, thus they lack the banded appearance of skeletal and cardiac muscle.

The muscular system serves many important functions in the body. Some functions are relatively superficial. The muscular system, in conjunction with the skeletal system, provides shape to our bodies. Muscles make voluntary movement possible, but they are also vital to involuntary processes, such as breathing and digestion. The muscular system contributes in other ways: muscles help provide support to other organs, they may help protect internal organs, and they can help generate warmth.

Because of the diverse roles served by muscles and their near ubiquitous distribution throughout the body, diseases and disorders can affect virtually any part of the body and can have a variety of effects, ranging from soreness to lethal effects, such as the loss of the ability to breathe alone as a result of the paralyzing effects of poliomyelitis.

Muscles are made of contractile fibers that shorten when stimulated by electrical signals from nerve cells or adjacent muscle fibers. The fibers contract in a coordinated fashion to produce a specific movement. For example, shortening of fibers in the biceps muscle (in the front part of the upper arm when the palms face forward) creates a coordinated contraction of the muscle that causes the arm to flex (bend); a corresponding shortening of fibers in the triceps muscle (in the back part of the upper arm) causes the arm to extend (straighten). Coordinated contractions of muscles lining the organs of the digestive tract cause food to move from the mouth through the esophagus, stomach, and intestines.

One type of muscle, skeletal muscle, produces voluntary movements, such as the hand and arm movements involved in typing. Skeletal muscle can also produce involuntary movements called reflexes, such as the jerking of the knee when a tendon below the kneecap is struck by a rubber hammer.

Most involuntary movements are produced by two other types of muscle. Cardiac muscle, which is similar in appearance to smooth muscle, is responsible for the

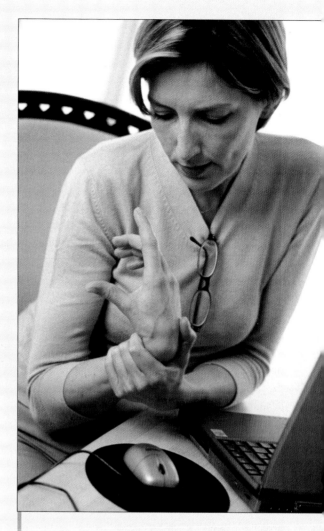

Using a computer involves repeating the same action again and again and can result in repetitive strain injury. The trauma may lead to carpal tunnel syndrome as a result of pressure on the nerve that passes through the wrist.

involuntary contractions of the heart, which pumps blood throughout the body. Smooth muscle, which is quite a bit different in appearance from skeletal and cardiac movements, is responsible for all other involuntary movements, such as the movement of materials through the digestive tract.

Because of the widespread distribution of muscular tissue throughout the body, diseases and disorders of the muscular system can have major effects on other systems. Diseases and disorders of the muscular system range from minor, acute injuries like strains, to chronic, genetic disorders like muscular dystrophy.

Acute disorders

Virtually everyone has experienced an acute muscle disorder at some point in their life. Among the most common are sports injuries and some involuntary contractions, such as muscle spasms. Sports injuries are typically caused by poor or inadequate training or warming up. Inadequate equipment or attire, such as shoes, may contribute. Sports injuries typically involve overstretching or even tearing of muscles or tendons, or both, that attach muscles to bone. Treatment for these injuries often includes rest and light exercise so that the damage is not increased. Surgery may be required in severe cases.

Autoimmune disorders

A number of autoimmune disorders, such as myasthenia gravis and multiple sclerosis, affect the muscular system. In myasthenia gravis, the immune system progressively destroys junctions between nerves and skeletal muscles. As a result, muscles with myasthenia gravis suffer from weakness, increasing fatigue, and possible paralysis. Fibromyalgia is more common in women. The muscles of the face and neck are most often affected. The ability to see, swallow, and breathe may be impaired as muscles involved become paralyzed. Drug therapies can reduce inflammation, suppress affected parts of the immune system, and counteract the chemicals involved in destruction of the nerve-muscle junctions.

In multiple sclerosis, the immune system attacks and destroys the myelin sheaths, which insulate the nerve cells that control muscles. As the myelin sheaths are destroyed, the muscles are indirectly affected. Some reflexes, such as in the knee, are exaggerated; while others, such as in the abdomen, are reduced. Tremors develop, as well as weakness and spasticity over time. Control over smooth muscles, such as the sphincters that control urination and bowel movements, may fail, leading to incontinence. Multiple sclerosis patients may become completely disabled. Corticosteroids and other drugs may help mitigate the symptoms and slow the progression of disease.

Fibromyalgias

Fibromyalgias are characterized by pain, tenderness, and stiffness of muscles and tendons. Women are most commonly affected. In addition to pain, those with fibromyalgias may be beset by fatigue, sleep difficulties, headaches, and depression. Stress reduction, exercise, physical therapy and massage, and drug therapy to control pain or depression, or both, may be used to treat fibromyalgia. Fibromyalgias may be triggered by certain autoimmune disorders, such as lupus.

Genetic disorders

Muscular dystrophy is a catchall term for several inherited, progressive disorders in which the muscle tissue weakens, possibly leading to destruction of muscle fibers and replacement by other types of tissue, such as fat tissue. The most common muscular dystrophy is Duchenne muscular dystrophy. It is a sex-linked trait, that is, the mutation that causes it is carried on one of the sex chromosomes (the chromosomes that determine whether someone is male or female). Most sex-linked traits, such as Duchenne muscular dystrophy, are carried on the X chromosome, of which females normally have two, while males have only one. Traits carried on X chromosomes can be passed by mothers to both sons and daughters, but can be passed by fathers only to daughters. Other types of muscular dystrophy include Becker muscular dystrophy and limb-girdle muscular dystrophy. A number of other disorders, such as some autoimmune disorders, fibromyalgias, and myopathies, may also be inherited.

Infectious and parasitic diseases

A number of infectious diseases affect the muscular system. Poliomyelitis is a viral disease that attacks nerve cells; in severe cases, muscle pain and paralysis may result. If respiratory muscles are affected, a polio patient may lose the ability to breathe without help. While treatments are available for polio, vaccination to prevent infection is most effective.

Tetanus is caused by a bacterium, *Clostridium tetanus*. The microbe releases a toxin that blocks signals that inhibit nerve transmissions. In the absences of such neuroinhibitors, the nerve cells are constantly switched on, triggering intense spasms of voluntary muscle. In many cases, the masseter muscles (of the cheek) are involved. As a result, the teeth are clenched so tightly the victim cannot eat, hence the name "lockjaw." The patient may not be able to eat, speak, cry, or breathe; death may eventually result. The best way to treat tetanus is to prevent it by vaccination.

A number of parasitic diseases cause muscle inflammation and pain. They include Chagas' disease, schistosomiasis, tapeworm, toxoplasmosis, and trichinosis, among others. In some cases, heart muscle tissue is affected; in others, skeletal muscle tissue is affected. When heart muscle is inflamed, heart function is impaired, and heart attacks may result. A broad range of other symptoms and signs may be present, depending on the infectious organism. A person may be infected by insect bites, as in Chagas' disease; wading in contaminated waters, such as in schistosomiasis; coming into contact with contaminated fecal matter, such as with tapeworms or toxoplasmosis; or by eating undercooked meat, as in toxoplasmosis and trichinosis. Some organisms, such as tapeworms, may form cysts inside muscle tissue. Therapies depend on the nature of the infectious agent.

Involuntary contractions

Spasms are sudden, involuntary contractions of muscle tissue. Cramps are painful, sustained involuntary contractions. A number of factors cause spasms and cramps, such as overuse, inadequate blood supply, dehydration, electrolyte imbalance, and injuries. Spasms and cramps may be treated by correcting the factors that contribute to them. Rest and light exercise may help as well. Drug therapy, such as muscle relaxers and painkillers, may help.

Other types of involuntary contractions include tics, which are spasmodic twitching of muscles normally under conscious control; tremors, which are rhythmic contractions that produce a quivering motion; fasciculations, that is, involuntary contractions of a muscle unit that do not involve movement of the affected part of the body; and fibrillations, which are spontaneous contractions of muscle fibers.

Tics are relatively minor and need little treatment. Tremors, fasciculations, and fibrillations may signal more serious disorders, such as Parkinson's disease in the case of tremors; multiple sclerosis and Lou Gehrig's disease, in the case of fasciculations; and degeneration of motor nerves, in the case of fibrillations. In the case of tremors, fasciculations, and fibrillations, the underlying disease must be treated.

Myopathies

Myopathies are disorders of muscle tissue in which the fibers fail to function properly, and the muscles eventually weaken. The term myopathy is a catchall term for many disorders. Some affect muscle tissue in infancy and childhood. In others—including the mitochrondrial myopathies, in which a defect in the mitochondria, the powerhouses of the cell, inhibits the ability to produce the energy required for movement—it may take years for the damage to accumulate before becoming noticeable. Glycogen storage disorders occur when glycogen, a carbohydrate used for energy storage in muscle tissue, accumulates in muscle tissue because of a breakdown in chemical pathways that convert glycogen to glucose, which is the carbohydrate that fuels muscle contractions.

Tumors

Tumors are caused by a breakdown in the regulation of cell growth and division. Some tumors have the potential to spread to other parts of the body, that is, they metastasize, and are called cancers. A cancer that originates in muscle tissue is called a myosarcoma. Leiomyosarcomas are malignant tumors of both smooth and cardiac muscle tissue. They are most often found in the abdomen and less often in deep soft tissues of the arms and legs. Cancers of cardiac muscle tissue are relatively rare.

Rhabdomyosarcomas, cancers of skeletal muscle, are typically found in the arms and legs, but the head, neck, and reproductive or urinary tract organs are also affected. Leimyosarcomas are more commonly found in adults, while rabdomyosarcomas are more commonly found in children.

Other tumors lack the potential to spread, thus are called benign. Cancers can be deadly if not treated. Benign tumors are often easily controlled or treated but may likewise be fatal depending on their location and the damage they cause to surrounding tissues. Leiomyomas are benign tumors that arise in smooth muscle tissue. They include fibroids, which are tumors of the muscles that form the wall of the uterus. They range in severity from those requiring little or no medical attention to those that require surgery. Rhabdomyomas, benign tumors of skeletal muscle tissue, are relatively rare.

David M. Lawrence

Muscular dystrophy

Muscular dystrophy is used to describe more than 30 different inherited diseases in which the muscles weaken over time and the muscle cells are unable to repair themselves after being damaged. Although each type of muscular dystrophy has a unique genetic cause, it is difficult to distinguish between them because many of the different types have similar clinical features. Important factors that help differentiate the types of muscular dystrophy include the age of onset and types of symptoms, which muscle groups are affected, and whether other members of the individual's family are affected or show signs of muscular dystrophy.

The muscular dystrophies are genetic diseases. They have been shown to be inherited in an autosomal dominant manner (in which only one copy of the defective gene is necessary to cause abnormality), in an autosomal recessive way (in which a pair of abnormal genes, one from each parent, causes the defect), and in X-linked recessive patterns (caused by defects on the X chromosome). It is therefore important to determine which type of muscular dystrophy affects an individual in order to know who else in the family is at risk.

Causes

Some muscular dystrophies are caused by a deficiency in the protein dystrophin, which provides stability to the muscle fibers. Dystrophin is reduced in Becker muscular dystrophy (BMD) and completely absent in Duchenne muscular dystrophy (DMD). The gene for dystrophin is located on the X chromosome, so these conditions show X-linked inheritance. Mothers and sisters of boys with these disorders have up to a 50 percent chance of having an affected son.

Myotonic dystrophy (DM) results from changes to a protein that is involved in the regulation of muscle cells. DM is inherited in an autosomal dominant pattern and affects both males and females equally.

There are 16 subtypes of limb girdle muscular dystrophy (LGMD). They are caused by changes to many different proteins that are associated with muscle stability and maintenance. Some types of LGMD are inherited in an autosomal dominant manner, while some of the others show an autosomal recessive pattern of inheritance.

There are other, more unusual types of muscular dystrophy, for example Emery-Dreifuss muscular dystrophy (EDMD). Around 300 cases have been identified in the United States. Oculopharyngeal muscular dystrophy (OPMD) causes weakness in the eyes and throat. It is prevalent in French Canadian families in Canada and in Spanish-American families in the southwestern United States.

Distal muscular dystrophy (DD) begins in middle age or later. It is most common in Sweden and rare elsewhere in the world.

The term *congenital muscular dystrophy* (CMD) refers to a group of inherited disorders. Muscular dystrophy is present from birth. It has a slow progression with generalized weakness. A variation is more common in Japan; this is called Fukuyama CMD.

Symptoms and disease progression

All muscular dystrophy types are characterized by progressive muscle weakness in different muscle groups. Onset of symptoms can range from infancy to adulthood. The rate of disease progression is dependent on the type of muscular dystrophy. Some types are mild, with slower progression of muscle weakness over an individual's life span. Other types are more severe, with rapid progression of muscle weakness resulting in death in infancy or childhood.

Signs of DMD usually present in early childhood. Symptoms include delays in sitting, walking, gait problems, muscular-looking calves (called pseudohypertrophy), and curvature of the spine (scoliosis). Affected boys are usually wheelchair-bound by early adolescence, and respiratory failure and cardiac problems result in death by their early twenties.

BMD is a milder form of DMD. The onset of symptoms is later than in DMD, and progress takes place at a slower rate. Many boys with BMD can still walk in their teens, and some even into adulthood. The average age of death in individuals with BMD is in the mid-forties.

Although BMD is associated with milder muscle weakness than DMD, heart failure is the most common cause of death for individuals with BMD. DM

KEY FACTS

Description

The term *muscular dystrophy* refers to more than 30 diseases characterized by progressive muscle weakness and wasting. Some of the more common muscular dystrophies include Duchenne muscular dystrophy (DMD), Becker muscular dystrophy (BMD), limb girdle muscular dystrophy (LGMD), and myotonic dystrophy (DM).

Causes

The muscular dystrophies are genetic diseases with various modes of inheritance. Many different genes have been implicated.

Risk factors

A family history of muscular dystrophy may indicate that other individuals in the family are at risk, depending on the mode of inheritance associated with the specific muscular dystrophy.

Symptoms

All muscular dystrophies are characterized by progressive muscle weakness. This may present as frequent falls, uncoordinated movements, or difficulty walking. However, which muscle groups are affected, the age of onset and severity of symptoms, and the rate of progression vary depending on the specific type of muscular dystrophy.

Diagnosis

Elevated creatine kinase levels in the blood, muscle biopsy, electromyography (a measurement of electrical activity in the muscles), and genetic testing.

Treatments

There is no cure for muscular dystrophy. Treatments such as physical therapy and orthopedic surgery may be used to slow the progression of disease and improve quality of life.

Pathogenesis

Changes in the DNA (mutations) lead to abnormal proteins that play important roles in muscle maintenance, stability, and structure. When damage occurs to the muscle cells, they are unable to repair themselves as they normally would. Muscle cells are eventually replaced with connective tissue and fat.

Prevention

There is no known prevention for any of the muscular dystrophies.

Epidemiology

The incidence differs with the type of muscular dystrophy. The most common, DMD, occurs in 1 in 4,600 to 5,618 male births. BMD is less common and occurs in approximately 1 in 30,000 male births. DM affects approximately 1 in 20,000 individuals. Other types of MD are much

generally has an onset of symptoms anywhere between 10 and 30 years of age. Infants who suffer from the disorder are likely to have limp limbs, without normal tension and tone, and fail to reach milestones in development. This type of dystrophy is characterized by muscle weakness in the face and digestive tract, an inability to relax muscles (for example, unable to let go of someone's hand after shaking it), cardiac and respiratory problems, and cataracts, endocrine problems, and mental retardation. The average age of death for these individuals is in their early fifties. The onset of DM tends to occur earlier and the symptoms are generally more severe with each generation of affected individuals in a family.

A more severe form of DM (called congenital DM) can present at birth in some individuals. These infants have severe muscle weakness, which leads to difficulties with feeding and breathing. Approximately 25 percent of these infants die in the first 18 months of life. For those that survive past the first several years of life, 50 to 60 percent have mental retardation. Congenital DM is most often inherited from the individual's mother.

All types of LGMD show symptoms of weakness of the muscles closest to the body, such as in the arms and legs. The bones of the shoulders abnormally protrude, known as scapular winging. Cardiac problems due to weakness in the cardiac muscle have also been identified in some types of LGMD. The severity of muscle weakness and the rate of progression of disease is variable, depending on the subtype of LGMD.

For some autosomal recessive types, symptoms can appear in childhood and clinically resemble DMD. However, onset of the autosomal dominant types of LGMD is often in adolescence or adulthood with slower progression of muscle weakness.

Diagnosis

For both DMD and BMD, a diagnosis can be made by seeing reduced or absent dystrophin on a muscle biopsy. For all types of muscular dystrophy, significant signs on a muscle biopsy include the breakdown of muscle tissue, and muscle cells replaced with connective tissue and fat. Individuals with DMD, BMD, and several other types of muscular dystrophy also have elevated levels of creatine kinase. This is a substance released into the bloodstream when the muscle cells break down, and it is a sign that there is muscle damage. Although both of these tests are useful for diagnosis of DMD and BMD, they are not as helpful for identifying female carriers of these diseases.

Electromyography is a test that measures the electrical activity of the muscles when they are at rest and contracted. Tiny needles with electrodes are inserted through the skin into the muscle. These electrodes then record the electrical activity. In muscular dystrophy, the electrical activity of the muscles is abnormal.

Genetic testing is currently available for DMD and BMD, DM, and certain types of LGMD in which the involved gene is known. Once a genetic mutation is identified in an affected individual, then carrier and prenatal testing can be made available to other family members to determine who else is at risk.

Treatments

There is currently no cure for MD. Treatments target the symptoms associated with the specific type of muscular dystrophy and aim to improve an individual's quality of life. Physical therapy helps maintain flexibility and allows patients to remain ambulatory (walk unaided) as long as possible.

Several types of medication have also been found to be effective in treating the symptoms associated with specific muscular dystrophies, such as pain and inflammation. For example, muscle relaxants are used in the treatment of DM. Another medication, prednisone, has been shown to delay the progression of disease and increase muscle strength in boys with DMD.

Orthopedic surgery is an option that can also be used to correct scoliosis or increase a patient's range of motion. Researchers are currently exploring the possibility of replacing the absent dystrophin through gene therapy in DMD and BMD.

Epidemiology

The incidence differs with different types of muscular dystrophy. The most common, DMD, occurs in 1 in 3,500 male births; it affects around 8,000 boys and young men in the United States. A few female carriers show mild symptoms.

BMD is less common and occurs in about 1 in 43,000 male births; this type of dystrophy tends to affect older boys and young men. BMD produces milder symptoms than DMD.

LGMD is difficult to diagnose, and estimates of the prevalence are not easy to produce, but it is believed that the number of people affected in the United States is in the low thousands.

DM affects about 1 in 20,000 individuals. Other types of MD are much rarer and tend to be common to certain areas of the world.

Brian Brost

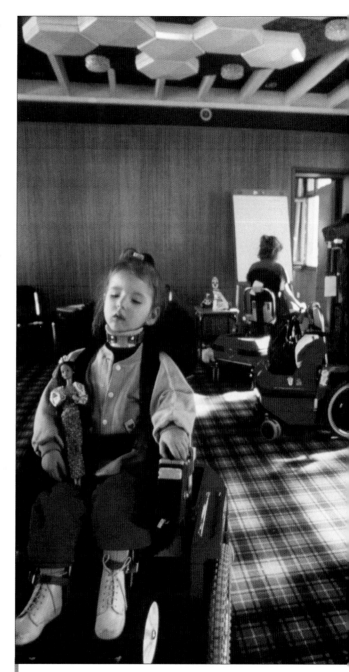

A young girl who suffers from muscular dystrophy attends a support center. She wears a neck brace and sits in a specially adapted wheelchair, in which she is securely strapped. The aim at the center is to maintain muscles not yet affected.

See also
- Genetic disorders • Learning disorders
- Spinal curvature

Myopia and hypermetropia

Myopia and hypermetropia are common refractive eye disorders. Light rays are bent and focused on the retina, which sends the images to the brain. Refractive errors are irregularities in the shape of the eye, causing the light to be refracted either in front of or behind the retina, so that the image appears blurred.

Light diverges from its source and converges to form an image. In a camera, light is bent or refracted by glass lenses which, in turn, refract the light passing through them because they have a greater optical density than the surrounding air.

Optical density is also referred to as the "index of refraction." Similarly, the cornea and lens bend light because they are denser than the surrounding air and the aqueous humor, respectively. The anterior surface of the cornea is the major refracting surface of the eye.

Causes

Myopia, or nearsightedness, is caused because the eye is longer or the cornea is steeper than normal, resulting in images being focused in front of the retina instead of directly on it. The image can be brought back onto the retina either by moving the object closer to the eye or by placing a lens that diverges light in front of the eye. Generally, people with myopia can see close objects clearly but have difficulty seeing distant objects. The degree of myopia determines the ability to focus. Severe myopia allows objects only a few inches away from the eye to be seen clearly, while mild myopia can allow objects a few yards away to be seen clearly. Large degrees of myopia (greater than 9 diopters) are called high myopia. The highly myopic eye is structurally abnormal: it becomes enlarged, with thinning of the retinal and sclera, which can predispose the individual to having a detached retina, especially if the eye is subjected to trauma.

Hypermetropia, or farsightedness, is caused by an eye that is shorter than normal, so that light rays focus behind, instead of on, the retina. People with hypermetropia have trouble focusing on nearby objects but can see distant objects clearly. As with myopia, the degree of hypermetropia determines the ability to focus. Severely hypermetropic eyes can only focus on objects a long distance from the eye. However, the average hypermetropic eye has good visual function until its accommodative reserves are depleted by age.

Risk factors

Both myopia and hypermetropia are inherited. Myopia may develop gradually or rapidly but generally worsens during adolescence, when the body grows quickly and there is increased focus on schoolwork. Hypermetropia is usually present at birth, but often young people's lenses are flexible enough to compensate for the error. However, as the person ages, the lens

KEY FACTS

Description
Refractive errors of the eye.

Causes
An eye that is longer than normal or a cornea that is steeper than usual.

Risk factors
Inherited trait. Asians and Caucasians are more likely to have myopia than other racial groups.

Symptoms
Blurred vision, excessive eyestrain causing discomfort and headaches.

Diagnosis
Standard eye examination.

Treatments
Corrective lenses, refractive surgery.

Pathogenesis
If it occurs in early childhood it can be severe.

Prevention
No proven method of prevention.

Epidemiology
In the United States, myopia is the most common of eye problems, present in 20–25 percent of all adults. Hypermetropia is also very common; it occurs in one-fourth of the population.

REFRACTIVE DISORDERS

In myopia, the eye is longer than usual, causing the light from distant objects to be focused in front of the retina; the image is blurred. In hypermetropia, the eye is shorter than normal, with the result that light from close objects is focused behind the retina, blurring the image.

light is refracted in front of retina

MYOPIA

cornea | retina

HYPERMETROPIA

light is refracted behind retina

Myopia or nearsightedness is an inability to see distant objects clearly; hypermetropia or farsightedness is an inability to see close objects clearly.

becomes less flexible and corrective lenses are generally required. The rapid increase in myopia among children emphasizes the importance of environment in the development of the disorder. China has reported that 50 percent of its teenagers are myopic, compared to 15 percent in the 1970s. This increase has been attributed to children focusing on near objects, including computers, computer games, and television.

Symptoms and diagnosis

A symptom of myopia is that distant objects appear blurry, and a symptom of hypermetropia is that nearby objects appear blurry. Common symptoms to both refractive errors are the need to squint in order to see clearly and excessive eyestrain, which causes discomfort and headaches. Both eye disorders are commonly diagnosed in a standard eye examination.

Treatments

Corrective lenses, which include eyeglasses and contact lenses, are the most common method of treating myopia and hypermetropia. Eyeglasses and contact lenses come in many different varieties to suit individual patients. Eyeglasses can also help protect the eye from harmful ultraviolet light rays. A special form of contact lenses is also available for a process called orthokeratology, in which hard lenses are used to flatten the cornea and reshape the cornea over time.

Refractive surgery is another common method for treating refractive errors. In LASIK (laser assisted in situ keratomileusis) surgery, an ophthalmologist makes a thin cut into the cornea, and then uses a laser to sculpt the central cornea. In LASEK (laser assisted subepithelial keratomileusis) surgery, a variant of LASIK surgery, an epithelial flap is cut instead of the much thicker stromal flap that is cut in the LASIK procedure. Since LASEK preserves more corneal tissue, the procedure may be safer for patients with thin corneas. PRK (photorefractive keratectomy) is a procedure that involves the removal of the eye's epithelium and the reshaping of the cornea, using a computer-controlled excimer laser. Finally, CK (conductive keratoplasty) is used for patients with hypermetropia who are more than 40 years old. CK uses radio frequency energy to reshape the cornea in order to make it slope more steeply.

Prevention

Myopia and hypermetropia are complex disorders involving both genetic and environmental factors. Researchers are attempting to identify the genes involved in order to better understand the pathogenesis and to develop diagnostic testing and, ultimately, treatment. Currently, there is no proven method of preventing myopia or hypermetropia, despite repeated attempts to halt or slow the process.

Epidemiology

Myopia is the most common of eye problems, present in 25 to 30 percent of all adults. Asian and Caucasians are generally more likely to have myopia than other racial groups. Hypermetropia is also very common, estimated to be present in approximately one-fourth of the population.

Josephine Everly and Herbert Kaufman

See also
• Eye disorders • Genetic disorders
• Glaucoma • Macular degeneration

Nervous system disorders

The nervous system includes the brain, spinal cord, and spinal and peripheral nerves. The brain and spinal cord comprise the central nervous system (CNS), and the spinal nerves and nerves of the body constitute the peripheral nervous system (PNS). Damage from disease or trauma to the peripheral nerves, spinal nerves, spinal cord, and brain can have profound consequences on homeostasis (the constant state of the internal environment) and bodily functions.

The brain and its disorders have been discussed in a separate section. Here, nervous system disorders will primarily include those with spinal cord or peripheral nerve involvement or both. The spinal cord is a thick whitish cord of nerve tissue that extends from the brain stem medulla oblongata through the foramen magnum of the skull, where it occupies the spinal canal and from which the spinal nerves branch off. The spinal cord, like the brain, is encased in a pair of membranes called the meninges, and the composite spinal cord and meninges are surrounded by the spine. The adult human spine usually contains 26 linked bones, 24 of which are called vertebrae, separated by cartilaginous disks that serve to cushion the spinal column and give it some flexibility. The spine consists of 7 vertebrae in the neck, called cervical vertebrae (C1 through C7), 12 thoracic vertebrae at the level of the chest (T1 through T12), and 5 lumbar vertebrae (L1 through L5) in the "small" of the back (where the spine

normally curves inward). The sacrum is composed of 5 fused vertebrae (S1 through S5) between the hip bones, and finally, there is the coccyx, which is the fusion of 3 to 5 bones at the lower end of the spine. Nerves from the cervical region, located in the neck, control the back of the head, the neck, shoulders, arms, hands, and diaphragm. The thoracic region controls the torso and parts of the arms. The upper lumbar region controls the hips and legs. The sacral region governs movement in the groin, toes, and parts of the legs. The adult spinal cord does not extend through the entirety of the spinal column. Instead, it terminates slightly above waist level. The collection of spinal nerves that lies below the spinal cord is called the *cauda equina* (Latin for "horse's tail").

The spinal cord has 31 pairs of spinal nerves that emerge from spaces between the vertebrae and connect with peripheral nerves throughout the body. Every spinal nerve but the first has two nerve roots: a motor root coming from the front, or frontal part, of the spinal cord; and a sensory root, coming from the back or dorsal part. The first spinal nerve has no sensory root. The motor root transmits signals from the spinal cord to the muscles. The sensory root transports nerve signals from sensory neurons in the skin and musculoskeletal system back to the spinal cord and brain.

The spinal cord is highly organized and, like the brain, consists of gray and white matter. Unlike the brain, the gray matter is mostly in the center of the

RELATED ARTICLES

STRUCTURE OF THE NERVOUS SYSTEM

The brain and spinal cord comprise the central nervous system, and all neural tissue outside that system is called the peripheral nervous system. The peripheral nervous system is divided into somatic and autonomic systems. The somatic nervous system regulates the skeletal muscles and collects sensory information from the skin and neuromuscular system. The autonomic nervous system governs involuntary actions such as heart beat, glandular secretions, blood vessel constriction, and peristalsis. It is controlled by the hypothalamus and is divided into two parts, the sympathetic nervous system and parasympathetic nervous system; the two systems work in tandem to regulate the body's physiological responses to the environment. Signals from sensory nerves in the periphery of the body send signals to the spinal cord and brain, where they are processed. Responses to environmental cues are elicited and communicated through motor neurons that control the muscles.

From the central nervous system (spinal cord and brain) nerves radiate all over the body to form the peripheral nervous system.

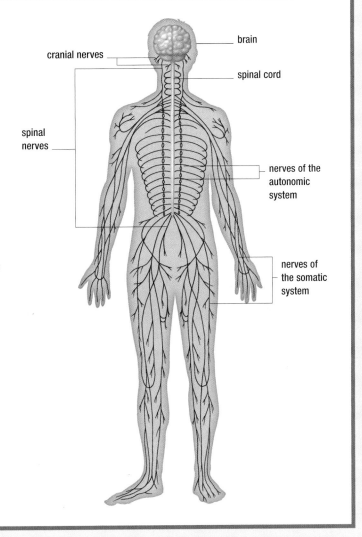

brain

cranial nerves

spinal cord

spinal nerves

nerves of the autonomic system

nerves of the somatic system

---

cord, and the white matter is mostly on the outer portion of the cord. The gray matter resides in a butterfly-shaped formation throughout the length of the spinal cord. The front wings, or lobes, are composed of motor nerves, and the dorsal lobes contain sensory nerves. The white matter contains columns of nerve fibers. Descending tracts transmit nerve impulses from the brain to the muscles; ascending tracts carry sensory information from the body to the spinal cord and brain.

The peripheral nervous system is divided into somatic and autonomic systems. The somatic nervous system regulates the skeletal muscles and collects

sensory information from the skin and neuromuscular system. It controls voluntary skeletal muscles and collects and transmits sensory information back to the spinal cord and brain, where it can be precisely located and processed in the cerebral cortex of the brain.

The autonomic nervous system governs involuntary actions such as the heartbeat, glandular secretions, blood vessel constriction, and peristalsis. It is controlled by the hypothalamus and is divided into two parts, the sympathetic nervous system and parasympathetic nervous system. Generally, the two systems work in tandem to regulate the body's physiological responses to the environment. The parasympathetic nervous system tends to stimulate digestive secretions, to dilate blood vessels, to constrict the pupils, and to slow the heart rate. The sympathetic nervous system tends to oppose the actions of the parasympathetic nervous system. It reduces digestive secretions, contracts blood vessels, enlarges the pupils, and increases the heart rate. Some consider the enteric nervous system as a separate entity within the autonomic nervous system. It comprises nerve fibers that supply the gastrointestinal tract, pancreas, and gallbladder.

In addition to the brain disorders previously discussed, the remainder of the nervous system also has a multitude of disorders that may or may not involve the brain. These include spina bifida, motor neuron disease, and multiple sclerosis.

Spina bifida

Spina bifida is a developmental disorder involving incomplete development of the neural tube into the brain, spinal cord, or the meninges. During the first month of gestation the spine fails to close properly. A child can have varying degrees of spina bifida, usually assigned to three different categories based on severity. These are occulta, meningocele, and myelomeningocele.

The mildest form is occulta, when there is no opening on the back but the outer part of some vertebrae are malformed. The meninges and spinal cord are not damaged and the nerves are usually intact. It rarely causes symptoms.

In meningocele spina bifida the spinal opening is severe enough that the meninges can protrude through it. The meninges are damaged and may appear as a cerebrospinal fluid-filled sac. The opening may not be covered by skin. The symptoms range from few or none to moderate. It is the form of spina bifida with the lowest incidence.

Myelomeningocele is the most severe form. The spinal opening is so severe that the spinal cord is exposed. This results in partial or complete paralysis of the body controlled by nerves distal (away from) the opening. Symptoms are highly variable. Depending on severity, the afflicted individual may show no sign of the disorder. Cases more severe than occulta may have an abnormal tuft of hair, birthmark, or dimple on the skin at the malformation site. Children with myelomeningocele

accompanied by hydrocephalus (buildup of fluid in the skull) may have learning disabilities. More serious symptoms also include severe or complete paralysis with urinary and bowel dysfunction.

There is no cure for spina bifida. Treatments are symptomatic and include surgery, medication, physiotherapy, and assistive devices such as braces, wheelchairs, or crutches.

Although the cause of spina bifida is not known, it is suspected that genetic, nutritional, and environmental factors may be contributing factors. There is evidence that the addition of the vitamin folic acid (0.4 mg daily) to the diet of women in their child-bearing years may significantly reduce the incidence of the disorder.

Motor neuron disease

Motor neuron disease (MND) is a group of four neurological disorders. These disorders are characterized by a steady degeneration of the motor neurons in the brain, brain stem, and spinal cord. Motor neurons send nerve impulses to the voluntary muscles; their degeneration leads to muscle weakness and wasting. MND usually affects the limbs. Weakness in the face and throat lead to problems with the functions of speech, chewing, and swallowing. It does not, for the most part, affect the senses, bladder and bowel control, sexual function, or intellect. The disorder usually manifests over the age of 40 years, with the highest incidence in the 50- to 70-year-old group. Men have a slightly higher incidence than women. The major site of motor neuron degeneration identifies the clinical subtypes. These include amyotrophic lateral sclerosis (Lou Gehrig's disease), spinal muscular atrophy, progressive bulbar palsy, and primary lateral sclerosis.

Amyotrophic lateral sclerosis (ALS) is a fatal neurological disease with a rapid regression of function upon disease onset. Both upper (brain) and lower (spinal cord) motor neurons degenerate, and the brain loses the capacity to control voluntary muscles. The muscles then weaken, atrophy (waste), and may ultimately twitch. Eventually, all voluntary muscles are affected, and the afflicted person loses the ability to move his or her arms and legs. Eventually, muscles in the diaphragm and chest wall are affected, and the patient cannot breathe without mechanical assistance (ventilator). Respiratory failure is the usual cause of death in these patients. Death usually occurs within five years of diagnosis, although some 10 percent of patients live for 10 or more years. Overt intellectual abnormalities are not obvious during the course of the disease, although new evidence indicates there may be minor cognitive impairment in some patients.

As with many neurological diseases, the cause of the most common form is not known. About 10 percent of ALS cases appear to have a strong genetic component that may be an autosomal dominant gene (see GENETIC DISORDERS). There are probably several genes that may contribute to ALS susceptibility. The diagnosis of ALS is difficult because early symptoms are shared by a variety of disorders. Early symptoms of muscle twitching, weakness, and cramping, eventually followed by slurred or nasal speech and difficulty chewing or swallowing, suggest ALS. Clinical tests are then performed that eliminate the presence of other diseases. There is no cure for the disease but recent experience indicates that Riluzole, which inhibits the release of the neurotransmitter glutamate, may prolong life by several months. This provides hope that more efficacious drugs will be found in the future. Additional current therapies address symptomatic relief and quality of life improvement.

Spinal muscular atrophy (SMA) is a disease with progressive degeneration of spinal-cord motor neurons. Often, the muscle wasting is more prevalent in the legs than in the arms, and it also affects the muscles used for crawling, walking, and control of the head and neck. There are different types of SMA, including those in children. Type I is the most severe (Werdnig syndrome), type II is of intermediate severity, and type III has mild symptoms (Kugelberg-Welander disease). The disease in children is usually acquired through autosomal recessive genes. There are also several adult onset forms of the disease that appear to be inherited by a variety of mechanisms.

In progressive bulbar palsy, the initial motor neuron degeneration is in the brain stem; in primary lateral sclerosis, degeneration is in the cortical neurons of the brain. The disease is usually not fatal and the patient can maintain some mobility with the use of ambulatory aids.

Meningitis
Meningitis is an acute infectious disease that causes severe inflammation of the brain and spinal cord. The infection is caused by a variety of agents, most often the bacterium *Neisseria meningitidis*, but may also arise from viruses or protozoa. The symptoms are flulike and include headache, vomiting, convulsion, stiff neck, light sensitivity, and small eruptions on the skin. If untreated, the disease can progress rapidly to death. Clinical signs and symptoms and analysis of cerebrospinal fluid obtained from a lumbar puncture are diagnostic for the disease. Treatment of the disease depends on the source of infection.

Multiple sclerosis
Multiple sclerosis is believed by many to be an autoimmune disease—a disease that occurs when the body is attacked by its own immune system. It can be relatively mild to severe. It affects the central nervous system (brain and spinal cord) and affects women more than men. The myelin sheath, the fatty insulation that surrounds axons, appears to be the primary tissue damaged. It is a slowly progressive disease, usually in a pattern of acute functional regression followed by periods of stability (remission). As a result of the autoimmune response and accompanying inflammation, segments of myelin are destroyed and replaced by sclerotic (scar) tissue. The damaged myelin impedes or blocks nerve signals, causing muscles to atrophy (waste). Overt symptoms vary from patient to patient, depending on the area affected. First symptoms are most often observed between the ages of 20 to 40 years and include blurred or double vision, red and green color distortion, or even blindness in one eye. In severe cases the patient experiences partial or complete paralysis. Most patients also experience numbness and prickling sensations (paresthesia), pain, difficulty with speech, tremors, and dizziness.

The initial cause of the disease and the factors that precipitate an attack are not clearly understood. Viruses, genetics, environmental factors, or combinations of them may increase susceptibility. The incidence is more prevalent in the United States, northern Europe, southern Australia, and New Zealand.

There is no cure for the disease. Many patients do reasonably well without therapy. The drug beta interferon reduces the number of attacks and may slow the progression of physical complications. Polymers may be given; they are substances that control drug release rate, enhance uptake of another drug, and limit toxicity. In addition, they may reduce the relapse rate and have few side effects. Immuno-suppressant treatment is being tested for use in advanced multiple sclerosis. Steroids also appear to reduce the duration and intensity of attacks. Treatment of the symptoms also helps improve quality of life.

Cervical spondylosis

Cervical spondylosis is caused by degeneration of the cartilage and bone in the cervical vertebrae (neck), often with mineral deposits in the cervical disks. The spinal canal may also become narrow (stenosed). Much of this simply may be a part of the aging process, although extreme degeneration is not. Neck injury can also cause the disorder. Pain, a first symptom of the disorder, may range from mild in the early phase to severe in the later stage. Other symptoms can include numbness or weakness in the arms, hands, and fingers, weakness in the legs, loss of balance, grinding or popping in the neck, muscle spasms in the neck, and headache. Sleep impairment may also cause additional symptoms such as fatigue or irritability. Diagnosis is by clinical observation of pain and follow-up tests, including X-ray, computed tomography (CT), magnetic resonance imaging (MRI), myelogram, or electromyography (EMG). Most patients will have some chronic symptoms that minimally affect activities of daily living. In more severe cases, drugs (nonsteroidal anti-inflammatory drugs), temporary traction, or surgery may be required.

Spinal cord injury

Spinal cord injury, or trauma, occurs when there is direct injury to the spinal cord or indirect injury to it from tissue or bone damage that may cause swelling, severing, or bruising of the spinal cord. If the spinal column is compromised in some fashion, for example, by age-related deterioration, an apparently minor injury can become severe. In addition to direct spinal damage from bone, the spinal cord can also be traumatized by being extended, compressed by fluid or physical pressures, or twisted. Many spinal cord injuries occur in young, active people, with the most commonly affected being males between the ages of 15 and 35 years old.

Symptoms vary in type and magnitude, depending on the location and severity of the spinal cord injury. Symptoms can include weakness or paralysis in both

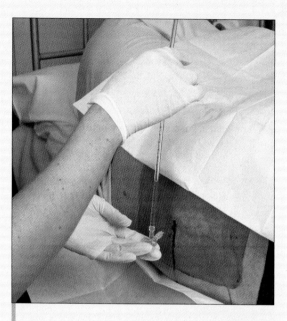

A doctor measures cerebrospinal-fluid pressure, to check for meningitis, after having performed a lumbar puncture. The clear spinal fluid in the pipette is being withdrawn by means of a needle inserted into the space between the third and fourth lumbar vertebrae.

the arms and legs, breathing difficulties, spasticity, sensory changes, numbness, pain, loss of bowel or bladder control, abnormal sweating, and difficulty in maintaining body temperature. Symptoms may manifest immediately or over time because of fluid accumulation around the spinal cord or swelling in the spinal cord proper. Spinal cord injury is an emergency, and recovery is improved when treated immediately or as soon as possible after the trauma. Diagnosis and treatment are similar to those described for cervical spondylosis above. Surgery may be required to relieve pressure, removing fluid or hematomas, or to remove objects such as bone, disc fragments, or foreign objects. Also, physical and occupational therapies are often required. The prognosis for affected individuals is greatly dependent on the severity of the trauma and the bodily functions that are affected.

Transverse myelitis

Transverse myelitis is an inflammatory disorder in which the inflammation occurs on both sides of one spinal cord segment. The affected area of the body is determined by the location of the inflammation.

Damage in one location affects the spinal cord from that point and below. The onset is usually rapid, most often with pain in the thoracic (upper back) region. This causes difficulties with leg movements and can progress to abnormal sensations in the feet, paralysis, urinary retention, and loss of bowel control. It may occur as the primary disorder (idiopathic) or as a result of some other illness. Idiopathic transverse myelitis may be due to an autoimmune response to the spinal cord. There is no cure, although corticosteroid treatment may help to reduce the intensity of the inflammation. Additional approaches include trying to keep the body functioning in the hope that spontaneous recovery will occur.

Neuropathy

The peripheral nervous system is susceptible to many neuropathies (nerve disease). Characteristic symptoms, developmental pattern, and prognosis are known for over one hundred peripheral neuropathies. The clinical manifestations of the particular disorders are dependent on the type of nerves affected (motor, sensory, or autonomic), and the severity of the damage. Symptoms can be mild (such as tingling, numbness, and pricking sensations) to severe (such as paralysis, burning pain, muscle wasting, and organ or gland dysfunction). There are inherited and acquired forms. Acquired peripheral neuropathy can be caused by physical trauma to a peripheral nerve, tumors, toxins, autoimmune responses, nutritional deficiencies, drug abuse, vascular disease, or metabolic disorders. Inherited forms can be acquired from genes passed down by parents or can develop from new mutations.

Some of the more common peripheral nervous system disorders include acrodynia, brachial plexus neuropathies, complex regional pain syndromes, Guillain-Barré, headache, trigeminal neuralgia, neuritis, neurofibromatosis 1, and congenital pain insensitivity or indifference.

Acrodynia

Acrodynia, also known as pink disease, Bilderbeck's, Selter's, Swift's, and Swift-Feer disease, is a painful condition. It is accompanied by a pinkish discoloration of the hands and feet and is most commonly found in children chronically exposed to mercury or, less commonly, other heavy metals. Mercury compounds used to be a component of many medicines such as laxatives, diuretics, antimicrobial agents, and teething powders. Although it has been recognized for decades that mercury is poisonous, acrodynia still occasionally occurs. Other symptoms include tingling or itching of the skin, burning pain, edema (swelling), and shedding of skin, ruddy complexion, profuse sweating, abnormally fast heartbeat (tachycardia), excess salivation, and elevated blood pressure.

Additional symptoms sometimes include red lips, hair loss, dental insufficiencies, nail loss, kidney dysfunction, and neuropsychiatric problems. Immediate cessation of exposure is imperative. Chelation therapy is helpful to reduce tissue stores of the heavy metal.

Brachial plexus neuropathy

Brachial plexus neuropathy entails decreased sensation or movement of the shoulder and arm. It is caused by damage to the brachial plexus, a nerve bundle that controls sensation and movement of the arm. The damage is usually due to direct trauma to the nerve, pressure from a tumor near the brachial plexus, or damage from radiation therapy used in the treatment of some cancers. It can also be a result of congenital abnormalities or inflammatory conditions.

Symptoms include: shoulder pain; shoulder, arm, or hand numbness or weakness; tingling or burning pain in areas dependent on the location of the injury; or Horner's syndrome (drooping eye, small pupil, decreased facial sweating). Clinical presentation, electromyography, and nerve biopsy may be used for diagnosis. Depending on the clinical picture, for example known trauma, treatment may involve watchful waiting, anti-inflammatory drugs, or surgery. Adjunct treatment such as painkillers or physical therapy may be helpful. Prognosis may vary from complete recovery to paralysis, depending on injury severity.

Complex regional pain syndrome

Complex regional pain syndrome (CRPS) is a condition in which the patient experiences continuous, intense pain beyond that expected for the observed injury, which gets worse over time. It usually affects one of the arms, hands, legs, or feet. The affected body part may display dramatic changes in color and temperature. The cause of CRPS is not known. It appears that the sympathetic nervous system may play a part in the disorder. It is also felt that an immune response may be involved that accounts for some disease consequences such as redness, warmth, and swelling. As with so many neurological disorders, there is no cure for CRPS. Treatment is directed to symptomatic relief. Some individuals may experience remission from the symptoms, while others experience irreversible outcomes.

Guillain-Barré syndrome

Guillain-Barré syndrome is an autoimmune disorder affecting the peripheral nervous system. Early symptoms include varying degrees of weakness and abnormal sensations spreading to the arms and upper body. Reflexes, such as knee jerk, are often lost because nerve conduction is slowed. In some cases, these symptoms can become so severe that the muscles cannot be used and the patient is nearly paralyzed. In that circumstance, the disorder is life threatening, and a respirator may be used to assist with breathing until function is regained. Most patients recover from even the most severe cases, although a few continue to have some degree of residual weakness. The onset of the disorder is fairly rapid (hours to days to weeks in some cases) and often occurs from a few days to a few weeks after symptoms of respiratory or gastrointestinal infection or, less commonly, after vaccinations or surgery.

Diagnostic procedures will usually include a determination of nerve conduction velocity and cerebrospinal fluid (CSF) analysis (patients often have elevated CSF protein levels). Treatment of the disorder can lessen disease severity and significantly decrease recovery time. Plasmapheresis (in which plasma is separated from the blood and the remaining components are returned to the patient) or high-dose immunoglobulin therapy is used. Plasmapheresis appears to lessen the intensity and duration of the disorder. Immunoglobulin therapy entails giving immunoglobulins acquired from normal donors. This seems to lessen the autoimmune attack on the peripheral nervous system. Of critical importance during the course of this disorder is maintaining body function, which is often accomplished by using a respirator and other instrumentation to aid normal body function.

Headaches and migraine

A headache is a pain localized to the head, usually above the eyes and ears, often in the back of the head or upper neck. Headaches have been categorized in several ways. Here, they will be described as primary or secondary. Primary headaches are not the result of other diseases. Secondary headaches are the consequence of some other primary disorder. Three types of primary headaches are migraine, tension, and cluster headaches.

Migraine headaches are vascular in origin due to the constriction and then expansion of blood vessels in the head. The pain is extremely severe and lasts from several minutes to several days. In adults, nearly three-quarters of the affected population are women. There are two types of migraine headaches: migraine with an aura (called "classic" by some), which involves visual disturbances such as flashing lights and blind spots, and migraines without an aura (called common), which do not have the visual affects. Susceptibility to migraines appears to run in families. Some scientists believe that migraines may be caused by low brain levels of the neurotransmitter serotonin. The best known preventive is to avoid materials that trigger attacks. Also, beta blockers, calcium channel blockers, antidepressants, serotonin antagonists, antiseizure medications, and biofeedback can be used to help prevent attacks. Pain relievers include over-the-counter analgesics and combinations of compounds such as aspirin, acetaminophen, and caffeine. Narcotic pain relievers, sedatives, ergot alkaloids, serotonin agonists (activators), and isometheptene-acetaminophen-sedative mixtures can also be used for treatment.

Tension headache is the most common and is more prevalent in women than in men. It is a condition that involves usually moderate pain in the head, neck, or scalp and is associated with muscle tightness or contractions in the affected areas. Circumstances in which the head and neck are held in one position for an extended time period, such as when using a computer or holding a telephone between the shoulder and head, tend to induce the disorder. Tension headache can also be a response to stress, depression, or anxiety. Additional causes appear to include fatigue, eye strain, drug abuse, especially alcohol, smoking, sinus infection, or nasal congestion. Analgesics such as aspirin or ibuprofen can be used to alleviate the pain. Stress management, biofeedback, and avoidance of precipitating factors are additional approaches to tension headache management.

Cluster headaches affect one side of the head and happen in clusters, occurring repeatedly at about the same time every day for weeks before they abate. They are more common between adolescence and middle age and occur in men more than women. The cause is unknown but suspected to be due to a sudden release of histamine or serotonin by body tissues. The headaches occur suddenly, often during the rapid eye movement (REM) phase of sleep. Glare, stress, certain foods, heavy smoking, or alcohol may contribute to the disorder. Treatment entails avoidance of triggers, prevention, and pain management.

Secondary headaches are the result of a primary disorder such as meningitis, brain tumors, stroke, or hemorrhage. Less serious conditions that can cause secondary headaches include caffeine withdrawal or abrupt analgesics withdrawal. Treatment of secondary headaches depends on the primary disorder.

Trigeminal neuralgia

Trigeminal neuralgia, also called tic douloureux, is a condition that causes recurring, episodic chronic face pain in the form of an extreme, sudden, sporadic burning sensation that lasts from a few seconds to a few minutes per occurrence. The pain can be so intense that it is debilitating. Typically, one side of the jaw or cheek is affected. Episodes can last for a few days to months, followed by a varying period of remission. Often, the attacks become worse over time and the pain-free periods are shortened. There are triggers for the onset of pain, such as, for example, physical contact with the cheek, brushing teeth, and talking. People over 50 years of age are more susceptible to the disorder, and the incidence is greater in women than in men. There is some evidence for a hereditary predisposition for the disorder. The cause is thought to be from a blood vessel impinging on the trigeminal nerve as it exits the brain stem. It may also be a secondary condition to a disorder such as multiple sclerosis in which the myelin sheath is damaged. If the cause of the pain can be found, treatment options might include anticonvulsants, tricyclic antidepressants, surgery, or combinations of all these. Although the disorder

can drastically affect the quality of life, it is not life threatening.

Neuritis is a condition in which the nerves are inflamed. The inflammation interferes with normal sensory and motor nerve function and alters the areas of tissue supplied by the affected nerves. Symptoms include numbness, tingling, prickling sensation, pain, weakness, and occasionally paralysis. The causes of this condition include local nerve trauma or irritation, autoimmune diseases, vaccine injury, exposure to cold, leukemia, diabetes, infections, vitamin deficiencies, alcohol abuse, arsenic, mercury or lead overexposure, and toxemia of pregnancy. Treatment is dependent on the primary disorder.

Neurofibromatosis 1

Neurofibromatosis 1 is an inherited, autosomal dominant disorder characterized by the presence of neurofibromas (nerve tissue tumors) in the cranial nerves, skin, spinal root nerves, and subcutaneous (beneath the skin) tissue. The disorder can also appear as a new mutation in one of the genes responsible for the disease. This gene encodes a protein known as neurofibromin. The disorder causes the growth of neurofibromatous tumors that compress affected nerves and cause pain, nerve damage, and loss of function. Overt neurological symptoms depend on the nerves affected. In addition to nodular and soft tumors of the skin, brownish (café-au-lait) spots on the skin are the hallmarks of neurofibromatosis 1. Other symptoms include impaired cognitive function, leg fractures, underarm or groin freckles, convulsions, and blindness. There is no cure for the disorder. Surgical removal of the tumors may be required on an individual basis, and rapidly growing tumors are removed immediately as they may become malignant. Life expectancy is nearly normal.

Congenital pain insensitivity and indifference

Congenital pain insensitivity and indifference are two separate entities. Pain indifference occurs when there is no obvious nerve pathology. The patient can perceive pain, but fails to have an appropriate response to it. Congenital insensitivity to pain is a rare disorder in which the patient has a nerve pathology that impedes pain perception.

David Ullman

Neuralgia

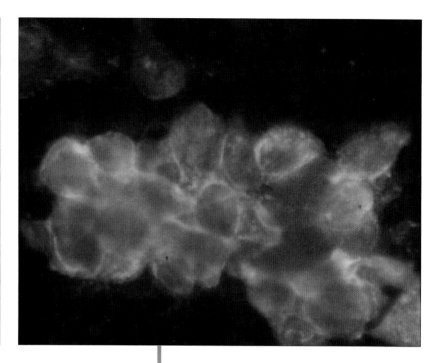

Neuralgia is pain that is often sharp, severe, and typically unilateral along an affected nerve. There are various types of neuralgia; trigeminal neuralgia and post-herpetic neuralgia are the most common, but neuralgia can arise from any sensory nerve root in the body. Other common forms of neuralgia include: glossopharyngeal neuralgia, geniculate neuralgia, and occipital neuralgia.

A colored photomicrograph shows the varicella-zoster virus magnified 200 times. After this type of infection, post-herpetic neuralgia sometimes develops in older people.

The cause of trigeminal neuralgia is thought to be vascular compression of the nerve root near its entry into the brain with subsequent focal demyelination (breakdown of fatty insulation around nerve fibers). Multiple sclerosis may cause trigeminal neuralgia; other causes are rare, but include tumors in the posterior fossa compressing the trigeminal nerve. The biggest risk factor for trigeminal neuralgia is advancing age, with female gender as a lesser predisposing factor. The cause of post-herpetic neuralgia is related to inflammatory changes that occur in the nerve and nerve root after infection (often decades earlier) with the virus that causes chicken pox and herpes zoster. The risk factors for post-herpetic neuralgia include preceding herpes zoster infection, advanced age at the time of infection, and location in the trigeminal nerve root.

Symptoms, signs, and diagnosis

The trigeminal nerve is responsible for sensation over the skin of the face and so, when individuals suffer from trigeminal neuralgia, they will complain of severe, paroxysmal pain in one side of the face. The pain is often reproduced by gentle stimulation of that area of the face, such as chewing or sometimes cold air. It lasts a few seconds to minutes in duration. Typically, trigeminal neuralgia is diagnosed based on the charac-

teristic history and normal examination. There are no laboratory, electrophysiologic radiologic abnormalities except in atypical cases associated with a structural lesion: demyelination or tumor. Pathological diagnosis of trigeminal neuralgia is not typically made, but when examined, histological changes can be seen in the gasserian ganglion.

Post-herpetic neuralgia (PHN) is diagnosed when pain continues more than three months after a herpes zoster infection (shingles). Herpes zoster infection is reactivation of a varicella virus (chicken pox) that remains dormant (inactive) in nerve cells. Herpes zoster manifests itself as a painful vesicular rash (fluid filled) in the distribution of the affected nerve root. The pain may be described as an unpleasant burning or tingling sensation in the distribution of the affected nerve root. Compared to trigeminal neuralgia, the pain is usually persistent. Most people who have a zoster infection will not develop PHN, but the older individuals are when they develop zoster, the greater the chances of PHN. Development of PHN is determined by the location of herpes zoster infection, with involvement of trigeminal and brachial plexus sites highest, followed in descending order by jaw, neck, sacral, and lumbar. The diagnosis is typically made based on the history of a painful herpes zoster eruption (shingles), with resolution of the vesicular rash but continued pain. Laboratory testing is not required, but examination of cerebrospinal fluid will often show an elevated number of lymphocytes and elevated protein due to inflammation in the nerve roots.

Other neuralgias such as glossopharyngeal neuralgia have symptoms similar to those in trigeminal neuralgia, but the symptoms occur in the distribution of the corresponding nerve root (that is, the pharynx).

Treatments and prevention

Medical treatment is generally the first line treatment for trigeminal neuralgia. The drug commonly used is carbamazepine. Other anti-epileptic drugs can also be used to treat neuralgia. A combination of two drugs may be required. Surgical options include local injections to anesthetize affected nerves or decompression of the nerve root in the case of trigeminal neuralgia.

Post-herpetic neuralgia is usually treated with anticonvulsants such as gabapentin, tricyclic antidepressants, analgesics, corticosteroids, or antiviral agents. These agents typically alleviate the neuropathic pain, allowing most people to function normally and participate in daily activities. In very severe and unremitting cases, surgical intervention with sectioning of the dorsal root ganglion may be helpful.

Pathogenesis

Trigeminal neuralgia is thought to result from vascular compression of the nerve as it enters the brain; age is therefore a risk factor. Trigeminal neuralgia may have typical exacerbations and remissions through life, but usually worsens with time and may require additional medications or surgical interventions as it worsens. Many individuals learn to avoid activities such as shaving, extreme temperatures, or smiling, or any conditions that worsen or bring on attacks. In extreme cases, the severe pain causes depression and suicidal tendencies.

Post-herpetic neuralgia is thought to result from inflammatory changes that occur in the nerves related to a prior herpes zoster infection. The inflammation affects and changes nerve fibers secondary to the preceding varicella virus infection. This manifests itself as a misperception of temperature or light touch. These pain sensations can be spontaneous or elicited with a light, nonpainful stimulus. Postherpetic neuralgia usually remits over time, but may occasionally worsen.

KEY FACTS

Description

Intermittent, severe pain in a single nerve.

Causes

Trigeminal neuralgia is thought to be due to vascular compression, but has not been definitively proven. PHN is due to inflammatory changes in the corresponding nerve and root.

Risk factors

Age and female gender are risk factors for trigeminal neuralgia. The risk factors for PHN include preceding herpes zoster infection, and advanced age at the time of the skin eruption.

Signs and symptoms

Unilateral pain in a nerve root such as the trigeminal, facial, or spinal nerves. A healing vesicular and painful rash is strong evidence for a post-herpetic neuralgia.

Diagnosis

History typical of a classic syndrome and corresponding exam findings.

Pathogenesis

Trigeminal neuralgia is lifelong but may have spontaneous exacerbations and remissions and is responsive to medical and surgical therapy. PHN occurs about one month after a herpes zoster skin eruption and typically persists indefinitely.

Prevention

No know prevention strategies for trigeminal neuralgia, but a recent vaccine can prevent zoster eruptions in those over the age of 60.

Epidemiology

More common in women over the age of 40. Affects about 5 in 100,000 people. PHN is reported in 3–15 percent of people.

Epidemiology

Trigeminal neuralgia is more common in women over the age of 40, and the incidence is estimated to affect 5 in 100,000 people. It is 200 times more common in patients with multiple sclerosis. PHN is reported in 3 to 15 percent of individuals after a herpes zoster infection, with an incidence of 500 in 100,000 in those over 50 years old; this more than doubles in people who are more than 80.

Meredith Roderick and Robert Daroff

See also
• Aging, disorders of • Chicken pox and shingles • Depressive disorders • Herpes infections • Multiple sclerosis • Nervous system disorders

Neural tube disorders

Although the exact cause of neural tube disorders is still under investigation, it is known that abnormal development of the nervous system in the first four weeks of embryonic development can have profound, lifelong effects. Just a simple change in a mother's diet, however, can make a dramatic difference in reducing the risk of developing this permanently disabling birth defect.

As early as the first few weeks of pregnancy, the neural tube of a developing embryo, destined to become the brain and spinal cord of a baby, should close completely along its length. If it does not, a neural tube disorder can result along any part of the tube.

Spina bifida is a common birth defect, affecting one of every 1,400 to 1,500 newborns in the United States. There are three types of spina bifida. In occulta or hidden spina bifida, there is only a small defect in the vertebrae. It causes symptoms in very few cases. Meningocele is the rarest form of spina bifida. The bones do not close around the spinal cord, and a fluid-filled sac protrudes through an opening in the spine. Surgery is often required. The third type of spina bifida, and the most common and most severe, is myelomeningocele. In this condition, part of the spinal cord protrudes through an opening in the spine, sometimes exposing skin and nerves. The position on the spine dictates the neurological disabilities; if the opening is low on the spine, there will be bowel and bladder problems, but if the opening is higher there also can be paralysis of the legs.

In severe cases of a neural tube disorder, membranes and the spinal cord protrude through a spinal opening. Skin usually grows over the opening, but telltale signs such as a fatty lump, hairy patch, or changes in pigmentation reveal the location of the defect. If the defect occurs at the head end of the embryo, severe brain malformations, including anencephaly, result.

In anencephaly, most of the brain and skull fail to develop. The condition causes death before birth or soon afterward. There are other neural tube disorders that disrupt brain development, but most are extremely rare.

Risk factors

The greatest risk factor appears to be a lack of the B vitamin folic acid in the diet before pregnancy and during the first 12 weeks of pregnancy. An adequate intake of folic acid is vital for fetal growth, the formation of blood cells, and the healthy development of the baby's nervous system. Deficiencies in women occur if they do not have a nutritionally balanced diet or if they drink large amounts of alcohol.

Neural tube disorders are more common in Hispanics and those of European descent, but in most cases, there is no family history of the disease. Other risk factors include diabetes, obesity, high body temperature, and some anti-seizure medicines.

Exposure to the herbicide Agent Orange is now officially recognized as a risk factor. If a parent was exposed while serving in Vietnam and has a child with spina bifida, the U.S. government will provide special disability payments, vocational training, and rehabilitation services to the family.

Diagnosis

Neural tube disorders are usually diagnosed before a baby is born. Doctors measure the level of alpha-fetoprotein (AFP) in the mother's blood 16 to 18 weeks into her pregnancy. An abnormally high AFP level indicates the possibility of a neural tube disorder. Ultrasound can be used to confirm the diagnosis. The alpha-fetoprotein test is often combined with two or three other tests to improve its accuracy. But these screening tests are not foolproof, and in some cases a neural tube disorder may be missed. Obvious deformities will be detected immediately after birth, but X-rays, magnetic resonance imaging (MRI), or computed tomography (CT) might be required to look for hidden damage.

Treatment and social impact

There is no way to cure neural tube disorders. Nerve damage is almost always permanent, so the goal of treatment is to prevent further damage and infections. The disease progression depends on the size, severity, and location of the defect. Spina bifida occulta or "hidden" spina bifida may go undiagnosed for years and cause no serious health impacts. At the other extreme, a child with a severe neural tube disorder may need surgery within the first 24 hours of birth to prevent paralysis and brain damage. Additional operations may be required as a child grows.

When the disease is diagnosed before birth, doctors are likely to recommend a cesarean section, to prevent damage that could occur during a vaginal delivery. In other cases, surgeons may actually perform corrective surgery before birth. It is believed that this surgery can improve brain function later in life, but fetal surgery is risky and not always an option.

Many children with neural tube disorders also develop hydrocephalus, commonly called "water on the brain." Cerebrospinal fluid is unable to drain normally, and the resulting pressure causes the head to swell. Shunts can be implanted surgically to restore normal drainage and prevent further damage.

KEY FACTS

Description
Disorder of the nervous system that can result in lifelong deformities or early death.

Causes
Unknown, but both genetic and environmental factors are suspected.

Risk factors
Insufficient folic acid in the mother's diet, family history, diabetes, obesity, and exposure to certain drugs or toxic agents.

Symptoms
Congenital malformations of the head and spine, pain or weakness in the back or legs, and changes in bowel or bladder function.

Diagnosis
Prenatal blood tests and ultrasound. Less severe cases are diagnosed by X-ray, magnetic resonance imaging, or ultrasound after birth.

Treatments
Vary widely depending on the severity of the disorder. Treatments can include surgery, medication, and physical therapy.

Pathogenesis
Some neural tube disorders may produce few or no symptoms, while others can lead to progressive neurodegeneration or death within the first year of life.

Prevention
Increased consumption of folic acid before and during pregnancy.

Epidemiology
One of the most common developmental disorders. Hispanics and Caucasians are at highest risk. African-Americans and Asians have a lower risk.

Pathogenesis

Children who have severe brain and spinal defects may have a shortened life expectancy; children with minor spinal defects will probably have a normal life expectancy. Care has improved so much that 90 percent of babies born with spina bifida will reach adulthood and about 80 percent have an intelligence quotient (IQ) in the normal range. However, these patients often face a number of related medical and social concerns, ranging from gastrointestinal problems and osteoarthritis to obesity and depression. Many will also require wheelchairs or braces to get around. The lifetime cost of treating a person with spina bifida in the United States is estimated at $600,000 to $1 million.

Prevention

The most effective way to reduce the risk of having a child with a neural tube disorder is to increase the amount of folic acid in a mother's diet before she becomes pregnant and continue the supplementation for at least 12 weeks into the pregnancy.

Sources of folic acid include dark green vegetables, dried beans, citrus fruit, and liver. The United States, Canada, and Chile all require cereals and flours to be supplemented with folic acid. In each country, there has been a significant decline in the number of neural tube disorders reported. Scientists believe the number of spina bifida cases could be reduced by 75 percent if all women took a multivitamin containing folic acid before becoming pregnant. Since folic acid is water soluble, it does not remain in the body long, so folic acid needs to be taken every day if it is to be effective against neural tube disorders. The recommended dose is 400 µg (micrograms) each day.

Because many pregnancies are unplanned, any woman of childbearing age with a possibility of conceiving should take a folic acid supplement.

Epidemiology

The most common neural tube disorder, spina bifida, affects about 1 in 1,400 to 1,500 newborns in the United States. The Spina Bifida Association estimates that there are around 70,000 people in the United States who have the condition.

Chris Curran

See also
- Birth defects • Brain disorders • Diabetes
- Obesity • Spina bifida • Spinal disorders
- Vitamin deficiency

Nutritional disorders

Nutritional disorders is a general term that describes a number of diseases or conditions that have some relationship to food or the nutrients contained in food. The term includes malnutrition (both too much and too little food), vitamin and mineral deficiencies.

Most people think of malnutrition as a condition caused by too little food. However, *malnutrition* literally means "bad" or "poor nutrition." It can be defined as any condition caused by excess or deficient food energy or nutrient intake or by an imbalance of nutrients. The term can describe not having enough to eat (undernutrition), eating too much food (overnutrition), or eating an imbalance of essential nutrients.

Undernutrition

Undernutrition is seen infrequently in the United States or the United Kingdom. However, individuals who live in poverty, as well as those suffering from severe chronic disease such as cancer, AIDS, tuberculosis, or anorexia nervosa (an eating disorder) are often undernourished. Undernutrition is a major problem in some of the less developed nations of Africa, Southeast Asia, the Middle East, and Central and South America. In these areas, as many as one-third of the population do not have enough to eat because of famine or other problems relating to access to food (food insecurity). Inadequate food intake leads to poor growth and development in children and weight loss in adults. When individuals do not get enough to eat over a long period of time,

the result may be protein-energy malnutrition (PEM). In this condition there is a lack of energy (kcalories) or protein, or both, in the diet. In the human body, energy in the form of food has a function similar to that of gasoline for an automobile. It provides the necessary fuel to allow internal organs (including the brain, heart, and muscles) to function. Thus, energy is necessary to sustain life. Protein is used in many ways: as building materials for growth and maintenance of muscles, blood, skin, and all other components of the body; as a component of enzymes (facilitators of chemical reactions) and hormones (chemical messengers); as a regulator of fluid and acid-base balance; as a transporter of other nutrients; as building blocks for antibodies; and as an energy source. Although adults can suffer from protein-energy malnutrition, it is more likely seen in childhood. It is estimated to afflict over 500 million children worldwide. Protein-energy malnutrition is seen in two forms: marasmus and kwashiorkor. The form it takes depends upon the balance among the limited amounts of protein, carbo-hydrate, and fat in the diet. Some authorities consider marasmus and kwashiorkor to be two stages of the same disease, since often a child who has marasmus later develops kwashiorkor. There may be a third form, marasmic-kwashiorkor, a clinical combination of the two conditions. If left untreated, many adults and children who suffer from any of the forms of PEM will die.

Marasmus

Marasmus, named from the Greek word meaning "drying away," results from near starvation with a

RELATED ARTICLES

MARASMUS AND KWASHIORKOR

Marasmus and kwashiorkor are two forms of protein-energy malnutrition, which differ only in the different balance of limited nutrients the child receives, such as protein, carbohydrates, and fat. Some experts have the theory that marasmus and kwashiorkor are stages of the same disease, because it has been observed that children with marasmus often develop kwashiorkor. Even if a child recovers from either of these diseases, his or her growth may be stunted, and learning difficulties are prevalent.

MARASMUS	KWASHIORKOR
Infants and toddlers 6 to 18 months	Toddlers and children 18 months and older
Near starvation with a deficiency of total food energy, vitamins, and minerals	Lack of protein in the diet
Develops slowly (chronic) over a long period of time	Develops rapidly (acute), often precipitated by an infection or measles
Severe weight loss	Some weight loss
Severe growth retardation	Some growth retardation
All "skin and bones" appearance	Swollen belly due to edema
Weakened immune system	Weakened immune system
Increased risk of death	Increased risk of death

deficiency of total food energy and micronutrients (vitamins and minerals) over a long period of time. It is the predominant form of protein-energy malnutrition found in most developing countries.

Marasmus is most common in children from 6 to 18 months of age. Children often develop the condition due to a lack of food energy, especially if their mother was unable to breast-feed and there was little other food available. Often these children have subsisted on only watery cereal drinks.

Since energy intake is insufficient for the body's needs, children must draw on their own body stores to meet their daily calorie requirements. Skeletal muscle and body fat are broken down to provide the fuel necessary to maintain life. However, the children pay a heavy price. Marasmic children look quite emaciated, presenting with gross weight loss, growth retardation, and a wasting of both muscle and body fat. They often look like little old people and are literally just skin and bones. If marasmus continues untreated, the children are stunted and can suffer from impaired brain development and learning problems.

These children are often anemic as a result of a lack of iron and B vitamins. The lining of their digestive tract has deteriorated, and often their heart and other organs are dramatically weakened.

Kwashiorkor

Kwashiorkor takes its name from the Ga language of Ghana and means "the evil spirit that infects the first child when the second child is born." It occurs when a mother who has been nursing her first child suddenly weans him or her after the birth of her next child. The first child's diet, which contained nutrient-dense breast milk with high-quality protein, is replaced with starchy, protein-poor foods such as yam, sweet potato, and green bananas. Children typically acquire kwashiorkor between 18 months and 2 years, a time frame compatible with the birth of the next child. The children develop the condition rapidly as a result of a protein deficiency. Often it is precipitated by an infection or illness such as measles. Frequently the children with kwashiorkor present with a swollen belly due to fluid retention in the abdomen because the low level of protein in the blood is not adequate to keep fluids from leaving the bloodstream and moving into the spaces between the tissues. As with marasmus, their weakened immune system make these children more vulnerable to death from various infectious diseases.

Marasmic-kwashiorkor

Marasmic-kwashiorkor is simply a combination of the two conditions. It is characterized by the edema of kwashiorkor superimposed on the tissue wasting of marasmus. Children with marasmic-kwashiorkor are usually suffering from both malnutrition and infections.

Infections

Children with protein-energy malnutrition and a concomitant weakened immune system are much more prone to develop life-threatening infections. In impoverished nations, infectious disease and pneumonia are the leading causes of death in children under five years of age. The relationship between malnutrition and infection is often deadly. Malnutrition reduces a child's general health, increasing the likelihood of acquiring an opportunistic infection. Infection negatively affects nutritional status by causing dysentery, an infection of the digestive tract, and diarrhea, which further depletes the body of fluid and nutrients. There follows a downward spiral of malnutrition, infection, worsening malnutrition, and more severe infections, which often culminates in death. In fact, malnutrition combined with infection is responsible for two-thirds of the deaths of young children in developing nations.

One example of a malnutrition- and infection-related disorder is a condition called noma. It is a gangrenous disease leading to tissue destruction of the face, especially the mouth and cheek, and later other tissues, including the bones and genitals. The mucous membranes (gums, lining of the cheeks) become inflamed, develop ulcers, and begin to break down. The infection spreads rapidly to the skin, which causes the cells of the lips and cheeks to deteriorate and die, often within days. Eventually, there is destruction of the bones around the mouth, which leads to deformity and loss of teeth. Noma occurs mostly in severely malnourished children aged two to six years in the poorest nations of Africa, Asia, and South America who

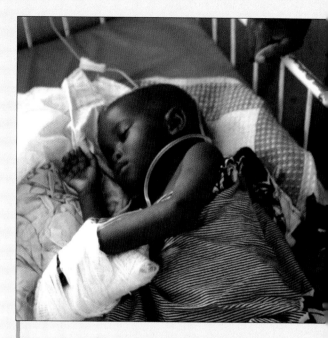

A young child suffering from malnutrition in Malawi is given intravenous fluids to combat dehydration.

have a weakened immune system. Usually they have had some preceding illness, such as measles, scarlet fever, or tuberculosis. Although the exact origin is unknown, doctors think it might be caused by bacteria, since poor sanitation is a known risk factor. Treatment with antibiotics and nutritional support will stop the progression of the disease. If left untreated, noma can be fatal. However, it may simply heal over time, though the tissue destruction may require plastic surgery and reconstruction of facial bones.

Treatment of protein-energy malnutrition in children or adults must be through nutritional and medical interventions. Initially, food intake should be limited until their digestive tract function is restored. The first step is to correct fluid and electrolyte (potassium, calcium, phosphorus, magnesium, sodium, and chloride) imbalances caused by diarrhea, and to treat infections with antibiotics. This nutrition is often given via intravenous fluids, although in some cases oral rehydration formulas may also be used. After 24 to 48 hours (a time frame used to avoid worsening the diarrhea), protein and food energy should be given in small quantities. Currently, milk-based formulas containing adequate amounts of vitamins and minerals are the treatment of choice. If necessary, liquid tube feedings can be used to enhance digestion and absorption of needed nutrients. The amount of formula or solid food should be gradually increased if it can be tolerated.

If caught early enough, the prognosis is quite positive. In children, mortality rates vary between 5 and 40 percent, with the lower rates observed in children who are given intensive care, such as antibiotics and appropriate medical nutrition therapy.

Anorexia nervosa

Anorexia nervosa is an eating disorder that is characterized by a refusal or inability to maintain a normal body weight in the face of abundant food availability. Individuals afflicted with anorexia nervosa have a distortion in their perception of body shape and weight; that is, they see themselves as too heavy in spite of a body mass index (BMI) that is in the underweight range (see the following section, overnutrition, for a discussion of BMI). The syndrome is potentially life threatening since those with the disorder engage in self-starvation, which leads to a deficiency in energy and essential nutrients as well as, ultimately, a number of health complications.

Overnutrition

Overnutrition is the nutritional disorder faced by more people in the United States, the United Kingdom, and the rest of the developed world, as well as by a growing number of individuals in developing nations. It is a type of malnutrition defined by an absolute excess of energy leading to overweight and obesity. More than two-thirds of adults in the United States are considered overweight or obese, a number that has increased dramatically over the past 20 years. The prevalence of overweight among children is also rising at a rapid rate.

A number of different indices are available to quantify adiposity. In the past, overweight and obesity were defined as a body weight of greater than 20 percent and 30 percent, respectively, above ideal or desirable weight on standard height-weight tables. Presently many authorities define it in terms of the body mass index (BMI), a measure derived by dividing weight (in kilograms) by height (in meters squared). A person is considered overweight when they have a BMI of 25 or greater, and obese when the BMI is

30 or greater. A better measure of obesity, especially for those who are very muscular, utilizes the percentage of body fat. Although guidelines vary, most agree that men and women who have more than 25 percent and 30 percent body fat, respectively, are obese. An easier measure is the waist-to-hip-ratio, wherein a ratio higher than 0.90 in men and 0.80 in women indicates obesity. Finally, some clinicians simply measure waist circumference. Risk of chronic disease is increased for males and females with a waist circumference above 40 inches (102 cm) and 35 inches (89 cm), respectively. Obesity is considered a major health problem. Of the six leading causes of death in the United States, obesity is linked to five of them: heart disease, cancer, stroke, chronic obstructive pulmonary disease, and diabetes mellitus.

Nutrient imbalance

Nutrient imbalance includes both consumption of too much or too little (nutrient deficiency) of the many vitamins and minerals needed for optimal body functioning. Although possible, it is extremely rare to find individuals who consume too much of either vitamins or minerals through food. There are cases in the medical literature of people who have consumed excessive amounts of vitamin A by eating polar bear liver, or who have had their skin turn slightly orange from drinking very large amounts of carrot juice, but that is certainly a rarity.

Generally, overconsumption of vitamins or minerals only takes place when an individual augments their diet with high potency dietary supplements (pills or potions). Most authorities agree that an individual who follows the dietary guidelines for Americans has little need for a supplement. However, taking a one-a-day multivitamin or mineral (or both) supplement that contains approximately 100 percent of the recommended dietary allowances (RDA) is a reasonable way to ensure that requirements are met. Use of individual supplements is not advised, unless recommended by a physician or registered dietitian.

Nutrient deficiencies are a problem both in the developed and developing nations of the world. This section will concentrate on mineral deficiencies. Minerals are micronutrients that do not contain carbon (inorganic elements). They are not digested but are absorbed intact. As a group, minerals assist in the regulation of many body processes. If dietary intake is limited, a deficiency of any mineral is possible, but in practice only a small number of minerals pose major problems for most people. The emphasis of this article will be on iron and iodine, but reference will be made to calcium, fluoride, and zinc.

Iron deficiency

Iron is part of hemoglobin and myoglobin, proteins that carry oxygen in the blood and muscle, respectively. It is found as a component of a number of enzymes in the body, where it assists in energy production and acts as an antioxidant.

Iron deficiency is the most common nutrient deficiency in the world. The World Health Organization (WHO) estimates that more than 30 percent of the earth's population is anemic due to inadequate iron intake. Thus, iron deficiency affects more than 1.2 billion people. In developing nations, it is estimated that almost half of the preschool children and pregnant women suffer from iron-deficiency anemia. In developed nations, iron deficiency is still a problem, but much less so. Approximately 10 percent of toddlers, adolescent girls, and women of childbearing age appear to be iron deficient.

Inadequate dietary intake (malnutrition) is the major cause of iron deficiency for children, adolescents, men, and postmenopausal women. In premenopausal women, blood loss through menstrual bleeding contributes to the problem. During pregnancy, the requirements of the growing fetus put women at increased risk. Malaria and parasitic infections of the digestive tract can also contribute to iron deficiency, especially in developing nations.

Without adequate iron, the body's energy metabolism is negatively impacted. The result is fatigue, weakness, apathy, and a tendency to feel cold. Additionally, iron deficiency is linked with increased risk of infection, premature birth, low birth weight, and learning problems, as well as reduced work capacity and decreased mental productivity. In some people, especially poverty-stricken women and children, iron deficiency appears to bring about an appetite for clay, paste, ice, or other nonfood substances. This condition is known as pica. In some but not all cases, pica responds to iron supplementation.

The World Health Organization (WHO) advocates increasing iron intake by supplemental iron (pills), promoting iron-rich diets, and iron fortification of foods (supplementing a food that is not naturally a good source of iron). The latter technique has been used very effectively in a number of developed nations, including the United States and the United Kingdom. Additionally, WHO encourages control of malaria and parasitic infections to help improve iron status in developing nations. Iron status in developed nations has improved over the past few decades. Increased numbers of women who breast-feed (which promotes iron absorption), increased use of iron-fortified infant formulas and cereals, and increased availability of products that are fortified with iron (including many ready-to-eat cereals and some orange juice), have all contributed to the improvement. The Special Supplemental Food Program for Women, Infants, and Children, which provides coupons for high iron foods, has also contributed to improving iron status in lower-income families.

Iodine deficiency

Iodine is involved in the synthesis of thyroid hormones and thus is involved in the maintenance of the metabolic rate (the rate at which energy is used to support body functions), temperature regulation, reproduction, and growth. Iodine deficiency is one of the world's most common and most preventable causes of mental retardation. According to the WHO, iodine deficiency affects 13 percent of the world's population, with another 30 percent at risk. Lack of iodine is associated with the development of goiter, an enlargement of the thyroid gland, which causes a visible lump in the front of the neck. The WHO has estimated that the world incidence of goiter is approximately 200 million people. In some nations it is so common that it is regarded as a normal feature.

Individuals with goiter often become sluggish and gain weight. Children with even a mild iodine deficiency usually have goiters and perform poorly in school. However, the effects of iodine deficiency are most devastating during pregnancy. Untreated infants born from iodine-deficient mothers may show irreversible mental and physical retardation known as cretinism.

Iodine occurs naturally in seafood and in foods grown on land that was once covered by oceans, so it is more of a problem in inland nations. Iodine deficiency was a major concern in the United States and Canada in the midwestern and mountain regions (the goiter belt). It has largely been eliminated with the addition of iodine to salt, along with the consumption of foods that are brought from iodine-rich areas.

A worldwide effort spearheaded by the WHO to provide iodized salt or administer a dose of iodized oil to individuals living in iodine-deficient areas has been quite successful. The latter technique corrects an iodine deficiency for about one year.

Calcium deficiency

Calcium is the most abundant mineral in the body, found mostly in bones and teeth. A low intake during childhood and early adulthood limits total bone mass and density. Since all adults begin to lose bone between the ages of 30 and 40, those with lower bone density due to less than optimal calcium intakes (both early on to build bone, and during adulthood to minimize bone loss) are more likely to suffer bone fractures.

When an individual has low bone mass and deterioration of bone tissue with an increased bone fragility and fracture risk, even under common, everyday stresses, they are said to have osteoporosis. This disease afflicts more than 25 million people in the United States, although it is found mostly in older women.

Fluoride deficiency

Fluoride is found in the body in teeth and bones. It combines with calcium and phosphorus to make teeth more resistant to decay from acid or bacteria. Many dentists recommend fluoride to protect against dental caries (cavities). Additionally, fluoride may prevent bone loss or stimulate new bone growth, or both, and thus may be useful to prevent or treat osteoporosis. Additional research in this area is currently being undertaken. Since a good dietary source of the mineral does not occur naturally (with the possible exception of seafood and tea), many children receive fluoride from fluoridated water or fluoridated dental products such as mouthwashes or toothpastes. Fluoride supplements are also available by prescription, but should only be used by children living in areas where the water has not been

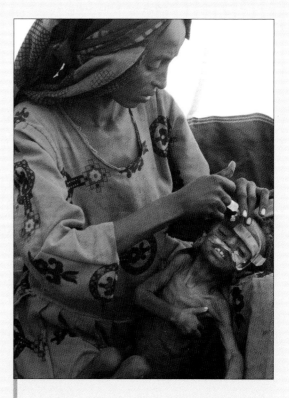

This dying child is a victim of a famine in Ethiopia. Although he is being given fluids, the treatment has come too late.

fluoridated. Consuming too much fluoride leads to fluorosis, a condition in which the teeth become discolored with small white specks and pitted.

Zinc deficiency

Zinc is a component of many enzymes in the body. It is also associated with the hormone insulin, plays a role in immune reactions, taste perception, wound healing, protein synthesis, transport of vitamin A, spermatogenesis, and fetal development. Severe deficiencies are uncommon in developed nations but may occur to groups at risk such as pregnant women, young children, the elderly, and those who live in poverty. In developing nations a zinc deficiency is more common and has been linked to growth retardation, short stature, and delayed sexual maturity. Chronic deficiency may also negatively impact the immune response and damage the central nervous system and brain. Children have especially high zinc requirements because of their rapid growth and need to synthesize many zinc-containing proteins.

Alan Levine

Obesity

Obesity is increasing at a rapid rate throughout both the developed and developing nations of the world. The World Health Organization (WHO) estimates that there are as many as 300 million obese people worldwide.

Obesity may be defined as an excess of body fat. WHO defines overweight as a body mass index (weight in kilograms divided by height in square meters) of at least 25 and obesity as a BMI of at least 30. Morbid obesity is defined as a BMI of 40 or greater. Both overweight and especially obesity are associated with increased risk of disease and death.

Epidemiology

In the United States, obesity afflicts approximately 33 percent of adults (28 percent of men and 34 percent of women) aged 20 to 74 years; this has more than doubled over the past two decades. Almost 10 percent of U.S. children between the ages of 5 and 17 are classified as obese. In Canada obesity rates have climbed to approximately 15 percent of adults, an increase of 150 percent since 1985. In Europe, most countries report adult obesity rates of more than 10 percent, with the United Kingdom, Ireland, Germany, Cyprus, Finland, Slovakia, Malta, and Greece reporting rates above 20 percent. The most rapid increase has been reported in England, where adult obesity rates tripled from 1980 to 2001. Rates for overweight and obesity (BMI of 25 or greater) among adults are as high as 65 percent in the United States and 60 percent in England. Although overweight and obesity levels are lower in most developing nations, WHO suggests that excess adiposity is a problem there as well.

Childhood overweight and obesity is also increasing in the United States and among European nations. Data from the United States and England suggests that 15 percent of children and adolescents are obese and almost 30 percent are included in the categories of overweight and obese. Children in other European nations show slightly lower levels but still show levels approaching 20 percent.

Causes

Most researchers agree that multiple factors contribute to obesity. These include a complex interface among genetic, physiological, metabolic, hormonal, sociocultural, environmental, behavioral, and psychological influences. More simplistically, there is an in-

teraction between an individual's genetic heritage and an environment that promotes excessive food consumption and a sedentary lifestyle. Thus, weight gain and, ultimately, obesity result from positive energy balance in susceptible individuals, that is, consuming more food energy than is utilized throughout the day.

Other factors influence the cause of obesity. Genetics most influences the risk for obesity. Theories include: possessing a thrifty gene, causing individuals to burn less energy at rest and during activity; maintaining weight at a predetermined set point, making it difficult to lose weight or maintain the loss; and alterations in various hormones, such as leptin, which influence energy intake. However, some people with overweight parents do not become obese themselves.

Overeating and eating foods that are highly calorific and contain a large amount of fat, as well as too little exercise, are contributory factors in causing obesity.

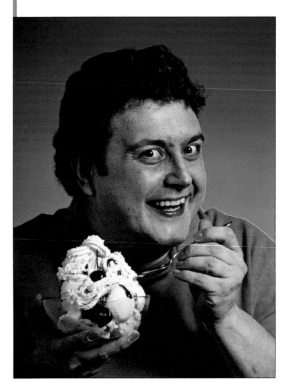

Risk factors

Beyond the genetic risk factor, a number of modifiable risk factors for obesity exist. Being overweight as a child can lead to adult obesity. It is estimated that about one-half of obese children will become obese adults. Substantial weight gain during gestation, early infancy, in the early schoolage years (five to seven years), and the adolescent period all increase the risk of adult obesity.

Lack of physical activity has been linked with greater body weight. Children and adults who watch excessive amounts of television or spend too much time in front of a computer have a greater risk of obesity. That, combined with eating a high-caloric diet, which causes increased storage of energy as body fat, has proved a potent risk factor for increased adiposity.

Psychological factors also influence the likelihood that an individual will become obese. In some, the sight or smell of foods may overstimulate the pleasure centers of the brain and trigger appetite and overeating, even when the individual is not very hungry.

Additionally, a number of social factors, including pressure to eat from family and friends, easy access to inexpensive and high-fat foods (often found at fast food restaurants), smoking cessation, excessive alcohol consumption, and an increased number of meals eaten away from home, often at establishments that serve large portions, are all linked to obesity.

Signs and symptoms

The most obvious sign of obesity is an individual who is overweight. However, excessive body weight does not necessarily correlate with obesity. Individuals who are very muscular (football or rugby players) may be overweight but may still be within recommended ranges for body fat. A measurement of stored fat will give a better indication of whether a person is obese.

A number of symptoms are associated with obesity. Those apparent with the onset of obesity include reduced physical agility, increased risk of accidents and falls, impaired heat tolerance (inability to stand or do well in hot weather), and in women menstrual irregularities and infertility.

Symptoms that are related to long-term obesity include: increased surgical risk attributed to increased anesthesia needs and greater risk of wound infections; pulmonary disease because of excess weight over the lungs and respiratory tract; type II diabetes as a result of insulin insensitivity of enlarged fat cells; hypertension (high blood pressure) owing to increased blood volume and increased resistance to blood flow

---

KEY FACTS

Description
An excess of body fat.

Causes
Multifactorial, including genetics, excessive food consumption, and sedentary lifestyle, coupled with sociocultural and psychological influences.

Symptoms
Excess body weight seen as abnormally large waist, hips, buttocks, and thighs. Obesity is associated with increased risk for many disorders, including high blood pressure, heart disease, type II diabetes, and some types of cancers.

Diagnosis
BMI more than 30 or body fat levels greater than 25 and 32 for males and females, respectively.

Treatments
Decreased food intake, regular exercise, and behavior modification. Drug therapy as an adjunct to diet, with surgery as a last resort.

Prevention
Lifestyle modifications include selecting limited amounts of nutritious foods, incorporating regular vigorous exercise into one's life, and practicing healthy food-related behaviors.

Epidemiology
Nearly one-third of U.S. adults and more than 20 percent of British adults are obese. Slightly lower or similar figures are found in most developed nations. The trend for overweight and obesity is increasing in both developed and developing nations.

---

throughout the circulatory system; cardiovascular disease as a result of increases in LDL-cholesterol (bad cholesterol) and triglycerides with concomitant decreases in HDL-cholesterol (good cholesterol) and physical activity; bone and joint disorders, including gout and osteoarthritis caused by increased uric acid levels and excess pressure on the hip, knee, ankle joints, respectively; gallstones due to increased cholesterol content of bile; skin disorders as a result of trapping of moisture and possibly microbes in tissue folds; various cancers (of the breast, colon, pancreas, and gallbladder) as a result of increased estrogen production by fat cells and possibly excess energy intake that encourages tumor development; pregnancy risks including more difficult delivery, increased number of birth defects, and increased toxemia of pregnancy; increased psychological problems associated with societal stigma attached to obesity; and increased mortality. The greater the degree of obesity, the more likely it is that someone will develop health problems.

CHILDHOOD OBESITY

Childhood overweight and obesity is increasing dramatically among U.S. children. It is estimated that around 18 percent of children between the ages of 5 and 18 are overweight, a number that has tripled since the late 1970s. Additionally, more than 10 percent of children between the ages of two and five are overweight or obese. Overweight in children and adolescents is generally caused by unhealthy eating patterns and lack of physical activity, with genetics and lifestyle both playing important roles. Being overweight or obese as a child is directly correlated to adult obesity. Childhood obesity has also been linked to increased and earlier onset of a number of diseases, including type II diabetes and heart disease, as well as premature death in adulthood. Prevention of obesity is of paramount importance. Ideally, parents and caregivers should offer a selection of nutritious food, while allowing children to decide how much they eat. Providing the opportunity for children to engage in physical activities that are fun, rather than competitive, should be a goal for both parents and schools. Modeling appropriate food- and exercise-related behaviors would also be quite useful in managing the childhood obesity epidemic.

Diagnosis

Obesity is commonly diagnosed by using BMI. However, body composition assessments that estimate the proportion of an individual's body fat, muscle mass, bone, and body water give a more accurate indication. Body composition methods commonly used include underwater weighing, skinfold measures, bioelectrical impedance analysis, near infrared reactance, dual-energy X-ray absorptiometry (DEXA), and computerized axial tomograpohy (CT or CAT scans). Although some disagreement exists, acceptable body fat ranges for adults are between 8 to 25 percent and 10 to 32 percent for males and females, respectively. Additionally, the location of body fat stores is quite important. Fat concentrated in the abdominal area (apple shape) is thought to be more problematic than that around the hips and thigh area (pear shape). Apple-shaped people have a higher risk for diabetes, hypertension, high blood cholesterol, and heart disease. Thus, some researchers assess obesity using the waist-to-hip ratio. Ratios of greater than 0.80 and 0.90 for women and men, respectively, are thought to increase the risk for health problems. Other researchers use waist circumference as an indicator of potential problems. A waist circumference of more than 40 inches (101 cm) in men and more than 35 inches (89 cm) in women is problematic.

Treatments and prevention

Weight loss treatment involves decreasing energy intake, increasing physical activity levels, and modifying behavioral problems. For success, the above triad must be coupled with a desire for change and self-acceptance (within reason) of body size. Diets should generally include a restriction of 500 to 1,000 kilocalories/day from the normal intake. This would allow for a weight loss of 1–2 pounds (0.5–1 kg) per week. Many nutritionists advocate total dietary fat intake below 30 percent of kcals, carbohydrate at 55 percent or more of kcals, and the balance from protein. Reducing saturated fat, cholesterol, and sodium are important, as well as eating foods high in fiber. Moderate exercise, initially 30 to 45 minutes three to five times per week (if tolerated), should later be increased to 30 to 60 minutes on most days.

Drug therapy has also been tried. A number of drugs, including orlistat (xenical), which blocks absorption of dietary fat, and sibutramine (meridia), which inhibits appetite, have met with some success.

Surgery should be used as a last resort due to the increased risks involved. A number of procedures, such as gastric bypass surgery, vertical banded gastroplasty, and laparoscopic adjustable gastric banding, are available to reduce the size of the stomach and limit the amount of food that can be eaten. Some individuals also use liposuction, a cosmetic procedure that removes fat deposits from the thighs, hips, arms, back, or chin. Both types of techniques are expensive and carry the risk of infections or other complications.

The rate of success for treating obesity is quite low, therefore prevention is the preferred strategy. Since little can be changed in terms of genetics, lifestyle changes are the keys to success. An eating plan that focuses on healthy nutritious foods, daily physical activities that are fun rather than competitive, and practicing healthful food-related behaviors would dramatically reduce the number of obese children and adults.

Alan Levine

See also
- Cancer • Diabetes • Eating disorders
- Heart disorders • Prevention

Resources for Further Study

General Reference Works

American College of Physicians. 2003. *Complete Home Medical Guide.* New York: DK Publishing.

American Medical Association. 2006. *Concise Medical Encyclopedia.* New York: Random House Information Group.

Clayman, Charles, ed. 2005. *The Human Body.* New York: DK Publishing, Inc.

Gray, Henry, and H. V. Carter (illustrator). 2000. *Gray's Anatomy.* New York: Barnes and Noble.

Labrecque, Mary C., Robert Pantell, Harold C. Sox, Timothy B. Walsh, and John H. Wasson. 2002. *Common Symptom Guide.* Columbus, OH: McGraw-Hill.

Marks, Andrea, and Betty Rothbart. 2003. *Healthy Teens, Body and Soul: A Parent's Complete Guide to Adolescent Health.* New York: Simon and Schuster.

Sultz, Harry A., and Kristina M. Young. 2005. *Health Care USA: Understanding Its Organization and Delivery.* Sudbury, MA: Jones and Bartlett Publishers, Inc.

Infections

Black, Samuel J., Peter J. Krause, Dennis J. Richardson, and Richard J. Seed, eds. 2002. *North American Parasitic Zoonoses.* Boston, MA: Kluwer Academic Publishers.

Bottone, Edward J. 2003. *An Atlas of Infectious Diseases.* Boca Raton, FL: CRC Press.

Callahan, Gerald N. 2006. *Infection: The Uninvited Universe.* New York: St. Martin's Press.

Chiodini, Jane. 2004. *Atlas of Travel Medicine and Health.* Ontario: B. C. Decker, Inc.

Fauci, Anthony S., John I. Gallin, and Richard Krause, eds. 2000. *Emerging Infections.* Burlington, MA: Elsevier Science and Technology.

Freeman-Cook, Kevin, Lisa Freeman-Cook, and Edward Alcamo, eds. 2005. *Staphylococcus Aureus Infections.* New York: Chelsea House Publishers.

Gittleman, Ann Louise, and Omar M. Amin. 2001. *Guess What Came to Dinner? Parasites and Your Health.* Wayne, NJ: Avery.

Gualde, Norbert, and Steven Rendall (translator). 2006. *Resistance: The Human Struggle against Infection.* Washington, DC: Dana Press.

Hart, Tony. 2004. *Microterrors: The Complete Guide to Bacterial, Viral, and Fungal Infections That Threaten Our Health.* Toronto: Firefly Books, Ltd.

Health Press. 2002. *Superficial Fungal Infections.* Abingdon: Health Press, UK.

Heelan, Judith Stephenson. 2004. *Cases in Human Parasitology.* Herndon, VA: ASM Press.

Henderson, Gregory, Allan Warshowsky, and Batya S. Yasgur. 2002. *Women at Risk: The HPV Epidemic and Your Cervical Health.* Wayne, NJ: Avery.

Irving, William L., John W. Rowlands, and Dave J. McCauley, eds. 2001. *New Challenges to Health.* NY: Cambridge University Press.

Molyneux, David H., ed. 2006. *Control of Human Parasitic Diseases.* Burlington, MA: Elsevier Science and Technology.

Regush, Nicholas. *The Virus Within.* 2000. New York: Penguin Group.

Richardson, Malcolm D., and David W. Warnock. 2003. *Fungal Infection: Diagnosis and Management.* Malden, MA: Blackwell Publishing.

Sherman, Irwin W. 2006. *Power of Plagues.* Herndon, VA: ASM Press.

Shmaefsky, Brian Robert, and Edward I. Alcamo, eds. 2004. *Meningitis.* New York: Chelsea House Publishers.

Noninfectious disorders

Addiction

Conyers, Beverly. 2003. *Addict in the Family: Stories of Loss, Hope, and Recovery.* Center City, MN: Hazelden.

Ehrlich, Caryl. 2003. *Conquer Your Food Addiction.* New York: The Free Press.

Griffin, Kevin. 2004. *One Breath at a Time: Buddhism and the Twelve Steps.* Emmaus, PA: Rodale.

Nakken, Craig. 1996. *The Addictive Personality: Understanding the Addictive Process and Compulsive Behavior.* Center City, MN: Hazelden.

Aging

Bullen, Timothy, and Anthony Campbell. 2004. *The Directory of Your Back, Your Bones, and Things That Ache.* Secaucus, NJ: Chartwell Books, Inc.

Whitbourne, Susan Krauss. 2004. *Adult Development and Aging: Biopsychosocial Perspectives.* New York: John Wiley and Sons, Inc.

AIDS

Greene, Warner C., Merle A. Sande, and Paul Volberding, eds. 2007. *Global HIV/AIDS Medicine.* St. Louis, MO: Saunders Publishing.

Allergies

Mitchell, Dean. 2006. *The Allergy and Asthma Cure: A Revolutionary New Treatment Program for All Airborne Allergies and Asthma.* New York: Marlowe & Company.

Arthritis

O'Driscoll, Erin Rohan. 2004. *Exercises for Arthritis.* New York: Hatherleigh Press.

Vad, Vijay. 2006. *Arthritis Rx.* New York: Penguin Group.

Backache

Freedman, Janet, and Elaine Petrone. 2003. *The Miracle Ball Method.* New York: Workman Publishing Company, Inc.

Katz, Jeffrey N., and Gloria Parkinson. 2007. *Heal Your Aching Back.* Columbus, OH: McGraw-Hill.

Kubey, Craig, and Robin A. McKenzie. 2001. *Seven Steps to a Pain-Free Life.* New York: Penguin Group.

Blood disorders

Sutton, Amy L. 2005. *Blood and Circulatory Disorders Sourcebook.* Detroit, MI: Omnigraphics, Inc.

Cancer

Tsupruk, Pavel. 2005. *Prevent Cancer Today.* Frederick, MD: PublishAmerica.

Weinberg, Robert A. 2006. *Biology of Cancer.* Oxford, UK: Taylor & Francis, Inc.

Diabetes

Becker, Gretchen E. 2001. *The First Year–Type 2 Diabetes: An Essential Guide for the Newly Diagnosed.* New York: Avalon Publishing Group.

Endocrinology

Gordon, John D., Dan I. Lebovic, and Robert N. Taylor. 2005. *Reproductive Endocrinology and Infertility.* Glen Cove, NY: Scrub Hill Press.

Eye disorders

Billig, Michael D., Gary H. Cassel, and Harry G. Randall. 1998. *Eye Book: A Complete Guide to Eye Disorders and Health.* Baltimore, MD: Johns Hopkins University Press.

Shaw, Kimberley Williams, and Amy L. Sutton. 2003. *Eye Care Sourcebook.* Detroit, MI: Omnigraphics, Inc.

Genetic disorders and birth defects

Iannucci, Lisa. 2000. *Birth Defects.* Berkeley Heights, NJ: Enslow Publishers, Inc.

Wynbrandt, James. 2007. *Encyclopedia of Genetic Disorders and Birth Defects.* New York: Facts On File.

Heart disease

Esselstyn, Caldwell. 2007. *Prevent and Reverse Heart Disease.* New York: Penguin Group.

Katzenstein, Larry, and Ileana L. Piñan. 2007. *Living with Heart Disease.* New York: Sterling Publishing.

Hepatitis

Wright, Lloyd. 2002. *Triumph over Hepatitis C.* Malibu, CA: Lloyd Wright Publishing.

Herpes

Connolly, Sean. 2002. *STDs.* Portsmouth, NH: Heinemann.

Stanberry, Lawrence. 2006. *Understanding Herpes.* Jackson, MS: University Press of Mississippi.

Immune system

Sompayrac, Lauren. 2003. *How the Immune System Works.* Malden, MA: Blackwell Publishing.

Lupus

Wallace, Daniel J. 2005. *Lupus Book: A Guide for Patients and Their Families.* Oxford, UK: Oxford University Press.

Motor neuron disease

Eisen, Andrew, and Pamela Shaw, eds. 2007. *Motor Neuron Disorders and Related Diseases.* Philadelphia, PA: Elsevier Health Sciences.

Multiple sclerosis

Blackstone, Margaret. 2003. *The First Year–Multiple Sclerosis: An Essential Guide for the Newly Diagnosed.* New York: Avalon Publishing Group.

Psychotherapy and psychology

Leszcz, Molyn, and Irvin D. Yalom. 2005. *The Theory and Practice of Group Psychotherapy.* New York: Basic Books.

Reproductive system

Heffner, Linda J., and Danny J. Schust. 2006. *The Reproductive System at a Glance.* Malden, MA: Blackwell Publishing.

Manassiev, Nikolai, and Malcolm I. Whitehead. 2003. *Female Reproductive Health.* Boca Raton, FL: CRC Press.

Sexually transmitted diseases

Parker, James N., and Philip M. Parker, eds. 2002. *The Official Patient's Sourcebook on Bacterial STDs.* San Diego, CA: ICON Health Publications.

Urinary system disorders

Datta, Shreelata. 2003. *Crash Course: Renal and Urinary Systems.* Philadelphia, PA: Elsevier Health Sciences.

Mental disorders

Andrews, Linda Wasmer, and Dwight L. Evans. 2005. *If Your Adolescent Has Depression or Bipolar Disorder: An Essential Resource for Parents.* Oxford, UK: Oxford University Press.

Barkley, Russell A., and Eric J. Mash, eds. 2006. *The Treatment of Childhood Disorders.* New York: Guilford Publications, Inc.

Brown, Thomas. 2005. *Attention Deficit Disorders: The Unfocused Mind in Children and Adults.* New Haven, CT: Yale University Press.

Brownell, Kelly D., and Christopher G. Fairburn. 2005. *Eating Disorders and Obesity: A Comprehensive Handbook.* New York: Guilford Publications, Inc.

Le Grange, Daniel, and James Lock. 2004. *Help Your Teenager Beat an Eating Disorder.* New York: Guilford Publications, Inc.

Miklowitz, David J. 2002. *The Bipolar Disorder Survival Guide.* New York: Guilford Publications, Inc.

Notbohm, Ellen. 2005. *Ten Things Every Child with Autism Wishes You Knew.* Arlington, TX: Future Horizons, Inc.

WEB RESOURCES

The following World Wide Web sources feature information useful for students, teachers, and health care professionals. By necessity, this list is only a representative sampling; many government bodies, charities, and professional organizations not listed have Web sites that are also worth investigating. Other Internet resources, such as newsgroups, also exist and can be explored for further research. Please note that all URLs have a tendency to change; addresses were functional and accurate as of April 2007. More extensive lists of Web sites appear in Volume 3.

American Academy of Family Physicians

www.familydoctor.org
The Web site supplies health information and an A–Z index of conditions with links that can be accessed for different groups of people.

American Cancer Society

www.cancer.org
A self-help Web site for patients, family, and friends to learn about cancer, various treatment options and choices, clinical trials, and coping with the disease. There are links to connect patients with cancer survivors and support programs.

American College Health Association

www.acha.org
ACHA aims to provide advocacy, education, communications, products, and services, as well as to promote research and culturally competent practices to enhance its members' ability to advance the health of all students and the campus community.

American Heart Association

www.americanheart.org
Web site includes suggestions for a better lifestyle to reduce the risk of a heart attack; warning signs; and explanations of diseases and conditions.

American Social Health Association

www.ashastd.org
ASHA aims to improve the health of individuals, families, and communities, with emphasis on the prevention of sexually transmitted diseases and infections (STDs/STIs). The site lists information about specific STDs/STIs, tips for reducing risk, and ways to talk with health care providers and partners.

Birth Defect Research for Children

www.birthdefects.org
This resource provides free birth defect information and details about parent networking and birth defect research through the National Birth Defect Registry.

Centers for Disease Control and Prevention

www.cdc.gov
Government-compiled health information, including health statistics, links to other Web sites, and research and development.

Childhelp

www.childhelp.org
Childhelp is dedicated to meeting the physical, emotional, and spiritual needs of abused and neglected children by focusing on prevention, intervention, and treatment. The Childhelp National Child Abuse Hotline, 1-800-4-A-CHILD, operates 24 hours a day, 7 days a week.

Mayo Clinic

www.mayoclinic.com
A site produced by a collective of medical experts with the aim of helping people manage their health. Information is up-to-date and all health issues are discussed.

National Institutes of Health (U.S. Department of Health and Human Services)

www.nih.gov
Health information with an A–Z index of NIH resources, clinical trials, health hotlines, and drug information. Also includes Medlineplus.

National Mental Health Information Center

www.mentalhealth.samhsa.gov
All aspects of mental health are covered on this site, which provides links to a large spectrum of topics. A drop-down menu allows users to look for mental health and substance abuse services by state.

Nutrition Source

www.hsph.harvard.edu/nutritionsource
The site supplies clear tips for healthy eating and dispels nutrition myths. There is useful advice on what to eat and why.

TeenGrowth

www.teengrowth.com
Health information specifically for teens; debates on relevant topics.

U.S. National AIDS Hotlines and Resources

www.thebody.com/hotlines/national.html
This Web site supplies hotline numbers for every group of people affected by AIDS or HIV.

U.S. National Library of Medicine (National Institutes of Health)

www.nlm.nih.gov
This Web site provides links to authoritative health information resources on hundreds of diseases, conditions, and health topics.

Glossary

acute
A term that describes an illness of sudden onset, which may or may not be severe but is usually of short duration.

AIDS
Acquired immunodeficiency syndrome. Caused by HIV (human immunodeficiency virus), AIDS leads to potentially fatal depression of the immune system. See encyclopedia entry.

albinism
A condition characterized by a lack of pigment in the hair, eyes, and skin.

alcoholism
Addiction to alcohol, which can lead to deterioration in physical and psychological health, family life, and social position.

allergen
A substance that causes an allergy.

allergy
Hypersensitive reaction, such as wheezing or a rash, to a foreign substance that stimulates the immune system.

alopecia
A lack or loss of bodily hair that is most obvious on the scalp, which tends to develop patchy hair loss.

alternative medicine
Medical systems, therapies, or techniques that are used in place of conventional medicine.

amenorrhea
Lack of menses (the flow of blood that occurs during menstruation).

amniocentesis
A procedure in which a sample of the amniotic fluid that surrounds the fetus is removed from the mother's uterus for testing.

analgesic
A drug that relieves pain.

anaphylactic shock
Severe allergic reaction.

anemia
A disorder of the blood in which there is a deficiency or disorder of hemoglobin, the oxygen-carrying pigment in red blood cells. See encyclopedia entry.

anorexia nervosa
Anorexia nervosa is an eating disorder in which people with the disorder perceive that they are too heavy, even though they are underweight. This perception results in a refusal or inability to maintain a normal body weight.

antibiotic
A drug that selectively attacks microorganisms by breaking down bacteria and prevents the growth of bacteria. Specific antibiotic drugs will work only against certain bacteria, leaving other bacteria unharmed.

antibody
A protein produced in the blood that inactivates invading organisms (or other foreign substances) and makes them susceptible to destruction by immune system cells such as phagocytes.

anticoagulant
Any drug that delays or prevents coagulation (clotting) of the blood.

antigen
A substance that can trigger the immune system into producing antibodies as a defense against infection and invading organisms.

antipruritic
A drug that relieves persistent itching, or pruritis, by reducing inflammation or numbing nerve impulses.

arthritis
Inflammation leading to pain and swelling of joints. See encyclopedia entry.

astigmatism
A condition that occurs because the cornea (outer lens of the eye) is not the correct spherical shape. Light rays from an object do not focus on the retina; they focus in front of or behind the retina, so the object appears blurred. See encyclopedia entry.

atheroma
Fatty deposit, also called arterial plaque, which is laid down in the inner lining of the artery walls. Atheroma causes narrowing and reduced blood flow, leading to heart attacks or strokes.

autoimmune
The term refers to any disorder caused by the body's immune system reacting against its own tissues and cells.

autosome
Any chromosome that is not a sex chromosome; in each human cell, 22 pairs of chromosomes are autosomes; the remaining pair of the 23 are the sex chromosomes.

bacteria
Small unicellular microorganisms. Bacteria exist in many areas in the body, but they are usually restrained by the immune system. Many bacteria cause serious, life-threatening infections.

bipolar disorder
Also called manic depression. Someone with this disorder fluctuates between feeling deep depression and excessive euphoria. See encyclopedia entry.

bladder
The hollow, muscular organ situated in the lower abdomen and protected by the pelvis holds urine until it is excreted.

botulism
A dangerous form of food poisoning that is caused by a toxin produced by the bacterium *Clostridium botulinum.* Botulism can occur in preserved food contaminated by the toxin and can cause paralysis of the muscles.

calorie
A unit used by dieticians to express the amount of energy taken into the body from digested food. A calorie is defined as the amount of heat that will raise one gram of water by one degree Celsius.

cancer
A group of diseases in which there is unrestrained growth of abnormal cells in tissues and organs of the body. See encyclopedia entry.

celiac disease
A condition, caused by sensitivity of the intestinal lining to gluten, that leads to malabsorption of food from the intestines. See encyclopedia entry.

central nervous system
The brain and the spinal cord comprise the central nervous system (CNS), which receives sensory information from organs in the body, analyzes the information, and produces an appropriate response.

cervical smear
A test in which a small sample of cells is removed from the surface of the cervix to detect abnormal changes in the cervix.

cervix
The lower part and neck of the uterus. The cervix separates the uterus from the vagina. The cervix is composed of smooth muscle tissue to form a sphincter that expands during childbirth.

chemotherapy
Treatment using anticancer drugs to destroy cancer cells. Normal tissues are also affected.

chicken pox
A common infectious disease usually contracted during childhood. The symptoms are fever and a rash of fluid-filled spots.

cholesterol
A fatty substance that is essential to the structure of cell walls. However, when cholesterol is present in the blood in excessive quantities (usually a result of a diet too rich in animal fats), there is the risk of atherosclerosis. Cholesterol can also crystallize as gallstones in the bladder.

chromosomes
Structures in the cell nucleus that carry genetic information. Each human cell has 23 pairs of chromosomes; 22 pairs are autosomal, that is, they are the same in both sexes. The other pair are sex chromosomes, which are either XX (female) or XY (male).

chronic
Term used to describe an illness that persists over a long period of time.

complementary medicine
Therapies or treatments used in conjunction with conventional medicine. An example is massage after surgery.

compound fracture
A fracture in which a broken bone breaks through the skin.

concussion
A brief loss of consciousness owing to a head injury; often followed by temporarily disturbed vision and loss of memory.

congenital
Term used to describe a disease or abnormality that is

present from birth but not necessarily hereditary.

cystic fibrosis
A genetic disorder that affects the lungs and digestive system. Cystic fibrosis appears in infancy and is characterized by excessive mucus, breathing difficulties, and abnormal secretion and function of many of the other secretory glands of the body. Treatments alleviate the condition, but so far there is no cure. See encyclopedia entry.

depression
This state of mind, characterized by a loss of interest in life and feelings of sadness, may be caused by a life event, such as a bereavement, or may be a symptom of a depressive disorder.

diabetes
A disease in which the cells of the body do not get enough insulin, usually because the pancreas is producing too little or no insulin. In other cases, the pancreas produces sufficient insulin but the cells in the body become resistant to its effects. There are two types of diabetes: type 1, which is insulin dependent, and type 2, which is noninsulin dependent. See encyclopedia entry.

Diagnostic and Statistical Manual of Mental Disorders
Also known as the DSM-IV, this reference work is published by the American Psychiatric Association and gives information on mental health disorders. It supplies lists of causes of disorders, useful statistics, and prognoses. The DSM-IV is used

by professionals to make psychiatric diagnoses in the United States and in other countries.

dilation
A condition in which an opening of the body is stretched, during childbirth, during a medical procedure, or as a result of disease.

DNA (deoxyribonucleic acid)
DNA is the genetic material from which chromosomes are formed. DNA is involved in protein synthesis and in inheritance. Because of DNA's structure (a double helix), exact replication occurs during cell division.

ECG
See electrocardiography.

eczema
Any superficial dermatitis, characterized by a red, scaly, itchy, and sometimes weeping skin rash.

EEG
See electroencephalography.

electrocardiography (ECG)
A technique that records the electrical activity in the heart.

electroencephalography (EEG)
A technique that is used to diagnose abnormal electrical activity in the brain.

endemic
Term used to describe a disease that is native to a particular area or population. Compare with epidemic.

endocrine system
The system of endocrine

glands (pituitary, thyroid, parathyroid, and adrenal) that produces the body's hormones.

enzyme
A protein molecule that acts as a catalyst in chemical reactions in the cells of the body without being altered itself.

epidemic
Term used to describe a widespread outbreak of an infectious disease. Compare with endemic.

epidemiology
The study of the incidence and prevalence of disease among a population. Statistical markers such as the variables of gender, age, race, and occupation are counted. Over a period of time, changes are calculated and information is gathered about the distribution of disease.

epilepsy
A disease of the nervous system that causes recurrent convulsions as a result of an overwhelming electrical discharge in the brain. See encyclopedia entry.

fetus
Human conceptus growing in the uterus—usually called a fetus from the seventh or eighth week of pregnancy.

fever
A high body temperature, above the normal 98.6°F (37°C). Most infectious illnesses cause fever, which is a sign that the body's temperature-regulating mechanism has been affected by the infection.

fracture
Term used to describe an injury to a bone in which the continuity of the tissue is broken. See encyclopedia entry.

gallbladder
A saclike organ, attached to the liver, that collects bile and then discharges it into the intestine in response to a fatty meal.

genes
Biological units that contain hereditary information. A gene is a tiny segment of DNA. The chainlike structure of DNA is composed of intertwined strands; each strand has thousands of pairs of genes, which are arranged on 23 pairs of chromosomes.

genetics
Genetics is the science of genes, heredity, and the variation of organisms. Modern genetics is based on the understanding of genes at the molecular, or DNA, level.

German measles
A viral infection. Also called rubella.

glucose
A simple sugar produced by the digestion of starch and sucrose. Glucose is the main source of energy for the body's cells.

glycogen
A form of glucose stored in the liver and muscles. Glycogen is released when the body requires it for for energy.

goiter
A visible swelling of the thyroid gland.

gonorrhea
A sexually transmitted disease that produces a greenish yellow urethral or vaginal discharge. See encyclopedia entry.

greenstick fracture
A partial fracture of a child's bone, which, because the bone is so pliable, splits rather than breaks.

gynecologist
A specialist in the diseases of the female reproductive system.

hallucination
An imaginary sensation perceived through any of the five senses; the result of alcohol withdrawal, drug use, severe illness, or schizophrenia. It occurs without any outside stimulus.

hay fever
Runny nose and coldlike symptoms owing to pollen allergy. See encyclopedia entry.

hepatitis infections
Inflammation of the liver, usually caused by one of the hepatitis viruses. See encyclopedia entry.

herpes infections
A group of viruses responsible for cold sores, chicken pox, shingles, and genital sores. See encyclopedia entry.

HIV
The human immunodeficiency virus (a retrovirus), which can lead to AIDS. The immune system makes antibodies in an attempt to combat the virus; the presence of these antibodies in the blood confirms the presence of HIV.

holistic
An approach that attempts to treat the whole body and mind.

homologue
Any organ that is similar to another organ, for example, the hands and feet.

hormone
A chemical messenger released from tissue or a gland to alter the activity of tissues elsewhere in the body. Hormones control metabolism, sexual development, and growth.

hyperactivity
A term used to describe excessive activity in children. Associated with brain damage, epilepsy, and psychiatric trouble, but only very rarely with food allergy. Also known as attention deficit hyperactivity disorder.

hyperparathyroidism
An excessive production of parathyroid hormone that is often caused by a noncancerous tumor called an adenoma.

hypoglycemia
An abnormally low level of sugar in the blood, which can cause such symptoms as confusion, coma, trembling, sweating, and even death.

immune system
The complex system of cells and proteins that the body uses to protect itself from harmful microorganisms, such as viruses, bacteria, and fungi.

immunization
A process that prepares the body to fight and prevent

an infection through the injection of material from the infecting organism, or by using an attenuated (non-disease-causing) strain of the organism itself.

immunoglobulin
See antibody.

immunomodulatory
An agent that can stimulate or reduce the body's immune responses.

infectious mononucleosis
Viral infection that causes swollen lymph nodes and a sore throat. Also called glandular fever.

inflammation
A reaction of the body's tissues to injury or illness, characterized by redness, heat, swelling, and pain. A mechanism of defense and repair.

inoculation
Administration of a vaccine in order to stimulate the immune system to produce antibodies and, hence, immunity to disease.

insulin
A hormone, secreted in the pancreas, that regulates blood sugar levels.

intravenous (IV)
Within or into a vein. For example, fluids or drugs are administered intravenously.

irritable bowel syndrome
A common condition that is characterized by episodes of abdominal pain and disturbance of the intestines (such as constipation or diarrhea). See encyclopedia entry.

keyhole surgery
Surgery performed using an endoscope and small incisions rather than one large incision. Also known as minimally invasive surgery.

laparoscopy
The use of a special endoscope that is passed through the abdominal wall in order to view the abdominal organs.

lymphatic system
A network of vessels that transfers lymph from the tissue fluids to the bloodstream. Lymph nodes occur at intervals along the lymphatic vessels.

lymphocyte
A type of white blood cell that is produced in bone marrow. Lymphocytes are present mainly in lymph and blood. Lymphocytes are part of the immune system and respond to fight infections and cancer.

malnutrition
A nutritional deficiency due to the lack of the basic elements of a balanced diet. Usually brought on by a severe food shortage, malnutrition can also be caused by inadequate absorption of food or an intake of inappropriate food. The term *malnutrition* also increasingly refers to the kind of excessive eating that causes obesity.

malocclusion
Improper alignment of the upper and lower teeth when biting.

measles
An acute, highly contagious viral disease that occurs principally in childhood and is characterized by red eyes, fever, and a rash. Also called morbilli and rubeola. See encyclopedia entry.

meninges
The three membranes that surround the brain and spinal cord.

meningitis
Any infection of the meninges. See encyclopedia entry.

meningocele
A hernial protrusion of the meninges, or covering of the spinal cord. A congenital defect of the spine (spina bifida) causes meningocele.

menorrhagia
Heavy menstrual periods.

menses
The flow of blood that occurs during a menstruation period.

menstruation
Periodic bleeding as the uterus sheds its lining each month during a woman's reproductive years. Begins at puberty and ends at menopause.

metabolism
The various vital processes that are necessary for bodily functions. These processes include breaking down complex molecules to produce energy (catabolism) and building up complex molecules, such as proteins, from simpler components (anabolism).

microsurgery
Surgery on tiny structures, which are not easily accessible, such as blood vessels, nerves,

or eyes. Microsurgery is carried out using a microscope and specially adapted miniature instruments.

migraine
Recurrent severe headaches that are associated with nausea and visual disturbance. See encyclopedia entry.

MMR vaccine
A combined vaccine that protects children against measles, mumps, and rubella. The MMR vaccine is first given to a child between 12 and 15 months. Follow-up booster doses occur when the child is between three and five years. Administration of the MMR vaccine on a large scale in the developed world has greatly reduced the occurrence of mumps.

MRSA (methicillin-resistant *Staphylococcus aureus*)
A bacterium that is difficult to treat, particularly in hospitals, where it may be fatal for already ill patients.

mumps
An acute viral disease that primarily affects the parotid glands in the cheeks, causing swelling and discomfort when eating. Other symptoms are fever and headache. Mumps usually occurs in childhood and one attack gives lifelong immunity. Since the advent of the MMR vaccination, mumps epidemics no longer occur in the developed world. See encyclopedia entry.

narcotic
A drug that dulls the senses. Used to induce sleep or as a painkiller.

over-the-counter (OTC) drug
A drug that is sold lawfully without a prescription in a pharmacy or drugstore. Common painkillers such as paracetamol and aspirin are available in this way.

pap smear
A method of detecting abnormal changes in the cells of the cervix that could lead to cervical cancer. The test involves staining a sample of exfoliated cells taken from the cervix. *See* cervical smear.

pediatrics
The branch of medicine concerned with the treatment of children and childhood diseases.

phocomelia
A defect in which the legs or hands are joined to the body by short stumps. The condition occurred in many children as a result of women taking the drug thalidomide during pregnancy.

psychosis
Any psychiatric disorder, such as schizophrenia or bipolar disorder, in which the person has distorted beliefs that are inappropriate and disconnected from reality. Delusions or hallucinations can occur.

retrovirus
A type of virus that has RNA (ribonucleic acid) as its genetic material and that uses an enzyme (reverse transcriptase) to produce DNA from the RNA. The viral DNA thus produced is then incorporated into the DNA of the host cell. HIV is an example of a retrovirus.

scarlet fever
An acute, but now rare, infectious childhood illness characterized by a sore throat, fever, swollen lymph nodes, and a pronounced red rash. Also called scarlatina. See encyclopedia entry.

schizophrenia
A group of psychiatric disorders in which thinking, emotions, and behavior are disrupted and the person is often delusional. A symptom of schizophrenia is hallucination, which is often auditory ("hearing voices") rather than visual. See encyclopedia entry.

septicemia
A condition in which bacteria multiply in the bloodstream. Also called blood poisoning.

side effect
An unwanted consequence that occurs, as well as the desired effect, of a medication or therapy.

syncope
A loss of consciousness. *Syncope* is the medical term for fainting.

syndrome
A collection of symptoms or signs that occur together to indicate a specific disorder.

synthesize
To produce a substance by building it from smaller components. Proteins are synthesized in the body from smaller units called amino acids.

trisomy
The condition of having three of a certain chromosome instead of just two.

Index